Practice and Science of Standard Barbering;
a Practical and Complete Course of Training
in Basic Barber Services and Related Barber
Science. Prepared Especially for use by
Barber Schools, Barber Students, Barber
Apprentices, Practicing Barbers in Preparat

Practice and Science

of

STANDARD BARBERING

A practical and complete course of training in
basic barber services and
related barber science.

Prepared Especially For Use By

- BARBER SCHOOLS
- BARBER STUDENTS
- BARBER APPRENTICES
- PRACTICING BARBERS

IN PREPARATION FOR
BARBER STATE BOARD EXAMINATIONS

1953 Printing

MILADY PUBLISHING CORP.

3837-3839 WHITE PLAINS AVENUE   ::   NEW YORK 67, N. Y.

FOREWORD

"The Practice and Science of Standard Barbering" marks a major advance in barber training. With the help of leading barber schools, instructors and educators, all the essential fundamentals and know-how of barbering have been combined into one comprehensive textbook.

Step-by-step instructions are clearly described for basic barber services. Many illustrations, charts, examinations and a glossary have been included. The regular study of this text assures complete training and thorough preparation for State Board Examinations.

Every barber who wants to combine professional skill with modern, scientific knowledge, and desires to maintain high standards of service will find that this text answers a real need.

THE AUTHOR.

CONTENTS

PART I

PART II

HISTORY OF BARBERING

HISTORY OF BARBERING

The history of barbering is deeply rooted in the progress
of mankind. As civilization advanced, barbering developed
from an insignificant practice to a recognized vocation. To
study the history of barbering is to appreciate the accom-
plishments and the role of the barber in early times. This
rich cultural heritage should be the basis for prestige and
respect in serving the public.

Primitive man had to devise rather crude instruments
with which to cut the hair. Simple cutting implements were
usually prepared from sharpened flint or oyster shells. To
this very day, the savages of Polynesia still use similar
objects in cutting the hair.

Superstitions

The beginning of barbering was steeped in strange super-
stitions. There was a general belief among savages that people
could be bewitched by hair clippings. Hence, the privilege of
hair cutting was designated to the priest or medicine man of
the tribe. The Irish peasantry believed that if hair cuttings
were burned or buried no evil spirits would haunt the
individual.

Among the American Indians, the belief existed that the
hair had a vital connection with the body, and that "any-
one possessed of a lock of hair of another might work his
will on that individual."

It was the widespread ancient belief in the magic influence of long-haired persons which caused Roman judges
to order the hair of Christian martyrs cut before putting
them to death.

Origin of the Barber

As far back as four hundred years before Christ, shaving
was introduced by the Macedonians. Later it spread to
Egypt and all Eastern countries, including China. The word
barber is derived from a Latin word "barba" meaning

beard. The word tonsorial in Latin means the cutting, clipping and trimming of hair with shears or cutting with a razor.

Beautifying the Body

The Egyptians were the first to cultivate beauty in an extravagant fashion. Excavations from tombs have brought to light such relics as combs, brushes, mirrors and cosmetics. Eye paint was the most popular of all cosmetics. Slaves enhanced the beauty of the Egyptian ladies by applying perfumed oil to their skins and henna to their hair.

Significance of the Beard

Although the importance of the beard belongs more with the past than to the present, nevertheless, it is interesting to note the various fashions and customs associated with it. A curious custom of the Middle Ages was that of imbedding three hairs from the king's beard in the wax of the seal. During the reign of Queen Elizabeth in England, it was fashionable to dye the beard and cut it into a variety of shapes.

In early times, the beard was considered by almost all nations as a sign of wisdom, strength and manhood, and was carefully cherished as being almost sacred. Among the Jews, the beard was regarded as a symbol of manliness; to cut off another man's beard was an outrage. According to the Greek philosopher, Pythagoras, the hair was the source of the brain's inspiration and the cutting of the hair decreased intellectual capacity In Rome, the first day of shaving (22nd birthday) was looked upon as a sign of manhood and was celebrated with great festivities.

The commands of certain rulers were at times responsible for the removal of beards. For instance, Alexander the Great ordered his soldiers to shave so that their enemies might not seize their beards in battle. After the Gauls were conquered, Julius Caesar compelled them to cut off their beards. Peter the Great made shaving compulsory by imposing a tax on beards.

In the spread of the Christian faith, long hair gradually became to be despised because it was considered sinful. Hence the clergy were directed to shave their beards. Among the Jews, shaving of the beard was forbidden, but they used the scissors to remove all excess hair. The Moslems observed great care in trimming the beard after prayer, and the hairs that fell out were carefully picked up and preserved for subsequent burial with the owner.

Barbers first became popular in Rome about the year 296 B.C. In Greece, barbers became popular as early as 500 B.C.

Greek and Roman Influence

In Greece and Rome, barbering was a highly developed art. Persons of means were shaved by their valets. The common people frequented the barber shops which were the resorts of loungers and newsmongers.

The Greeks and Romans gave considerable attention to beautifying the hair. Sparkling gems and hairpins of silver and gold adorned the elegant hair styles of the Greek women. The Roman women often dyed their hair, and some replaced the hair with fashionable wigs.

In ancient Rome, the color of a woman's hair indicated her rank. Women of the nobility tinted their hair red; those of the middle class colored their hair yellow; while women of the poorer classes were compelled to dye their hair black.

The Greeks were noted for the cultivation of health by natural methods. They realized the value of exercise and massage for building a strong body. Hippocrates, the father of modern medicine, advocated the use of sunlight, water and diet, as important aids to recovery from illness. The motto of the Greeks was "a sound mind in a sound body".

Some of the finest bathing establishments were erected in Rome. Soap was first discovered and came into common usage there. Later, with the decay of Rome and the rise of Christianity, the use of soap and bathing was banned because these practices were associated with the cruelty and wickedness of Roman rulers.

RAZORS OF THE PAST

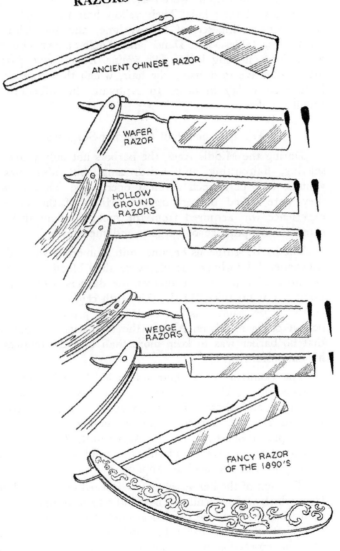

ANCIENT CHINESE RAZOR

WAFER RAZOR

HOLLOW GROUND RAZORS

WEDGE RAZORS

FANCY RAZOR OF THE 1890'S

English Influence

The ancient Britons were extremely proud of the length and beauty of their hair. Their yellow hair was brightened with washes composed of tallow, lime, and the ashes of certain vegetables. The Danes and Anglo-Saxons also admired long, flowing locks. The young Danes were particularly attentive to dressing the hair, which they combed at least once a day in order to captivate the affections of English ladies.

The Rise and Fall of Barber-Surgeons

During the Middle Ages, the barbers not only practiced shaving, haircutting and hairdressing, but also dressed wounds and performed surgical operations. That is why they were called barber-surgeons. Much of the barbers' experience was acquired from the monks, whom they assisted in the practice of surgery and medicine.

The barber-surgeons became quite numerous when Pope Alexander III forbade the clergy to shed blood in surgical operations. To protect themselves, the Barbers' Company of London was organized in the thirteenth century. The object of the trade guild was to regulate the profession for the benefit of its members. Among the regulations passed was that no barber was to keep more than four apprentices in his establishment.

The Company of Barbers was ruled by a Master, and consisted of two classes of barbers, viz: those who practiced barbering and those who specialized in surgery. Under Edward III, the barbers made a complaint against unskilled practitioners in surgery. As a result, the court chose two Masters to inspect and rule the guild and give examinations to test the skill of applicants.

The sign of the barber-surgeon consisted of a striped pole from which was suspended a basin: the fillet around the pole indicating the bandage twisted around the arms previous to blood-letting and the basin the vessel for receiving blood. Another interpretation of the colors in the barber's pole was that red represented the blood, blue the veins, and white the bandage. This sign, without the basin, has been generally retained by the modern barber.

Besides the Barbers' Guild, there was also a Surgeons' Guild in England. There was reason to believe that competition and antagonism existed between these two organizations. In 1450, both groups were united by law for the purpose of fostering the science of surgery. A law was enacted that no one doing surgery should practice barbering and that no barber should practice any point in surgery except the pulling of teeth. The long slumbering jealousy between the two guilds soon reached a climax. The surgeons harbored a dislike for a system under which the diplomas were signed by Governors, two of whom were always barbers. Finally, in 1745 a bill was passed separating the barbers from the surgeons.

The barber-surgeons also flourished in France and Germany. In 1371, a corporation was organized for the French barber-surgeons under the rule of the King's barber. With the advent of the French revolution, the corporation was dissolved. Wigs became so elaborate in the nineteenth century that a separate corporation of barbers was formed in France. Not until 1779 was a corporation formed in Prussia. This was disbanded in 1809 when new unions were started.

The Dutch and Swedish settlers in America brought with them barber-surgeons from their native countries to look after the well being of the colonists. They not only shaved but performed everyday medical and surgical procedures.

Modern Trends

By the nineteenth and twentieth centuries, barbering was completely separated from religion and medicine, and began to take on an independent position. Rapid strides have been made in barbering since the invention of electricity, the development of better instruments for cutting and shaving the hair, and the discoveries in hygiene, chemistry and medicine.

With the exception of Virginia and certain counties in

Alabama, the remaining states have passed laws regulating the practice of barbering. The state boards are primarily interested in maintaining high standards of education and training in order to assure competent and intelligent service. The barber schools, barber unions, and Master Barbers Association, have cooperated in the enforcement of state laws and in the protection of the barbers' rights and privileges.

Important discoveries which have improved the practice of barbering in recent times are as follows:

1. The use of electricity and electrical appliances in the barber shop.

2. The use of better barber implements.

3. The practice of sterilization and sanitation in the barber shop.

4. The study of anatomy dealing with those parts of the body (face, head and neck) which are served by the barber.

5. The study of preparations used in connection with facial, scalp and hair treatments.

Historical Notes on Barbering

The Journeymen Barbers' Union was organized 1887, and the first convention was held on November 5, 1887, at Buffalo, New York.

The first barber school in the United States was started by A. B. Moler in Chicago, in 1893.

The first state to pass a barber license law was Minnesota, in 1897.

The Associated Master Barbers of America was organized in 1924, at Chicago, Illinois.

HAIRCUTS AND BEARDS IN VOGUE
AT THE ONSET OF THE 20th CENTURY

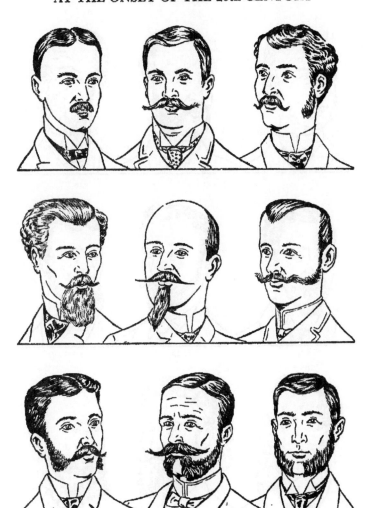

HAIRCUTS AND BEARDS IN VOGUE
DURING THE 19th CENTURY

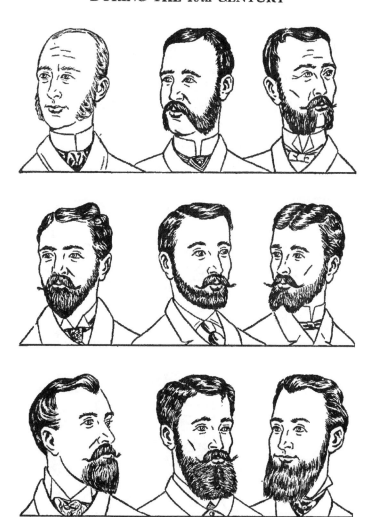

HISTORY OF BARBERING

1. What is the origin of the word "barber"?	"Barba" is a Latin word meaning beard.
2. Why did men wear beards in ancient times?	They were signs of wisdom, strength and manhood.
3. Name two ancient nations which practiced barbering.	Ancient Egypt and China.
4. When did the Macedonians introduce the practice of shaving?	About 400 years B.C. (before the birth of Christ).
5. In what year did barbers become known in Rome?	About 296 B.C.
6. When did barbers become popular in Greece?	About 500 B.C.
7. Who were the barber-surgeons?	Barbers who assisted the clergy in the practice of surgery and medicine.
8. a) When did the barber-surgeons start their practice?	About 110 A.D. (after the birth of Christ).
b) When did the barber-surgeons end their practice?	In the year 1745.
9. What were the duties of the barber-surgeons?	Besides being a barber, they did blood-letting, performed operations, pulled teeth and dressed wounds.
10. Describe the barber's sign used by the barber-surgeons.	The barber's sign consisted of a striped pole, from which was suspended a basin. The white band around the pole indicated the ribbon for bandaging the arm, the red band indicated the bleeding and the basin was intended to receive the blood.
11. What was the origin of the modern barber pole?	The modern barber pole started in the days when the barber-surgeons bled their patients in treating disease.
12. What kind of organization was the Barbers' Company of London?	A trade guild or society for the protection of barber-surgeons.
13. When was the Barbers' Company organized in London?	During the thirteenth century.
14. When was the first school for barber-surgeons opened in France?	In the middle of the thirteenth century.
15. Who brought the barber-surgeons to America?	The early Dutch and Swedish settlers.
16. In what year did A. B. Moler open the first barber school in America?	In 1893.
17. In what year did the State of Minnesota pass the first barber license law?	In 1897.

18. What are three important advantages of having barber license laws?	1. Elevates the standards and practice of barbering. 2. Eliminates incompetent barbers who lack the required training and experience. 3. Protects the public health and assures better service.
19. In what year were the Master Barbers of America organized?	In 1924.
20. When was the Journeymen Barbers' International Union organized in America?	In 1887.
21. Which important discoveries improved the practice of barbering in recent years?	1. The use of electricity and electrical appliances in the barber shop. 2. The use of better barber implements. 3. The practice of sterilization and sanitation in the barber shop. 4. The study of anatomy dealing with those parts of the body (face, head and neck) which are serviced by the barber. 5. The study of preparations used in connection with facial, scalp and hair treatments.

PART I

HYGIENE, SANITATION AND

STERILIZATION

PERSONAL HYGIENE

Good health is a valuable asset to the barber. It permits him to function efficiently and render satisfactory service to his customers. **Poor health** is a serious handicap which interferes with the best work of the barber. A sick person, having a contagious disease, tends to spread it to others. Any bacterial disease which affects the body should be sufficient to disqualify the barber from doing his work. An **annual physical examination** will help to discover the presence of any communicable disease.

Personal hygiene concerns the intelligent care given by the individual to preserve health. This requires a knowledge of good eating and drinking habits, and a wholesome mental attitude. A good balance between work, sleep and play, is fundamental to hygienic living.

Public hygiene or sanitation refers to the measures used by governmental agencies to preserve the health of the community. It is the responsibility of the barber to know sanitation and sterilization rules so that he may cooperate with the Board of Health and the State Board of Barbering in the maintenance of a high standard of public health.

Mental Hygiene

The mind and body operate as a unit; and the neglect of either must be to the detriment of both. Optimistic and encouraging thoughts promote good health. Healthy mental attitudes can be cultivated by self-control and practice. Make up your mind as to what is right and then continue to do it until a habit is established. In place of worry and fear, the health-giving qualities of cheerfulness, courage and hope, should be promoted. Outside interests and recreation tend to relieve the strain of monotony and hard work.

Thoughts and emotions influence bodily activities. A thought may cause the face to turn red and increase the heart action. A thought may either stimulate or depress the functions of the body. Strong emotions such as worry and fear have an injurious reaction on the heart, arteries and glands. Mental depression impairs the functions of these organs, thereby lowering the immunity of the body to disease.

Cleanliness

Cleanliness is an important factor in maintaining personal hygiene. It is essential to the preservation of health and the prevention of disease. A clean person is careful not only with his body but also with his clothing and surroundings. The barber must be dressed in a clean, washable outer coat or uniform. Shoes should be neat and comfortable. Clean personal habits reflect themselves in the physical condition of the barber shop.

For the body to be truly clean, only pure food, water and air should be consumed, and the waste products should be regularly eliminated. Otherwise, self-poisoning will ensue. Since constipation is a hindrance to internal cleanliness, it should be remedied by a change in eating and living habits.

The skin must be kept clean for hygienic as well as aesthetic reasons and to keep the pores open to allow the impurities to be excreted. Bathing with soap and water assists in the removal of surface dirt.

Body odor or foul breath is an indication of faulty personal hygiene and diet. The use of deodorants helps to counteract a disagreeable body odor.

To keep the teeth and mouth in a healthy condition, adequate mouth hygiene is required. Brush the teeth at least twice daily. Rinse the mouth with water after each meal. All decayed teeth should be either filled or removed.

Adequate personal hygiene demands appropriate attention to the needs of the body. Six requirements are essential to good health:

1. Breathe clean air.
2. Eat wholesome food.
3. Drink pure water in sufficient quantity.
4. Keep the body clean, both internally and externally.
5. Be moderate in work, play, exercise and sleep.

6. Stand, sit and walk correctly and maintain good posture.

Air

The quality of air a person breathes is important to health. Whereas warm, dry air is depressing, cool air with the proper amount of moisture is stimulating to the functions of the body. Country air is purer than city air because plants remove carbon dioxide and give off oxygen in the presence of the sun. Excess moisture, especially in hot air, causes great discomfort and renders the body susceptible to colds upon exposure to a draft. On hot and humid days, the body cannot readily dispose of the accumulated perspiration.

The air within a barber shop should be neither dry nor stagnant. Stagnant air has a stale, musty odor. Room temperature should be about 70 degrees Fahrenheit. Dry air in a heated room can be overcome by placing a water pan on the radiator or by having plants in the barber shop. Opening of the windows, one at the top and another at the bottom, helps to secure good ventilation. The impure air containing the carbon dioxide leaves through the top of the window, whereas the fresh air enters through the bottom. Drafts must be avoided. Fresh air is refreshing, not so much because of less carbon dioxide and more oxygen, but because it is usually cooler and less laden with moisture.

Food

Since no one food is in itself adequate for the nourishment and growth of the body, it becomes necessary to properly select and combine various foods so as to yield a balanced diet. The individual's choice should be guided by the purity, wholesomeness and freshness of foods. Contaminated water and food contain many harmful bacteria. Proper sanitation of water and food is supervised by governmental agencies.

Individuals differ in their nutritive needs and in their ability to digest and assimilate foods. A strong, healthy person, living an outdoor and active life, can easily digest

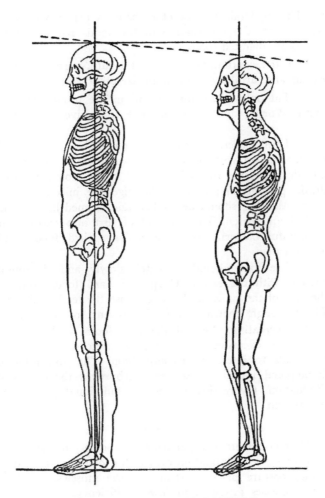

TYPES OF STANDING POSTURE

Excellent Mechanical Use
of the Body

1. Head straight above
   chest, hips and feet.
2. Chest up and forward.
3. Abdomen in or flat.

Poor Mechanical Use
of the Body

1. Head forward of chest.
2. Chest flat.
3. Abdomen relaxed and
   forward.

any kind of food. On the other hand, a person who works with his mind more than with his hands requires simple and easily digested foods.

For the continuance of sound health, certain hygienic eating and drinking rules must be observed.

1. Eat only when hungry and in the proper frame of mind. Worry and fatigue are not conducive to good digestion.

2. Drink several glasses of water daily. Do not gulp the food down with water. Iced water chills the stomach and decreases the rate of digestion in the stomach. Warm drinks promote the flow of the digestive juices.

3. All foods should be washed and cleaned before being cooked and eaten. The removal of dirt also carries with it harmful bacteria. Decomposed or spoiled food should not be eaten.

4. The food should be eaten slowly and thoroughly chewed with the saliva. Crisp and hard foods stimulate the flow of the saliva and also exercise the teeth and gums. The thorough chewing of foods prevents overeating.

5. Overeating, even of the best foods, is harmful to health. An excessive intake of food stretches the stomach and leads to intestinal decomposition. The absorption of decomposed intestinal residues overburdens the organs of elimination. Overeating makes the individual put on excess weight.

Posture

Correct posture is of particular importance to the barber, who is required to stand on his feet for long periods of time. Faulty posture places a strain on the muscles, which in turn increases fatigue and lowers efficiency.

To stand or walk correctly, the shoulders should be kept straight and backward while the abdomen is retained inward. Drooping shoulders limit the action of the lungs, which results in deficient aeration of the blood. Correct posture gives balance to the body and evenly distributes body weight.

Exercise

Exercise has a beneficial effect on the metabolic functions of the body. During exercise, the rate of breathing is increased, thereby supplying the blood with more oxygen with which to oxidize the food. The circulation of the blood and the nutrition of the cells are likewise improved.

Mild exercise is preferred to any violent exercise which may be a strain on the heart To get the best results from exercise it should be conducted in the open air, should bring a large number of muscles into play and should be pleasurable. Do not start any exercise when tired nor continue it if fatigued. Strenuous exercise after a hearty meal impairs digestion. The best kinds of exercise are sports, walking, swimming, and dancing.

Sleep

Sleep is necessary in order to revitalize the body and to neutralize and eliminate the products of mental and physical fatigue. During waking hours, the end products of metabolism accumulate faster than can be eliminated. Sound sleep permits the body to neutralize the waste products and discharge them from the system. During sleep, the body is recharged with energy. A clear mind and refreshed body are signs of adequate sleep.

Good Health Habits

1. Eat three good meals a day. Include the necessary variety of wholesome foods such as milk, eggs, fruit, vegetables, meat or fish and cereals.
2. Have regular times for meals, sleep and elimination.
3. Get sufficient sleep every night to feel rested and alert the next day.
4. Use leisure time for rest and recreation.
5. Avoid unnecessary infection by washing hands before and after serving customers, and by treating cuts and scratches promptly.
6. Steer clear of excesses in food, alcohol, sex or tobacco.
7. Adopt a cheerful attitude towards life and conquer the temptation to worry when things go wrong.
8. Have periodic check-ups by your doctor and dentist.

YOUR PERSONAL HYGIENE
IS VERY IMPORTANT

To keep your appearance at its best, give daily attention to correct posture, cleanliness and neatness.

Daily Bath and Deodorant

Keep the body clean and fresh by having a daily shower or bath, and if necessary by using an underarm deodorant.

Teeth and Breath

Clean and brush the teeth regularly. Use mouth wash to sweeten the breath.

Face

Shave the face daily. If worn, keep the mustache trimmed neatly.

Hair

Keep the hair clean, properly trimmed and dressed.

Hands and Nails

Keep the hands clean and smooth, and have the nails manicured.

Clothes

Wear clean pants and uniform that is properly fitted and pressed. Keep barber implements out of pockets. Wear shoes that are well-fitted and shined.

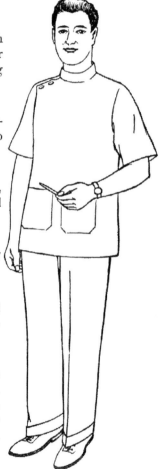

A Well-Groomed Barber

YOUR PERSONALITY CHART

No barber can hope to have or maintain a successful career in barbering unless he develops a pleasing personality.

Personality is your greatest asset in life It can be cultivated by giving careful attention to details in grooming and the forming of good habits and desirable traits.

Try to make this personality chart a true picture of yourself. Consult your teacher, friend or doctor, to find out what can be done to improve your personality. Check yourself every three months to find out what progress you are making.

PERSONAL INVENTORY

To determine to what extent you posses each of the traits or qualities listed, place a check in the proper box.

Body Cleanliness	Excellent 100%	Good 75%	Fair 50%	Poor 25%
Hands and Nails:				
Hands clean and free from nicotine stains	☐	☐	☐	☐
Nails cleaned and properly trimmed	☐	☐	☐	☐
Face:				
Face properly shaved	☐	☐	☐	☐
Mustache properly trimmed	☐	☐	☐	☐
Nostrils and ears clean and free from protruding hairs	☐	☐	☐	☐
Hair:				
Hair clean and properly trimmed	☐	☐	☐	☐
Hair properly groomed	☐	☐	☐	☐
Offensive Odor:				
Body odor	☐	☐	☐	☐
Breath odor	☐	☐	☐	☐
Clothing Cleanliness				
Uniform:				
Uniform clean and pressed. (Pockets free of implements.)	☐	☐	☐	☐

Pants:
Pants clean and pressed .... ☐ ☐ ☐ ☐
Shoes and Socks:
Shoes shined .... ☐ ☐ ☐ ☐
Socks clean ....:.........................: ☐ ☐ ☐ ☐

Clothing Habits:

Uniform and working apparel neat,
well fitted and properly worn .... ☐ ☐ ☐ ☐

Personal Habits

Sanitary Habits:
Handkerchief clean and pressed .... ☐ ☐ ☐ ☐
Manner of blowing and wiping nose. .. ☐ ☐ ☐ ☐

Posture Habits:

Erect standing posture .... ☐ ☐ ☐ ☐
Proper walking posture without
shuffling the feet .... ☐ ☐ ☐ ☐

Speech Habits:

Tone of voice .... ☐ ☐ ☐ ☐
Ease in talking .... ☐ ☐ ☐ ☐

RATING YOUR PERSONALITY

Add percentages for each trait or quality and get totals
for each column. Add combined totals to get grand total. Divide grand total by 20 to get average percentage for all.

To evaluate your personality, compare the final rating with
the following standards:

        Excellent Personality .... 85 - 100%
        Good Personality .... 75 - 85%
        Fair Personality .... 50 - 75%
        Poor Personality .... 40 - 50%

PERSONALITY IMPROVEMENT

After finishing this personal inventory, take stock of your
good and bad traits. Make a list of those traits in need of
correction or improvement. Select the most glaring fault first.

Each day make a conscious effort to do the right thing. Do not give up until you have formed the desirable habit. When one good habit has been formed, then follow the same procedure for the correction of another personal trait.

Every three months check your personal inventory to note what progress has been made towards your personality improvement.

RECORD OF PERSONALITY IMPROVEMENT

	Now	After 3 Months	After 6 Months	After 9 Months	After 1 Year
RATING					

PERSONAL HYGIENE

1. Why is the practice of personal hygiene important to the barber?	In order to keep the body clean, healthy and free from disease.
2. What is hygiene?	The science which treats of the prevention of disease and the improvement of health.
3. Name two important branches of hygiene. How is each applied?	Personal hygiene and public hygiene. Personal hygiene is applied to the individual. Public hygiene or sanitation is applied to the community.
4. Name six requirements of good health.	1. Breathe clean air. 2. Eat wholesome food. 3. Drink pure water in sufficient quantity. 4. Keep the body clean, both externally and internally. 5. Be moderate in work, play, rest and sleep. 6. Stand, sit and walk correctly.
5. How should the barber be dressed?	Wear a clean, washable outer coat or uniform.
6. What are three signs of a correct standing posture?	Keep head up, chest up and forward, abdomen flat.
7. How can body odors and foul breath be eliminated?	Bathe daily and if necessary use a deodorant under the armpits. Gargle the mouth with an antiseptic solution.
8. What hygienic care should be given to the teeth?	Brush and clean them each day. Visit the dentist to fill or remove bad teeth.
9. Why are regular physical examinations necessary?	To check the condition of the body and treat any disease that is discovered.

BACTERIOLOGY

Bacteriology is that science which deals with the study of micro-organisms called bacteria. In order for the barber to understand the importance of sterilization, it is necessary that he first make a study of bacteria.

While it is true that the barber is not concerned with the treatment of disease, he must understand how the spread of disease can be prevented, and become familiar with the precautions which must be taken to protect his own, as well as his customer's health Contagious diseases, skin infections and blood poisoning are caused either by the conveyance of infectious material from one individual to another, or by using contaminated implements (such as combs, brushes, razors, etc.) on an individual without being sterilized.

Bacteria are minute one-celled vegetable micro-organisms. They are especially numerous in dust, dirt, refuse and diseased tissues. Ordinarily, bacteria are not visible except with the aid of a microscope. Fifteen hundred rod-shaped bacteria will barely reach across a pinhead. It is only when thousands of them have grown in one spot to form a "colony" that they become visible as a mass. Harmful bacteria are also known as germs, or microbes.

Bacteria are **classified** as to their **harmful** or **beneficial** qualities. It must be borne in mind that not all bacteria are harmful; in fact, a great majority are helpful and useful.

There are two types of bacteria.

1. **Non-pathogenic organisms** constitute the majority of all bacteria and perform many useful functions such as decomposing refuse and improving the fertility of the soil. To this group belong the **saprophytes** which live on dead matter.

2. **Pathogenic organisms (microbes or germs)**, although in the minority, produce considerable damage by invading plant or animal tissues. Pathogenic bacteria are harmful because they produce disease. To this group belong the **para-**

sites which require living material for their growth.

It is due to the pathogenic bacteria that the practice of sterilization and sanitation is necessary in a barber shop.

Structural Classification of Bacteria

There are many hundreds of different kinds of bacteria which ·may be classified according to their shape or form Each bacterium has a specific structure and definite characteristics. They are arranged into three main classes as follows:

1. **Cocci** (singular, **coccus**) are round-shaped organisms which appear singly or in groups as follows:

    a) **Staphylococci** (singular, **staphylococcus**) are pus-forming organisms which grow in bunches or clusters, and are present in abscesses, pustules and boils.

    b) **Streptococci** (singular, **streptococcus**) are pus-forming organisms which grow in chains, and are found in such diseases as erysipelas and blood poisoning.

    c) **Gonococci** (singular, **gonococcus**) grow in pairs and are responsible for gonorrhea (clap).

    d) **Diplococci** (singular, **diplococcus**) grow in pairs, and cause pneumonia.

2. **Bacilli** (singular, **bacillus**) are rod-shaped organisms which present either a short, thin or thick structure. They are the most common and produce such diseases as tetanus (lockjaw), influenza, typhoid, tuberculosis and diphtheria. Many bacilli are **spore** producers.

3. **Spirilla** (singular, **spirillum**) are curved or corkscrew-shaped organisms. They are further subdivided into several groups, of chief importance being the spirochaetal organisms. The **spirochaeta** or **Treponema pallida** is the causative agent in syphilis.

Movement of Bacteria

The ability to move about is limited to the bacilli and spirilla, for the cocci rarely show active motility. Wherever any motility of bacteria is shown, we find hair-like projec-

THREE GENERAL FORMS OF BACTERIA

Cocci Bacilli Spirilla

GROUPINGS OF BACTERIA

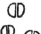

Diplococci Tetracocci Streptococci Staphylococci

SIX DISEASE-PRODUCING BACTERIA
(PATHOGENIC BACTERIA)

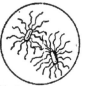

Typhoid Bacillus showing Flagella | Tubercle Bacillus (Tuberculosis) | Streptococcus

Diphtheria Bacillus | Cholera (Microspira) | Tetanus Bacillus with spores

tions, known as **flagella** or **cilia,** extending from the sides, end or sides and end, of certain bacteria. By moving these fine hairs with a whip-like motion, these bacteria propel themselves about through a liquid.

Bacterial Growth and Reproduction

Bacteria consist of an outer cell wall and internal protoplasm. They manufacture their own food from the surrounding environment, give off waste products and are capable of growth and reproduction.

Bacteria may exhibit two distinct phases in their life cycle.

1. **The active or vegetative stage** in which the bacterial cell grows and reproduces.

2. **The inactive or spore stage** in which the bacterial cell remains dormant and does not grow or reproduce itself.

Germs live and multiply best in warm, dark, damp and dirty places where sufficient food is present. Many parts of the human body offer a suitable breeding place for bacteria.

When conditions are favorable, bacteria reproduce with marvelous rapidity. As food is absorbed and converted into protoplasm, the bacterial cells increase in size. When the limit of growth is reached, it divides crosswise into halves, thereby forming two daughter cells. From one bacterium, as much as sixteen million germs may develop in half a day.

Spore-forming bacteria. When favorable conditions cease to exist, bacteria either die or cease to multiply. To withstand periods of famine, dryness and unsuitable temperature, certain bacteria such as the anthrax and tetanus bacilli can form spherical spores having a tough outer covering. In this stage, the spore can be blown about in the dust and is not harmed by disinfectants, heat or cold.

When favorable conditions are restored, the spore changes into the active or vegetative form and then starts to grow and reproduce.

Infections

Pathogenic bacteria become a menace to health when they successfully invade the body. An infection occurs if the body is unable to cope with the bacteria or their harmful poisons. At first, the infection may be localized as in a boil. A **general infection** results when the blood stream carries the bacteria and their poisons to all parts of the body

The presence of pus is a sign of infection. Found in pus are bacteria, body cells and blood cells, both living and dead.

An infectious disease becomes **contagious** because it tends to spread more or less readily from one person to another by direct or indirect contact. The most common contagious diseases met in the barber shop are **ringworm, favus, scabies,** and **head lice.**

In addition to these contagious diseases, a barber is not allowed to work in a shop if he has either diphtheria, influenza, typhoid fever, tuberculosis, gonorrhea or syphilis. Severe coughs and colds also prevent the barber from working in the shop, as they are contagious and may be spread to customers.

The chief sources of contagion are: unclean hands, unclean instruments, open sores and pus, and mouth and nose discharges. Uncovered coughing and sneezing in public also spreads germs. Through personal hygiene and public sanitation, infections can be prevented and controlled.

The body attempts to fight infections by using its defensive forces. The first line of defense is the unbroken skin In a healthy person, bodily secretions such as perspiration and digestive juices discourage bacterial growth. Within the blood, there are white blood cells to destroy harmful bacteria, and anti-toxins to counteract the poisons produced by the bacteria.

Bacteria enter the body through the following routes:
1 Through the mouth (with food, water and air).
2. Through the nose (with air).
3. Through the eyes (on dirt).
4. Through cracks or wounds in the skin

Immunity is the ability of the body to resist invasion and destroy bacteria once they have gained entrance. Immunity against disease is a sign of good health. It may be natural or acquired. **Natural immunity** is partly inherited and partly developed by hygienic living. **Acquired immunity**, being artificial, is secured after the body has by itself overcome certain diseases, or when it has been assisted by animal injections to fight bacterial attacks.

A person may be immune to a disease and yet carry germs which can infect other people. Such a person is called a **human disease carrier.** The diseases most frequently spread in this manner are typhoid fever and diphtheria.

The destruction of bacteria may be accomplished by physical agents such as heat (boiling, steaming or baking) ; and chemical agents such as antiseptics, disinfectants or germicides.

BACTERIOLOGY

1. What is bacteriology?	The science or study of bacteria.
2. What are bacteria?	Bacteria are minute one-celled vegetable organisms.
3. Where are bacteria generally found?	In the air, water, dust, dirt, and in diseased and decayed tissues.
4. Classify and describe bacteria according to their shape.	1. Cocci (sing., coccus) are round-shaped and appear in groups, pairs or clusters. 2. Bacilli (sing., bacillus) are rod-shaped and have a short, thin or thick appearance. 3. Spirilla (sing., spirillum) are corkscrew-shaped, having from one to eight curves.
5. Name and distinguish between two types of bacteria.	Pathogenic bacteria are harmful and produce disease. Non-pathogenic bacteria are beneficial and do not produce disease.
6. By what other names are pathogenic bacteria generally known?	Germs and microbes.
7. Name two common pus-forming bacteria.	Staphylococcus and streptococcus.
8. Which substances are usually found in pus?	Bacteria, body cells, blood cells, both living and dead.
9. Which kind of bacteria causes boils and pimples?	Staphylococcus.

10. Which kind of bacteria causes blood poisoning?	Streptococcus.
11. Which kind of bacteria causes gonorrhea (clap)?	Gonococcus.
12. Name four requirements for the growth of bacteria.	Warm, dark, damp and dirty places where sufficient food is present.
13. How do bacteria multiply?	Each bacterium lengthens and divides in the middle, thus forming two bacteria.
14. How fast do bacteria generally multiply?	From one bacterium, as many as sixteen million germs may develop in half a day.
15. What causes an infection?	The invasion of harmful bacteria into a weakened body.
16. Distinguish between a local infection and a general infection.	A local infection such as a boil is confined to a small part of the body. A general infection such as blood poisoning results when bacteria or their poisons enter the blood stream.
17. Through which four routes do bacteria enter the body?	1. The mouth (with air, water, or food). 2. The nose (with air). 3. The eyes (on dirt). 4. The skin (through cracks or wounds in the skin).
18. Which blood cells destroy bacteria in the body?	White blood cells.
19. How can infection be prevented in the barber shop?	By the practice of personal hygiene, sterilization and sanitation at all times.
20. What is immunity?	The ability of the body to fight and overcome certain diseases caused by germs and their poisons.
21. What is a human disease carrier? Give two examples.	A human disease carrier is a person who, although immune to the disease himself, can infect other persons with the germs of the disease. Two examples are diphtheria and typhoid fever.
22. What is a communicable or contagious disease?	A disease which can be readily spread from one person to another by direct or indirect contact.
23. Name ten communicable diseases that prevent a barber from working.	diphtheria gonorrhea influenza ringworm typhoid fever favus tuberculosis scabies syphilis head lice
24. Why should severe colds or coughs prevent a barber from working?	Because the germs of coughs due to colds are easily spread.

STERILIZATION

Sterilization is of practical importance to the barber because it deals with methods employed to check or destroy all kinds of micro-organisms, particularly those which are responsible for infections and communicable diseases.

The barber should know the local regulations of the Health Department and Board of Barbering regarding acceptable methods of sterilization.

Sterilization is the process of making an object germ-free by the destruction of all micro-organisms, whether beneficial or harmful.

~ Methods of Sterilization

There are four methods of sterilization with which the barber should be familiar. These may be grouped under two main headings:

1. **Physical agents:** ´
    a) Moist heat (boiling or steaming.)
    b) Dry heat (baking in an oven).
2. **Chemical agents:**
    a) Antiseptics and disinfectants.
    b) Vapors (fumigation) to keep articles sterile.

The choice of the sterilizing agent will depend to a very large extent on its effectiveness and cost and the available facilities in the barber shop.

Forms of Heat

Moist heat. An effective and relatively inexpensive method of sterilizing implements in a barber shop is boiling or steaming. The temperature and duration of heat are important considerations. The time is counted not from the moment the flame is lighted or the switch turned on, but from the time the particular temperature or pressure has been reached. To avoid cracking fragile objects and burning fingers, implements must never be placed in or removed from heated sterilizers with the hands; use forceps to insert and remove objects from the receptacles.

Instruments and glassware for immediate use are readily sterilized by boiling or steaming as follows:

1. **Boiling.** Boiling water at 212° Fahrenheit (100° centigrade) is germicidal in action, and will completely destroy all bacteria except spores. Instruments, glassware, towels, or headbands, should be placed in boiling water and allowed to remain for at least twenty minutes.* Adding a small quantity of sodium carbonate (washing soda) to the water will keep the instruments bright.

2. **Steaming.** Exposure to direct steam is probably one of the most effective methods of sterilization. Steam at ordinary atmospheric pressure never exceeds a temperature of 212° Fahrenheit (100° Centigrade), but if it is confined within a given area, the temperature will rise with increased pressure. The average steam pressure sterilizer is an air-tight chamber in which steam is generated from water by the application of heat. All forms of micro-organisms, including spore-forming bacteria are completely destroyed at 15 lbs. pressure (equivalent to a temperature of 250° Fahrenheit (121° Centigrade) for 20 minutes.*

Dry heat. This method of sterilization is not practical in the barber shop and is therefore rarely used. However, it is employed by hospitals to sterilize sheets, towels, gauze, cotton and similar materials.

Light. Bacteria cannot tolerate the effect of direct sunlight for more than a few hours. Almost all bacteria may be killed or weakened by **ultra-violet irradiation.**

Antiseptics and Disinfectants

Next to heat, chemical agents are most effective in destroying or checking bacteria. The chemical agents used for sterilizing purposes are either antiseptics or disinfectants (germicides) A distinction is usually made between an antiseptic and disinfectant.

The boiling or steaming time of water should conform to State Board regulations issued by your state.

1. An **antiseptic*** is a substance which may kill, or retard the growth of bacteria without killing them. Antiseptics can be used with safety on the skin.

2. A **disinfectant** destroys bacteria and is used for the sterilization of instruments.

A chemical such as formalin can be classed under both heads: a **strong solution** of it acting as a disinfectant; a **weak solution** acting only as an antiseptic.

Wet Sterilizer

A wet sterilizer is any receptacle large enough to hold the disinfectant solution and completely immerse the objects to be sterilized. A cover is provided to prevent contamination of the solution. Various sizes and shapes of wet sterilizers can be purchased from the barber supply dealer.

Before immersing objects in a wet sterilizer containing a disinfectant solution, they should be thoroughly cleansed with soap and water. This procedure prevents contamination of the solution. Besides, soap suds actually kill ordinary germs except the typhoid bacilli and staphylococci.

The kind and strength of chemical solution to use depends on the objects to be sterilized. The implements are usually immersed for a period ranging from 10 to 20 minutes.

After the barber implements are removed from the disinfectant solution, they should be rinsed in clean water, wiped dry with a clean towel and stored in a dry sterilizer until ready to be used.

Combs and **brushes** will be completely sterilized by immersion into a 10% formalin solution for 20 minutes.

Metallic instruments will be completely sterilized and will not corrode if they are immersed for 10 minutes in a 25% formalin solution to which glycerine has been added.

---

*The Federal Food, Drug and Cosmetic law interprets the meaning of an antiseptic as follows: If an antiseptic is intended for short contact on body surfaces, it should possess the effectiveness of a disinfectant and be able to kill germs. For prolonged contact as in the case of an antiseptic dusting powder, the product may exert an inhibiting effect on bacteria.

Using Alcohol As A Sterilizing Agent

Instruments having a fine cutting edge, such as razors, shears and clipper blades, may be sterilized either by immersion into 70% alcohol or by rubbing the surface with a cotton pad dampened in 70% alcohol which prevents the cutting edges from becoming dull.

Electrodes may be safely sterilized by gently rubbing the exposed surface with a cotton pad dampened in 70% alcohol.

Floors, Sinks, Toilet Bowls and Cuspidors

The disinfection of floors, sinks, toilet bowls and cuspidors in the barber shop calls for the use of such commercial products as lysol, CN, pine needle oil or similar disinfectants. Deodorants are also useful to combat offensive odors and for imparting a refreshing odor. Whatever disinfectant is being used, make sure that it is properly diluted as suggested by the manufacturer.

Dry Sterilizer

Dry sterilizer is an air-tight cabinet containing an active fumigant (formaldehyde gas). The sterilized implements are kept sterile by placing them in the cabinet until ready for use.

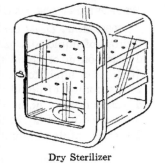

How fumigant is prepared. Place one tablespoonful of borax and one tablespoonful of formalin on a small tray or blotter on the bottom of the cabinet. This will form formaldehyde vapors. Replace chemicals periodically to insure effectiveness of the fumigant.

Dry Sterilizer

Formalin

Formalin is a safe and effective sterilizing agent which can be used either as an antiseptic, disinfectant or deodorant, depending on its percentage strength. As purchased, formalin is approximately 37% to 40% of formaldehyde gas in water.

When properly diluted with water, formalin serves many useful purposes in the barber shop.

Formalin is used in various strengths, as follows:

25% solution—(equivalent to 10% formaldehyde) used to. sterilize instruments, by allowing them to remain in the solution for at least ten minutes. (Preparation: 2 parts formalin, 5 parts water, 1 part glycerine).

10% solution—(equivalent to 4% formaldehyde) used to sterilize articles such as combs and brushes, by allowing them to remain in the solution for at least twenty minutes. (Preparation: 1 part formalin, 9 parts water).

5% solution—(equivalent to 2% formaldehyde) used to cleanse the hands in extreme measures, i.e., when they have been in contact with wounds or skin eruptions. It is also used for the sterilization of shampoo boards and chairs. (Preparation: 1 part formalin, 19 parts water).

2½% solution—(equivalent to 1% formaldehyde) used as a deodorant for sponging the armpits. (Preparation: 1 part formalin, 39 parts water).

PROPORTIONS FOR MAKING PERCENTAGE SOLUTIONS

100% *Active Liquid Concentrate*	*Strength*
5 drops of liquid to 1 oz. water or	
1 teaspoonful of liquid to 12 oz. water	1%
10 drops of liquid to 1 oz. water or	
2 teaspoonfuls of liquid to 12 oz. water	2%
4 teaspoonfuls of liquid to 12 oz. water	4%
5 teaspoonfuls of liquid to 12 oz. water	5%
10 teaspoonfuls of liquid to 12 oz. water	10%

TABLE OF EQUIVALENTS

60 Drops	1 teaspoonful
8 Teaspoonfuls	1 oz.
Ordinary Measured Glass	8 oz.
One Pint	16 oz.
One Quart	32 oz.
Half Gallon	64 oz.

HOW TO CLEAN AND STERILIZE
COMBS AND BRUSHES

1. **Arrange necessary supplies.**
   a) Prepare bowl of warm, soapy water to which is added a little ammonia (proportion of 1 tablespoonful to 2 quarts of water).
   b) Prepare bowl of warm water for rinsing purposes.
   c) Prepare sufficient quantity of 10% formalin solution or other approved disinfectant and place it into wet sterilizer.
   d) Prepare dry sterilizer. Mix 1 tablespoonful of borax with 1 tablespoonful of formalin in a small tray, and place into dry sterilizer.
   e) Have ready a supply of clean towels and individual envelopes.

2. **Clean combs and brushes.**
   a) Remove hair from combs and brushes.
   b) Immerse combs and brushes (with bristles down) into bowl of soapy water for several minutes.
   c) Clean each comb separately with a small brush.
   d) Clean the brushes two at a time by rubbing the bristles against each other.
   e) When thoroughly cleansed, rinse combs and brushes in bowl of clear, warm water.
   f) Drain off water and remove any adhering hairs.

3. **Sterilize combs and brushes.**
   a) Immerse combs and brushes into formalin solution for 20 minutes.
   b) Remove combs and brushes, rinse in clean water, and dry them thoroughly with a clean towel.
   c) Rest comb and brushes (with bristles down) on a clean towel in an airy, dust-free place, and allow them to dry thoroughly.

4. **Store combs and brushes.**
   a) When completely dry, place combs and brushes into dry sterilizer, or wrap in sealed individual envelopes, until ready for use.

HOW TO CLEAN AND STERILIZE
METALLIC IMPLEMENTS
(Razors, Shears, Tweezers and Comedone Extractors)

1. Arrange necessary supplies.
   a) Prepare a bowl of warm soapy water.
   b) Prepare disinfectant in wet sterilizer (25% formalin) to which a small amount of glycerine has been added, or use any other type of disinfectant approved by the State Board.
   c) If necessary, replace chemicals in dry sterilizer.
   d) Have ready a supply of clean towels and individual envelopes.
2. Clean metallic implements.
   a) Clean implements with warm soapy water.
   b) Dry them thoroughly in a clean towel.
3. Sterilize metallic implements.
   a) Immerse implements in disinfectant solution for 10 minutes, or follow your State Board requirements. **Caution:** In sterilizing razors or shears, it is advisable that only the blades be dipped into the solution, the handles should remain suspended in specially constructed sterilizers.
   b) Remove implements, rinse them in clean water and dry thoroughly.
4. Store metallic implements.
   a) Place sterilized implements in dry sterilizer or wrap them in individual envelopes until ready for use.

Moist Heat Sterilization

Moist heat (either boiling water or steam under pressure) can be used to sterilize barber implements, glassware, towels and linens. Objects that are readily destroyed by heat cannot be sterilized by this method.

The following procedure is recommended:

1. Cleanse the sterilizing kettle with soap and warm water.

2. Cleanse the implements and articles with warm water and soap.

3. Fill sterilizing kettle with sufficient water for articles to be sterilized. Add some sodium carbonate to the water in order to prevent the rusting of metallic implements.

4. Turn on the heat and bring the water to a boil.

5. Grasp articles with a forceps and immerse them into boiling water for the required time.

6. Allow water to cool, remove articles with forceps and dry them in clean towels.

7. Place sterilized articles into dry sterilizer until ready for use.

To use steam sterilization in the barber shop requires special apparatus. Follow the manufacturer's instructions for the particular steamer being used.

HOW TO CLEAN AND STERILIZE ELECTRODES

1. **Clean electrodes.**
    a) Clean surface of electrodes with warm, soapy water. **Caution should be taken** so that wires and metal attached to the electrodes do not come in contact with the water, as they may corrode or cause a short circuit.
    b) Dry thoroughly.

2. **Sterilize electrodes.**
    a) Dip a piece of cotton pad into 70% grain alcohol, or other approved disinfectant, and rub over the surface of the electrodes.
    b) Re-apply disinfectant.
    c) Dry electrodes thoroughly.

3. **Store electrodes.**
    a) Place electrodes in dry sterilizer or wrap in individual envelopes until ready for use.

ANTISEPTIC PREPARATIONS USED IN BARBER SHOPS

NAME	FORM	STRENGTH	USES	ADVANTAGES	DISADVANTAGES
Formalin	Liquid	5% solution	Cleanse hands, shampoo board, cabinet, etc.	Cheap. Effective.	Poison; pungent. Hardens skin.
Formalin	Liquid	2½% solution	Deodorize the armpits and feet.	Cheap. Effective.	Poison; pungent. Hardens skin.
Ethyl or Grain Alcohol	Liquid	60% solution	Cleanse hands, skin and minute cuts. Not to be used if irritation is present.	Safe. Effective.	Expensive. Hardens skin.
Chloramine-T (Chlorazene; Chlorozol)	White crystals	½% solution	Cleanse skin and hands and for general use.	Safe. Effective.	Unstable. Bleaches.
Sodium Hypochlorite (Javelle water; Zonite)	White crystals	5% solution	Rinse the hands.	Cheap. Powerful.	Unstable. Bleaches.
Boric Acid	White crystals	2-5% solution	Cleanse the skin and eyes.	Safe. Cheap.	Limited action.
Tincture of Iodine	Liquid	2% solution	Cleanse cuts and wounds.	Safe. Reliable.	Stains skin. Corrosive.
Cresol (Lysol)	Liquid	2% soap solution	Rinse hands.	Cheap. Powerful.	Poison; pungent.
Hydrogen Peroxide	Liquid	3-5% solution	Cleanse skin and minor cuts.	Cheap. Effective.	Unstable. Bleaches.

Other improved antiseptics are being used in barber shops. Consult the State Board of Barbers or the Health Department.

DISINFECTANT PREPARATIONS USED IN BARBER SHOPS

NAME	FORM	STRENGTH	USES	ADVANTAGES	DISADVANTAGES
Formalin	Liquid	25% solution	Immerse instruments into solution for 10 minutes.	Cheap. Effective.	Poison; pungent Hardens skin.
Formalin	Liquid	10% solution	Immerse instruments, combs, brushes, etc. into solution for 20 minutes.	Same as above.	Same as above.
Ethyl or Grain Alcohol	Liquid	70% solution	Same as above	Safe. Effective.	Expensive. Hardens skin.
Chloramine-T (Chlorazene; Chlorozol)	White crystals	2% solution	Same as above.	Safe. Effective.	Unstable. Bleaches.
Sodium Hypochlorite (Javellewater; Zonite)	White crystals	1-2% solution	Same as above	Cheap. Powerful.	Unstable. Bleaches.
Phenol (Carbolic acid)	White crystals	3-5% solution	Immerse instruments into solution for 30 minutes.	Cheap. Powerful.	Poison; pungent. Corrosive
Mercury bichloride (Corrosive sublimate)	White crystals	1/10% solution	Same as above.	Cheap. Effective	Poison; pungent. Corrosive.
Cresol (Lysol)	Liquid	10% soap solution	Cleanse floors, sinks and toilets.	Cheap. Powerful.	Poison, pungent

Other approved disinfectants are being used in barber shops. Consult the State Board of Barbers or the Health Department

Definitions Pertaining to Sterilization

1. **Sterilize**—to render sterile; to make aseptic.

2. **Sterile**—free from all living organisms.

3. **Antiseptic**—a chemical agent having the power to kill or prevent the growth of bacteria.

4. **Germicide or Bactericide (Disinfectant)**—a chemical agent having the power to destroy germs or microbic life.

5. **Deodorant**—a chemical agent having the power to destroy offensive odors.

6. **Asepsis**—freedom from disease germs.

7. **Sepsis**—poisoning due to pathogenic organisms.

8. **Styptic**—an agent causing contraction of living tissue, such as powdered alum, used to stop bleeding in cases of small cuts.

9. **Prophylaxis**—an agent used in the prevention of disease.

10. **Fumigant**—a vapor used to keep disinfected objects sterile.

Safety Precautions

The use of sterilizing agents involves certain dangers, unless safety measures are taken to prevent mistakes and accidents.

1. Purchase chemicals in small quantities and store them in a cool, dry place; otherwise they deteriorate due to contact with air, light and heat.

2. Weigh and measure chemicals carefully.

3. Keep all containers labeled and covered under lock and key.

4. Do not smell chemicals or solutions, as many of them have pungent odors.

5. When dissolving or diluting chemicals, avoid spilling on clothing or furniture. .

6. Wear rubber gloves to protect the skin from stains or burns. Burns resulting from touching hot objects can be prevented by using a forceps to insert or remove the objects from the source of heat.

Sterilization Rules

1. **Solutions or chemicals** in sterilizers must be changed regularly.

2. **All articles** must be clean and free from hair before being sterilized.

3. **Combs, brushes, razors, shears, clipper blades, and tweezers** must be sterilized after each customer has been served.

4. **Shampoo boards and bowls** must be cleaned and sterilized before using again.

5. **All cups, bowls or similar objects** must be sterilized with yellow soap, lysol, chlorozol or similar disinfectant, prior to being used for another customer.

STERILIZATION

1. What is sterilization?	Sterilization is the process of completely destroying all kinds of bacteria, whether infective or not.
2. Name four methods of sterilization.	Moist heat, dry heat, disinfectants, and vapors.
3. Which type of bacteria makes necessary the practice of sterilization and sanitation in the barber shop?	Pathogenic bacteria.
4. What are the dangers of using unsterilized barber implements and linens on customers?	Infectious diseases may be spread from one person to another.
5. Distinguish between asepsis, sterile and sepsis.	Asepsis—freedom from germs. Sterile—free from all living organisms. Sepsis—poisoning due to germs.
6. Which forms of heat will kill bacteria?	Boiling, steaming and dry heat.
7. Which groups of chemicals will check or destroy bacteria?	Antiseptics, disinfectants, and fumigants.
8. What is an antiseptic?	A chemical agent which may kill or prevent the growth of bacteria.
9. What is a disinfectant?	A chemical agent which destroys harmful bacteria.
10. What is a fumigant?	A chemical vapor used to keep disinfected objects in a sterile condition until ready for use.
11. Which kind of objects are best sterilized by means of moist heat (boiling water or steam)? How long?	Objects which can withstand heat such as metallic instruments and glassware. Twenty minutes.

12. What are the disadvantages of sterilizing barber implements with boiling water?	Implements may become tarnished and dull.
13. Which chemical added to boiling water keeps metallic instruments bright?	A small quantity of sodium carbonate (washing soda).
14. Where is the dry heat method of sterilization mostly used? For which objects?	Dry heat is used mostly in hospitals for the sterilization of linens, sheets, gauze, cotton and similar articles.
15. Which objects are best sterilized with a disinfectant solution?	Objects which cannot be boiled or steamed such as combs, brushes, razors, clipper blades, and shears.
16. When using a disinfectant, how are objects sterilized?	Clean each object with soap and hot water and place it into a suitable disinfectant solution for about twenty minutes.
17. What should be done with barber implements after sterilization in a disinfectant solution?	Rinse implements in clean water, dry them in a clean towel and place them in a cabinet sterilizer until ready to be used.
18. How should combs be kept after sterilization?	Wrap them in an individual paper envelope and place them into a dust-proof cabinet or cabinet sterilizer until ready for use.
19. What is a dry sterilizer?	A closed air-tight cabinet containing an active fumigant (formaldehyde gas).
20. What is the proper way to produce formaldehyde vapors in a cabinet sterilizer?	Place one tablespoon of borax and one tablespoon of formalin solution on a small tray or blotter in the cabinet sterilizer.
21. What is the composition of formalin?	Formalin is a 37% to 40% solution of formaldehyde gas dissolved in water.

SANITATION

Sanitation is the application of hygienic measures to promote public health and prevent the spread of infectious diseases. Various governmental agencies protect community health by providing for a wholesome food and water supply and the quick disposal of refuse. These steps are only a few of the ways in which the public health is safeguarded.

In many states and localities, the **Board of Health** and the **State Board of Barbering** have formulated sanitary regulations governing the barber shop. The barber must be familiar with these regulations so that he may obey them.

Sanitary conditions cannot be maintained in the barber shop in the presence of any infectious disease. **A person with an infectious disease** is a source of contagion to others. Hence, barbers having colds or any communicable disease must not be permitted to handle customers. Likewise, customers obviously suffering from an infectious disease must not be served in a barber shop. In this way, the best interests of other customers will be served.

The public has learned the importance of sanitation and is now demanding that every possible sanitary measure be used in the barber shop for the promotion of public health. Barbers who desire to attract public patronage should aim to conduct their shops in a clean and orderly manner. A high standard of sanitary efficiency should be practiced. Adopting the sanitary rules on page 48 will result in cleaner and better service to the public.

Water

Since water is used internally and externally for personal hygiene and as an aid in the barber's work, it becomes necessary to know more about the properties of water. Water for drinking purposes should be odorless, colorless and free from any foreign matter. Crystal clear water may still be unsanitary because of the presence of pathogenic bacteria which cannot be seen with the naked eye. The transmission of disease by water depends upon the introduction of germs or refuse into the water. Local health boards exercise control over the purity of the water supply.

Even though water may be suitable for drinking purposes, it may still be unsatisfactory for use with soap. When used externally for shaving or bathing, the water should be soft so that it will easily lather with the soap. Hard water produces an insoluble curd which wastes soap and interferes with its cleansing action. Water is said to be "hard" when it contains the soluble compounds of calcium and magnesium. Temporary hard water can be overcome by boiling which converts the soluble salts into insoluble compounds. The precipitate is removed mechanically. When permanent hard water is not softened by boiling, it can be rendered soft either by distillation or by chemical treatment. Hard water can be softened by using borax or washing soda. Besides softening the water, these agents make the water alkaline in reaction.

Sanitary Rules

1. Every barber shop must be well lighted and ventilated in order to keep it in a clean and sanitary condition.

2. The walls, curtains and floor covering must be washable and kept clean.

3. All barber shops must be supplied with running hot and cold water.

4. The barber shop is not to be used for eating, sleeping or living quarters, unless a special room is provided for that purpose.

5. All hair, cotton or waste material, must be removed from the floor without delay, and deposited in a closed container.

6. The washroom should be kept in a sanitary condition and be provided with individual towels and drinking cups.

7 Each barber must wear a uniform or coat while working on customers.

8. The barber must cleanse his hands throughly before and after serving a customer.

9. A freshly laundered towel must be used for each customer. Towels ready for use must be stored in clean, closed containers.

10. Neck-strips and headrest covering must be changed for each customer.

11. The use of the same neck duster and styptic pencil on more than one customer is prohibited, for they may spread infection.

12. Liquids, creams and powders must be kept in clean, closed containers, and used individually for each customer. Use clean spatula instead of fingers to remove cream from container. Use sterile cotton pledgets to apply or remove facial creams.

13. Objects dropped on the floor or kept in the pocket are no longer sterile and are not to be used again until sterilized.

SANITATION

1. What is sanitation?	Sanitation is the application of hygienic measures to promote public health and prevent the spread of infectious diseases.
2. Which unsanitary practices may spread disease in the barber shop?	Contact with a person having an infectious disease, unclean hands, use of unsterilized instruments and the common use of towels, combs, brushes, drinking cups, shaving mugs or styptic pencils.
3. How should the hands be treated after touching a customer suspected of having a skin or scalp infection?	Wash hands with tincture of green soap and water, apply 60% alcohol or rinse hands in an antiseptic solution.
4. What are five sanitary requirements of a barber shop?	1. Keep the barber shop well ventilated and lighted. 2. Keep the walls, curtains and floor coverings in a clean condition. 3. Have running hot and cold water in a barber shop. 4. The barber must cleanse his hands thoroughly before and after serving a customer. 5. Keep all waste materials in closed containers and have them removed regularly.
5. Which sanitary rule should be observed regarding the use of headrests?	Cover the headrest with a clean towel or paper tissue and change it for each customer.
6. Why are neck-strips or towels required?	To prevent the shaving cloth or hair cloth from touching the customer's neck.
7. What is the sanitary way to keep lotions, ointments, creams and powders?	Keep them in closed, dust-proof containers.
8. What is the sanitary way to remove creams and ointments from their containers?	With a spatula or wooden tongue blade.
9. Where should towels be kept after laundering?	In closed, dust-proof cabinet or towel cabinet.
10. Where should dirty towels be kept?	In closed containers, separate from the clean towels.
11. Which barber supplies must be changed for each customer?	Neck-strip, headrest covering, and towels.
12. Why should styptic pencils never be used in common?	The use of the same styptic pencil on more than one person may spread infection in the barber shop.

PART II

BARBER PRACTICE

WILL YOU BE A SUCCESS .. OR .. FAILURE?

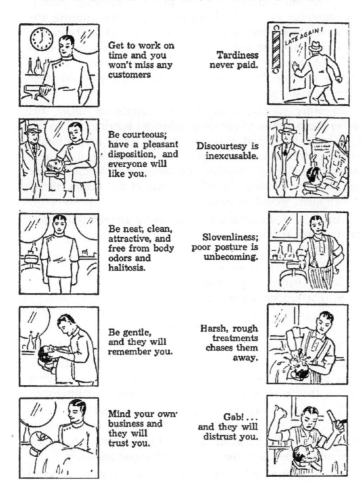

Get to work on time and you won't miss any customers	Tardiness never paid.
Be courteous; have a pleasant disposition, and everyone will like you.	Discourtesy is inexcusable.
Be neat, clean, attractive, and free from body odors and halitosis.	Slovenliness; poor posture is unbecoming.
Be gentle, and they will remember you.	Harsh, rough treatments chases them away.
Mind your own business and they will trust you.	Gab! ... and they will distrust you.

TO BE SUCCESSFUL—you must learn to do the little things that will make people like you

BARBER IMPLEMENTS

A barber can be no better than the tools he selects and uses. Limitations and defects in equipment are not only hazardous but usually give rise to work of poor quality. The purchase of standard materials helps to improve the quality of the barber's work. To do his best work, the barber should buy and use only superior implements obtained from a reliable manufacturer. Uninformed and improper use will quickly destroy the efficiency of any implement, however perfectly made at the factory.

In order to give a satisfactory haircut or shave, the barber has occasion to use three principal instruments, namely, razors, shears and clippers. Besides these major implements, certain accessory implements are employed such as hones, strops, combs, brushes and latherizers. Without these accessory implements, the effective use of the razors, shears and clippers, would be impaired.

Among the important facts to know about each implement are the following:

1. The main parts.
2. The material composition.
3. The various types and sizes.
4. The proper use and care.

Straight Razors

The straight razor is one of the most important implements used by the barber. Over the years the razor has undergone improvement in quality and design. For superior service, the barber should use only the highest quality razor.

The barber's tool kit should include several high grade razors. Should one razor become unfit for use, an immediate replacement will be available Besides, razors receive less wear and better care when they are changed regularly.

Selecting the right kind of razor is a matter of personal choice. The best guides for buying high quality razors are:

1. Consult with reliable company or salesman who can

recommend the type of razor best suited to the barber's work.

2. Consult with more experienced barbers as to which razors they have found best for shaving.

Judging the value of a razor in any other ways may be misleading. Merely observing the color or design of a razor does not reveal the true quality of the implement. Nor does the ring of a razor have any significance as far as its hardness or softness is concerned. Ornamental handles on razors sometimes hide inferior quality.

The important points to know about a straight razor are: the main parts, the balance, the temper, the size, the grind, the style, and the finish.

The straight razor is constructed of a hardened steel blade attached to a handle by means of a pivot. The handle

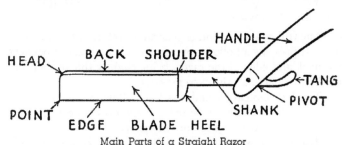

Main Parts of a Straight Razor

is made of either hard rubber, celluloid or bone. When the blade is closely examined, the following parts can be seen, namely: the head, back, shoulder, tang, shank, heel, edge and point.

The balance of a razor refers to the relative weight and length of the blade as compared with that of the handle.

A straight razor is properly balanced when the weight of the blade is equal to that of the handle. Proper balance means greater ease in shaving with the straight razor.

The grind of razor represents the shape of the blade after it has been ground over a stone. The most common types of grinds are: the full concave, the half concave and the wedge grind.

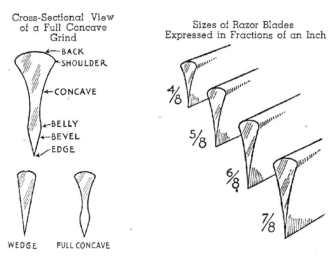

Cross-Sectional View
of a Full Concave
Grid

BACK
SHOULDER
CONCAVE
BELLY
BEVEL
EDGE

WEDGE   FULL CONCAVE

Sizes of Razor Blades
Expressed in Fractions of an Inch

⁴⁄₈ ⁵⁄₈ ⁶⁄₈ ⁷⁄₈

The full concave grind is generally preferred by most barbers. It presents a hollow appearance when observed between the back and edge of the razor, being slightly thicker between the hollow part and the extreme edge.

The half concave grind has less hollowness than the full concave. There will not be more thickness between the concave and the extreme edge of the razor.

The wedge grind has no hollowness or concavity, both sides of the blade forming a sharp angle at the extreme edge of the razor. The old type razors were made with a wedge grind. For most barbers, learning how to sharpen a wedge grind is quite difficult. Once barbers get accustomed to using the wedge grind, they usually find that it produces an excellent shave.

Tempering the razor involves a special heat treatment given by the manufacturer. When razors are properly tempered, they acquire the proper degree of hardness and toughness necessary for good cutting quality. Razors can be purchased with either a hard, soft or medium temper. From this assortment, the barber can select the kind of temper which produces the most satisfactory shaving results. Generally, the medium temper of razor is preferred by barbers.

The size of the razor deals with the length and width of the blade. The width of the razor is measured in eighths or sixteenths of an inch, most generally in eighths such as 4/8, 5/8, 6/8 and 7/8. The 5/8 inch size is the one most frequently used. It is not advisable to purchase a smaller size razor, as repeated honings will wear out the blade and render the razor valueless.

The style of a razor indicates its shape and design. The modern razor has such features as a straight, parallel back and edge, a round heel, a square point, and a flat or slightly round handle. To prevent scratching of the skin, the barber usually rounds off the square point of the razor.

The finish of a razor is the condition of its surface which may be either plain steel, crocus (polished steel) or metal plated (nickel or silver). Of these types, the crocus finish is the choice of the discriminating barber. Although the crocus finish is more costly, it usually lasts longer and does not show any signs of rusting. The metal plated razors are undesirable because they wear off quickly and often hide a poor quality steel.

Care of razors. Razors will maintain their cutting quality if care is taken to prevent corrosion of the extremely fine edge. After use, they should be stropped and a little castor oil applied over the cutting edge, thus preventing the corrosive action of moisture. Be careful not to drop the razor as the blade may be damaged.

Haircutting Shears

The two most general kinds of shears used by barbers are the German type, without a finger brace, and the French

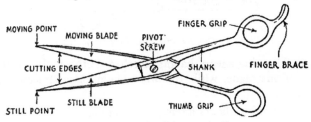

The Main Parts of a Haircutting Shears

type, with a brace for the small finger. The French type is used to a greater extent than the German type.

The main parts. Barber shears are composed of two blades, one movable and the other still, fastened by a screw which acts as a pivot. Other parts of the barber shears are the cutting edges of the blades, two shanks, finger grip, finger brace, and thumb grip.

Size. Shears differ both in their length and size. The most popular length of shears is 7 and 7½ inches. The barber selects the one which is most convenient for easy handling.

Grinds. There are two types of shear grinds, the plain and the corrugated. The plain grind is most frequently used. It may be finished either smooth (knife edge), medium or coarse. The medium finish is usually preferred.

Thinning Shears

Thinning or serrated shears are used occasionally by the barber, particularly for ladies' haircutting. These shears serve to reduce the thickness of the hair or can be employed to taper the hair. There are two general types of thinning or serrated shears available.

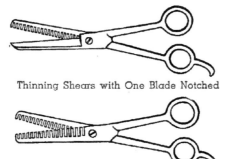

Thinning Shears with One Blade Notched

Thinning Shears with Both Blades Notched

1. Thinning shears having notched teeth on the cutting edge of one blade, while the other blade has a straight cutting edge.

2. Thinning shears having overlapping notched teeth on the cutting edges of both blades.

Thinning shears may also differ in respect to the number of notched teeth on the cutting blade. The greater the number of notched teeth, the finer the hair strands can be cut.

Clippers

Two types of hair clippers are often used by barbers. They are the hand clipper and the electric clipper.

The hand clipper. If the hand clipper is taken apart the following parts will be noted: cutting blade, still blade, finger guide, movable handle, still handle, thumb rest, thumb screw, set screw, and heel.

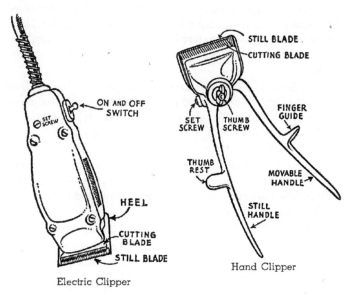

Electric Clipper

Hand Clipper

The electric clippers operate either by means of a motor or by magnetic action. They have either a detachable cutting head or a non-detachable cutting head. The magnetic electric clippers are the most popular among barbers. The visible parts of an electric clipper are: cutting blade, still blade, heel, switch, set screw and conducting cord.

Cutting thickness. The blades of both the hand and electric clippers are indicated in cutting thickness by ciphers.

The range in the cutting thickness of the clipper blade is from 0000 (the shortest cut) to 000, 00, 0, 1 and 2 (the longest cut).

Accessory Implements

The accessory implements include those aids which render the razor, shears and clippers, more effective in the process of shaving the beard and cutting and dressing the hair. The accessory implements include the hone, strop, comb, hair brush, hair duster, shaving brush, and latherizer.

Hones

Various types of hones are available for the purpose of sharpening a razor. A hone is primarily a rectangular block composed of abrasive material. Being harder than steel, the abrasive in the hone is capable of cutting an edge on the razor.

The final choice of hone rests mainly with the barber. The question often arises as to which type of hone will best serve to sharpen a razor. As a general rule, any type of hone is satisfactory, provided it is properly used and produces a sharp cutting edge on the razor.

As a result of their experiences, barbers may prefer one type of hone to another. The student barber usually practices with a slow cutting hone; while the experienced barber generally prefers a faster cutting hone.

Depending on their source, hones are classified as:

1. **Natural hones** such as the water hone and the Belgian hone, derived from natural rock deposits. These hones are usually used wet with either water or lather.

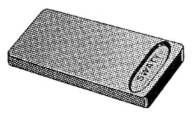

Synthetic or Manufactured Hone

2. **Synthetic hones** such as the Swaty hone and the carborundum hone are manufactured products. These hones can be used dry, or a lather can be spread over them before use.

Water hone. It is a natural hone usually imported from Germany. Accompanying the water hone is a small piece of slate of the same texture, called the rubber. As the rubber is applied over the water hone moistened with water, a proper cutting surface is developed. Care must be taken when using the rubber on the water hone not to work a bevel into the hone.

The water hone is primarily a slow cutting hone When used as directed by the manufacturer, a smooth and lasting edge is formed on the razor. Its color may be either grey or darkish yellow. Of the two colors, the greyish yellow water hone is considered to be a slightly better grade, and also exerts a slightly faster cutting action.

Belgium hone. It is a natural hone cut out of rock formation found in Belgium. It is a slow cutting hone, but a little faster than the water hone. It is capable of putting on a very sharp edge on the razor. Lather is generally applied to the hone when honing.

One type of Belgium hone consists of a light yellowish colored rock glued on to a dark red slate back. The principal advantage is to yield a keen cutting edge on the razor. It can be used either wet or dry.

Swaty hone. It is a synthetic hone usually imported from Austria. Because it cuts faster than the water hone, it has the advantage of yielding a keen cutting edge on the razor.

Carborundum hone. It is a synthetic hone produced in this country. The barber has a choice of several types, ranging from a slow cutting hone to a fast cutting hone. Many barbers prefer the faster cutting type of hone because of its quick sharpening action. In the hands of a beginner, the carborundum hone should not be used because it may produce a very rough edge.

General Information on Hones

Hones are to a large extent a matter of choice and the type of steel in a razor may make some difference as to whether a good edge can be put on it with a particular type of hone. There are a great many other hones on the market besides the several mentioned which will give very satisfactory results.

Care of hone. Whenever a hone fills with steel, it should be removed. The best method is by using water and a pumice stone. If a new hone is very rough, the same method can be used to work it into shape.

When wet honing is done, the hone should always be **wiped dry** after each usage. This aids in cleaning the hone and also wipes away the tiny particles of steel that adhere to its cutting surface.

Strops

A good strop is made of durable and flexible material, has the proper thickness and texture, and shows a smooth finished surface. Some barbers like a thin strop; whereas others prefer a thick heavy strop. Most barber strops are made in pairs, one side being leather and the other side being canvas. The best assurance for a good strop is the reliability of the manufacturer.

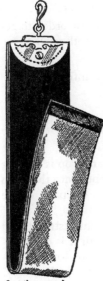

Leather and
Canvas Strop

For the barber's choice there are available various types of strops such as the canvas strop, and the Russian shell and the Russian strop. Leather strops are made out of cowhide, horsehide and pigskin. The better grade strops are broken in by the manufacturer before they are purchased by the barber.

Canvas strop. It is composed of high quality linen or silk woven into a fine or coarse texture. A fine texture linen strop is most desirable for putting a lasting edge on a razor.

To obtain the best results, a new canvas strop should be thoroughly broken in. A daily hand finish will keep its surface smooth and in readiness for stropping.

For a hand finish, the canvas strop is given the following treatment:

1. Attach swivel end of strop to a fixed point such as a nail.
2. Hold the other end tightly over a smooth and level surface.
3. Rub bar of dry soap over strop, working it well into the grain of the canvas.
4. Rub a smooth glass bottle several times over the strop each time forcing the soap into the grain and also removing any excess soap.

Russian strop. This strop was originally imported from Russia. Most of these strops are now made in this country from cowhide leather. The name Russian strop still persists, and usually signifies that the Russian method of tanning was employed.

The Russian strop is one of the best strops in use today. If new it requires a daily hand finish until suoh time as it is thoroughly broken in Thereafter, it will require an occasional servicing. There are several ways of breaking in a Russian strop. One method frequently used is as follows:

1. Rub dry pumice stone over the strop in order to remove the outer nap and develop a smooth surface.
2. Rub stiff lather into the strop.
3. Rub dry pumice stone over the strop until smooth.
4. Clean off the strop.
5. Rub fresh stiff lather into the strop.
6. Rub a smooth glass bottle several times over the strop until a smooth surface is developed.

Another method of breaking in a Russian strop is to omit the pumice stone. Instead, stiff lather is rubbed into the strop with the aid of a smooth glass bottle or with the palm of the hand.

Russian shell. This is a high quality horsehide strop taken from the rump muscle of the horse. Although it is quite expensive, it makes one of the best possible strops for the barber. It always remains smooth and requires very little, if any, breaking in.

Horsehide strop. This strop is of medium grade and has a fine grain. It has a tendency to become very smooth and in this condition does not readily impart the proper edge on the razor. For this reason, it is not recommended for the barber's use. However, it is suitable for private use.

Combs

. Combs are made of either hard rubber, celluloid or bone. The celluloid combs are undesirable for professional use as

Comb

they are combustible and not as durable as the other kinds of combs. Combs made of hard rubber are mainly used by barbers. The teeth of the comb may be fine (close together) or coarse (far apart). To keep combs in good condition, avoid contact with heat and moisture, and store them in a cool, dry place.

Brushes

The brushes that some barbers still use are the hair brush, the hair or neck duster, and the lather brush. The texture of brushes varies with the kind of brush, a hair brush is usually stiff, a hair duster is soft, and a lather brush is flexible.

The lather brush serves to apply the soap lather which softens the beard. Most barbers favor the number three type of lather brush. However, some barbers use the larger sizes.

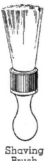

The vulcanized type of lather brush is the most durable, since its bristles will not fall apart in hot water.

To protect the public against contaminated brushes, many states have passed laws requiring that brushes made from animal hair be free from anthrax germs at the time of purchase. These brushes must contain the imprint "Sterilized" to show that the manufacturer has taken necessary steps to destroy the anthrax germs.

Shaving
Brush

Several states consider brushes to be unsanitary and do not allow them to be used at all.

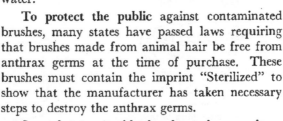

Lather Receptacles

Shaving receptacles are containers used to produce lather necessary for shaving. The most commonly used shaving receptacles are:

1. Electric latherizer.
2. Atomizer latherer.
3. Tube of shaving cream.
4. Lather mug.

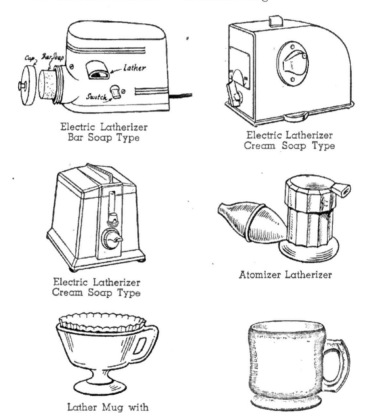

Electric Latherizer
Bar Soap Type

Electric Latherizer
Cream Soap Type

Electric Latherizer
Cream Soap Type

Atomizer Latherizer

Lather Mug with
Paper Lining

Lather Mug

LATHER RECEPTACLES

Lather mugs are gradually disappearing from the barber shop. Gaining in popularity and also replacing the lather mug to a large extent are the newer lather making machines. They offer many advantages to the barber in terms of greater convenience and better service to his customers.

Lather mugs are receptacles made out of glass or earthenware. When the lather mug is to be used, shaving soap and warm water are thoroughly mixed with the aid of the lather brush Since the lather mug is continually exposed and collects dirt easily, it requires a thorough cleansing regularly

To be sanitary, a separate paper lining should be used in the lather mug for each customer. Lather mugs come in handy in the absence or break down of lather electric equipment.

Lather making machines, such as the electric latherizer and the hand operated atomizer latherer, are far superior to the lather mug. Not only are these machines cleaner and more sanitary, but they are more convenient and easier to operate Customers are favorably impressed by the clean sanitary lather coming from these modern machines. For satisfactory performance, follow the manufacturer's instructions on proper use and care.

Shaving Soap

Shaving soap is available in the form of powdered soap, shaving stick or cake soap, and shaving cream (lathering and latherless).

Shaving soaps are preparations made by a chemical process When an alkali (potassium or sodium hydroxide) is mixed and heated with oils and fats, a soap is the final product. The addition of cocoanut oil to the soap improves its lathering qualities. Also present in the shaving soap are varying amounts of water and special ingredients.

Hard soap. The use of **sodium hydroxide** yields a hard soap which is available in the form of either powdered shaving soap, shaving stick or cake soap.

A **soft soap** is the result when **sodium hydroxide** is used. Lather shaving cream usually contains a soft soap and large quantities of water.

The **brushless or latherless shaving cream** differs from any other shaving preparation. Its principal ingredients are uncombined fatty acids (stearic and palmitic acids) together with large amounts of water. Other chemicals present in this type of shaving cream may be soda, potash and special agents.

Tweezer

The tweezer is a metallic implement having two blunt prongs at one end. The blunt prongs of the tweezer are used to pluck unsightly hair and to shape the eyebrows.

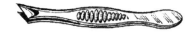

Tweezer

Comedone Extractor

The comedone extractor is a metallic implement having a screwed attachment at each end. The fine needle point at one end is used in piercing whiteheads. The rounded end on the other side is used to press out blackheads.

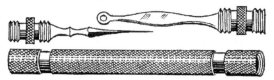

Comedone Extractor

BARBER IMPLEMENTS

1. Name the principal implements used in barbering.	Razors, shears and clippers.
2. Name the accessory implements used by the barber.	Hones, strops, combs, brushes, and lather receptacles.
3. What should the barber look for in the purchase of implements?	High quality, good workmanship, guarantee and reliability of the manufacturer.

Straight Razors

1. Name seven important points to be learned about razors.	The various parts, styles, widths, lengths, tempers, grinds, and finishes of razors.
2. Name the important parts of a razor.	The head, back, shoulder, pivot, blade, point, edge, heel, shank, tang, and handle.
3. Describe the standard style of a razor.	The back and edge are straight and parallel, the head and heel are rounded, while the point is square.
4. Why should the barber round off the sharp point of a razor?	To prevent scratching of the skin during shaving.
5. Which razor widths are commonly used by barbers? Which width is the most commonly used?	4/8, 5/8, 6/8 or 7/8 of an inch. 5/8 is the most commonly used.
6. Which part of the razor is ground by the manufacturer?	The blade.
7. Name two types of grinds found on razors.	The regular wedge and hollow or concave grind.
8. What is meant by the finish of a razor?	Its final polish.
9. Name three kinds of razor finishes.	Plain steel, crocus or nickel plated.
10. What is a crocus finish?	A steel surface polished with crocus or rouge powder.
11. Why is a nickel or steel-plated finish not to be recommended?	Such razors are usually made of inferior steel.
12. Why is balance important in a razor?	For efficient handling, the weight of the blade should be equal to that of the handle.
13. What is meant by the temper of a razor?	The proper degree of hardness and toughness imparted to the steel of the razor.
14. What is the proper way to care for razors?	After being used, strop and dry the razors and then apply a little castor oil over the blades.

Shears

1. Name the important parts of haircutting shears.	Moving point, moving blade, still point, still blade, two cutting edges, pivot screw, two shanks, finger grip, thumb grip and finger brace.
2. Distinguish between the German and French types of haircutting shears. Which one is mostly used?	The German type has no finger brace. The French type has a brace for the small finger. The French type is mostly used.
3. How is the size of the shears usually measured? Which sizes are mostly used?	Shears are usually measured by half inches. 7 and 7 1/2 inch sizes are mostly used.
4. What are the two main types of shear grinds, and which type is mostly used?	The plain edge and the corrugated edge. The plain grind is mostly used.
5. Give the finish of the various plain grinds. Which one is preferred by the barber?	Smooth, medium or coarse. The medium is preferred.

Clippers

1. Name two types of hair clippers.	The hand clipper and the electric clipper.
2. Name the parts of the hand clipper.	Cutting blade, still blade, finger guide, movable handle, still handle, thumb rest, thumb screw, set screw, and heel.
3. Name the visible parts of an electric clipper.	Cutting blade, still blade, heel, switch, set screw and conducting cord.
4. List six sizes of cutting blades used in hair clippers.	0000, 000, 00, 0, 1, 2.
5. Which size gives the shortest cut?	0000.

Accessory Implements

1. What is a hone?	A solid block containing an abrasive for sharpening razors.
2. Name two types of hones available to barbers.	The natural hone obtained from quarried rock and the synthetic or manufactured hone.
3. Name a popular synthetic hone used in the barber shop.	The Swaty hone.
4. Name two kinds of natural hones.	The water hone and Belgian hone.
5. Describe the water hone.	It is a slow cutting hone having a grey or darkish yellow appearance.
6. Describe the Belgian hone.	It is a slow cutting hone but a little faster than the water hone, whose upper surface is yellow and whose bottom portion is dark red.
7. Which natural hones are usually used wet, either with water or lather?	The water hone and Belgian hone.

8. Which hones may be used either dry or with lather?	Synthetic hones.
9. What is a slow cutting hone? Give an example.	A slow cutting hone takes time to produce a sharp razor. A water hone.
10. What is a fast cutting hone? Give two examples.	A fast cutting hone gives a sharp edge quickly. Swaty and carborundum.
11. Which strops are used by barbers?	A leather strop and a canvas strop.
12. Of what are combs made?	Bone, hard rubber and celluloid.
13. Which combs are best for the barber?	Hard rubber and bone combs.
14. Name three types of brushes that some barbers still use.	The hair brush, the hair duster and the lather brush.
15. What should the barber look for in the purchase of brushes?	Purchase brushes of good quality bristles capable of being easily sterilized without destroying the bristles.
16. Name four shaving soap receptacles.	1. Atomizer latherer. 2. Electric latherizer. 3. Tube of shaving cream. 4. Lather mug.
17. Name three types of shaving soap used in a barber shop.	Shaving cream (lathering or latherless), powdered soap and stick or cake soap.

HONING AND STROPPING

An expert barber who knows the right way to hone and strop razors is in a position to render satisfactory service to his customers. To acquire the right technique in honing and stropping requires constant practice and long experience under the guidance of an instructor or licensed barber.

Honing

Honing is the process of sharpening a razor blade on a hone. The main object in honing is to obtain a perfect cutting edge on the razor. For the beginner a slow cutting hone is preferable to the fast cutting hone. Use an old, useless razor for practicing the various movements.

Prepare hone for honing. Honing will be more satisfactory if the razor and hone are kept at room temperature. Depending on which hone is used, it may be moistened with water or lather, or kept dry. When in use, the hone must be kept perfectly flat. Sufficient space should be provided to permit free arm movements in honing.

Technique of honing. This is accomplished by honing the razor with smooth, even strokes of equal number and pressure on both sides of the blade. The angle at which the blade is stroked must be the same for both sides of the blade.

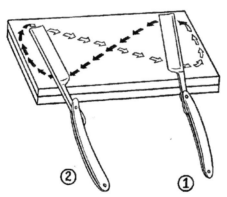

Proper Honing of a Razor

How to hold the razor. Grasp the razor handle comfortably in the right hand as follows:

1. Rest index finger on top of the side part of the shank.
2. Rest ball of thumb at the joint.
3. Place second finger back of the razor near the edge of the shank.
4. Fold remaining fingers around the handle to permit easy turning over of the razor.

First stroke in honing. The razor blade must be stroked diagonally across the hone, drawing the blade towards the cutting edge and heel of the razor, as in Fig. 1.

Second stroke in honing. After the completion of the first stroke, the razor is turned on its back with the fingers in the same manner as you would roll a pencil, without turning the wrist, and then the second stroke is made, as in Fig. 2.

From three to six strokes each way generally does a good job.

Testing razor on moistened thumb nail. Depending on the hardness of the hone and the number of strokes taken, the razor edge may be either blunt, keen, coarse or rough Different sensations are felt when the razor is passed lightly across the thumb nail which has been moistened with water or lather. (See Fig. 3.)

To test the razor edge, place it across the nail of the thumb and slowly draw it from the heel to the point of the razor.

1. **A perfect or keen edge** has fine teeth and tends to dig into the nail with a smooth steady grip.

2. **A blunt razor edge** passes over the nail smoothly, without any cutting power.

3. **A coarse razor edge** digs into the nail with a jerky feeling.

4. **A rough or overhoned edge** has large teeth which stick to the nail and produce a harsh, disagreeable feeling.

5. **A nick in the razor.** A feeling of a slight gap or unevenness in the draw will indicate a nick in the razor.

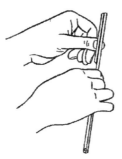
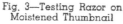
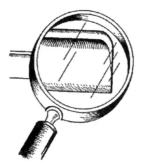

Fig. 3—Testing Razor on   Fig. 4—Magnified Razor Edge
Moistened Thumbnail

Correcting an overhoned razor. To eliminate an over-honed edge, draw the razor backward in a diagonal line across the hone, using the same movement and pressure as in regular honing. One or two strokes each way will usually remove the rough edge. Then, the razor is honed again, being careful to prevent overhoning.

Seldom does it become necessary to put an entirely new edge on the razor. If after repeated honings or abuse, the razor edge remains blunt, it may require a new edge. For this purpose, the razor should be forwarded to an expert sharpener of cutlery.

Magnified razor edge. While honing, the abrasive material makes small cuts in the sides of the razor blade. The small cuts resemble the teeth of a saw, and they point in the same direction as the stroke, as shown in Fig. 4.

Care of the Hone

The barber should know how to use and take care of the particular type of hone he has selected. The manufacturer's instructions offer a reliable guide for keeping the hone in a serviceable condition.

New hones may require a preliminary treatment to put it into good working shape. If a new hone is very rough, rub its surface with water and pumice stone. No preliminary treatment is required for the water hone as it is ready for immediate use.

Before using, make sure that the surface of the hone is smooth and clean. Use the hone either moist or dry, as directed by the manufacturer.

After using any kind of hone, always wipe the surface clean and cover it. Make sure that all adhering steel particles resulting from the honing are completely removed. Whenever a dry hone has been used, rub its surface with water and pumice stone.

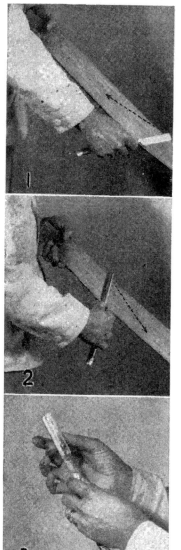

Stropping

Stropping a razor is a fine art developed by repeated practice. The aim in stropping is to smooth and shape the razor edge into a keen cutting instrument. After being honed, the razor seldom needs any stropping on the canvas. Instead, the honed razor is stropped directly over the surface of the leather strop. The time to use the canvas strop is when the razor develops a smooth edge from continued use.

The Technique of Stropping

Hold the end of the strop firmly in the left hand so it cannot sag. Hold it close to the side, and as high as it is comfortable. Take razor in right hand, well up into the hand, holding the shank of razor with the thumb and next two fingers so that the razor can be rolled in the same manner as a lead pencil.

In stropping the razor, use a long diagonal stroke with even pressure from the heel to the point.

Note: The direction of the razor in stropping is the reverse of that used in honing.

First stroke. Start about two-thirds down the strop, as in Fig. 1. Draw the razor edge perfectly flat and straight over the surface of the strop, proceeding towards the back of the razor for a distance of twelve to eighteen inches.

Second stroke. When the first stroke is completed, turn the razor on the back of the blade by rolling it in the fingers without turning the hand, as in Fig. 2. Now draw the razor twelve inches to eighteen inches away from you, thus completing the second stroke in honing.

Bear just heavy enough on the strop to feel the razor draw. Rapid movement is necessary, and this will come to you gradually as you practice.

Final testing of razor on moistened tip of thumb, prior to shaving. Touch the razor edge lightly and note the reaction, as in Fig. 3. A dull edge produces no drawing feeling. A razor that has the proper cutting edge produces a keen drawing feeling.

If the razor edge produces a rough, disagreeable feeling upon testing, it indicates that the cutting edge is still wiry. To correct this condition, additional finishing on the leather strop is necessary.

Should the razor edge yield a smooth feeling upon testing, finish it again on the canvas strop, followed by a few more strokes on the leather strop.

Care of Strops

A leather strop becomes better or worse according to the care it is given. Do not fold a strop, but keep it suspended or attached to a swivel, or laid flat. When a leather strop appears rough, it needs a hand finish to make it smooth. A canvas strop needs a daily hand finish to keep it in good condition. How to break in strops is described on pages 62 and 63.

A strop is sanitary if it is kept clean. Accumulated grit is removed from a canvas strop by rubbing it with lather. To remove imbedded dirt, the leather strop is softened with lather and then scraped with the back side of the shear blade or similar implement.

HONING AND STROPPING

1. What is the proper way to learn how to hone and strop razors in a barber shop?	By continued study, practice and experience.
2. What is accomplished by proper honing?	The razor acquires a perfect cutting edge.
3. Describe the manner of stroking a razor on a hone.	Hold the razor at the proper angle and use smooth, even strokes and pressure on both sides of the blade.
4. Describe the first stroke used in honing.	Stroke the razor blade to the left diagonally across the hone, from the heel to point towards the edge.
5. How is the second stroke performed in honing?	Turn the razor over on its back and stroke the blade to the right diagonally across the hone, from the heel to the point towards the edge.
6. What happens to the razor edge as it is honed?	The abrasive material on the hone makes small cuts in the sides of the razor's edge.
7. Why should the honed razor be tested on a moist thumb nail?	To determine if the razor edge is either blunt, keen, coarse or rough.
8. What are the signs of a keen edge or a properly honed razor?	It tends to dig into the nail with a smooth steady grip.
9. What are the signs of a blunt razor edge?	It passes over the nail smoothly without any cutting power.
10. What are the signs of a coarse razor edge?	It tends to dig into the nail with a jerky feeling.
11. What are the signs of a rough or overhoned razor edge?	It has large teeth which stick to the nail and give a harsh, cutting feeling.
12. What is the proper care of a dry hone?	Use hone as directed by manufacturer. After being used, rub its surface with water and pumice stone, then wipe clean and keep covered.
13. What is the proper care of a wet hone?	Use hone as directed by manufacturer. After being used, keep its surface clean, smooth and covered.
14. What is the purpose of stropping the razor after honing?	To smooth the razor's edge.
15. How does stropping differ from honing?	The stroking of the razor blade in stropping is just the reverse of honing.
16. Which strop is used on a freshly honed razor?	The leather strop.
17. What is the proper way to hold the strop?	Grasp the end of the strop with the left hand and hold it firm and tight.

18. How should the razor be held for stropping?	Hold the razor in the right hand with the fingers wrapped around the handle and shank.
19. Where should the first stroke be started?	Start about two-thirds down the strop.
20. Describe the movements used in stropping.	1. Place the razor flat against the strop with the back towards the barber about two-thirds down the strop. 2. Draw the razor towards the barber. 3. Turn the razor over on its back with the fingers. 4. Draw the razor away from the barber. 5. Repeat these movements until razor is properly stropped.
21. Which fingers are used in rolling and turning the razor in the hand?	The thumb and next two fingers of right hand.
22. How much pressure should be applied in stropping?	Use normal pressure at the point and heel for both sides of the razor.
23. How is the razor edge tested after stropping?	Touch the razor edge lightly over the cushion of the thumb.
24. What is the sign of a smooth, sharp razor edge?	It produces a keen, drawing sensation.
25. What is the sign of a dull razor edge?	It produces no drawing sensation.
26. How can the strop be kept clean and smooth?	Apply lather or soap to the strop, then wipe it clean to remove accumulated grit.
27. What is the purpose of stropping the razor before shaving?	To smooth and shape the edge of the razor into a keen cutting edge.
28. In what way should the strops be kept?	Either suspended or attached to a swivel, or laid flat.
29. What is used to remove accumulated grit from leather strops?	Rub lather into the strop, then remove lather and grit with back side of a shear blade or similar implement.

FACE SHAVING

Face shaving is necessary for hygienic, business or social reasons. To feel clean and look their best, most men require regular shaving. Since there is a universal need for face shaving, every effort should be made to attract men to the barber shop for this service.

Shaving is one of the basic services rendered in the barber shop. It deserves greater attention and skill than it has received in the past. With the introduction of the safety razor and now the electric razor, the income from shaving gradually declined in the barber shop. Instead of making a vigorous effort to offset this trend, the barber devoted less of his time to shaving. As a result, shaving soon became a lost art.

Barbers are now beginning to realize that they are losing a considerable amount of business that should rightfully be theirs. More and more barbers are now featuring shaving as a means of holding on to their customers. Men who make a regular habit of being shaved in the barber shop are likely prospects for other services such as haircuts, facials and scalp treatments The barber's prestige and earning power will be vastly increased if he is capable of giving the best shaves to his customers.

Fundamentals of Face Shaving

The object of shaving is to remove the visible part of the hair extending over the surface of the skin of the face and neck in such a manner so as not to cause irritation to the skin. For this purpose, a straight razor and lather are commonly used for shaving a man's beard.

Although there are certain general principles of shaving which apply to all men, there are nevertheless particular exceptions. Account should be taken of the texture of the hair (coarse, medium or fine), the grain of the beard and the sensitivity of the skin to the razor edge, shaving cream, hot towels and astringent lotion. Hot towels should not be used when the skin is chapped or blistered from heat or cold. **A person having any infection of the beard must not be shaved by a barber, as this may be the means of spreading the infection.**

Four Standard Shaving Positions and Strokes

To obtain the best cutting stroke, the razor must glide over the surface at an angle with the grain of the hair, and be drawn in a sawing movement with the point of the razor in the lead.

To shave the face and neck with the greatest of ease and efficiency, the barber employs the following standard positions and strokes:

1. Free Hand Position and Stroke.
2. Back Hand Position and Stroke.
3. Reverse Free Hand Position and Stroke.
4. Reverse Back Hand Position and Stroke.

Under each of the standard shaving positions and strokes, consideration should be given to:

1. When to use the shaving stroke.
2. How to hold the razor.
   a) Position of right hand with razor.
   b) Position of left hand.
3. How to stroke the razor.

Review the proper method of honing and stropping the razor before learning each shaving stroke.

Exercise No. 1

Free Hand Position and Stroke

In the first lesson, the barber student learns the correct way to perform the free hand position and stroke. To master this important shaving skill requires regular practice.

1. **When to use the free hand stroke.** The free hand position and stroke comprises six of the fourteen shaving areas. See Numbers 1, 3, 4, 8, 11, 12 on the accompanying illustration.

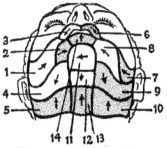

Diagram of Shaving Areas
The Free Hand strokes are shown
in white.

- 1. Free hand.
- 2. Back hand.
- 3. Free hand.
- 4. Free hand.
- 5. Reverse free hand.
- 6. Back hand.
- 7. Back hand.
- 8. Free hand.
- 9. Back hand.
- 10. Reverse free hand.
- 11. Free hand.
- 12. Free hand.
- 13. Reverse free hand.
- 14. Reverse free hand.

2. **How to hold razor.** The position of the right hand is as follows:

   a) Take the razor in right hand.

   b) Hold handle of razor between third and fourth fingers, the small finger-tip resting on the tang of the razor. Place tip of thumb on shank close to blade and rest tips of fingers back of the shank.

   c) Raise elbow of the right arm nearly level with the shoulder. This is the position used in the arm movement.

   (Note: Some barbers prefer to use the wrist movement, in which case the elbow is not raised as high.)

The position of the left hand is as follows:

   a) Keep the fingers of the left hand dry in order to prevent them from slipping on the wet face.

b) Keep left hand back of razor in order to stretch skin tightly under razor.

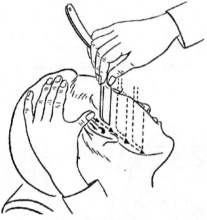

Free Hand Stroke
Area No. 1

3. **How to stroke the razor.** The free hand stroke is performed in the following manner:

a) Use a gliding stroke towards you.
b) Direct the stroke towards the point of the razor in a back and forth sawing movement.
c) Keep the length of the strokes from one inch to three inches, depending upon the location of the part of the face being shaved.

Exercise No. 2

Back Hand Position and Stroke

After the barber student has developed skill in performing the free hand position and stroke, he is now ready to proceed with the back hand position and stroke.

1. **When to use the back hand stroke.** The back hand stroke comprises four steps in the fourteen basic shaving areas. See Numbers 2, 6, 7, 9 on the accompanying illustration.

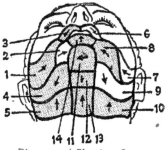

Diagram of Shaving Areas
The Back Hand strokes are
shown in white.

  1. Free hand.
• 2. Back hand.
  3. Free hand.
  4. Free hand.
  5. Reverse free hand.
• 6. Back hand.
• 7. Back hand.
  8. Free hand.
• 9. Back hand.
  10. Reverse free hand.
  11. Free hand.
  12. Free hand.
  13. Reverse free hand.
  14. Reverse free hand.

2. **How to hold razor.** The position of the right hand is as follows:

   a) Hold the shank of the razor firmly with the handle bent back.

   b) Rest the shank of the razor on the first two joints of the first two fingers. Hold thumb on the shank. Rest end of tang on inside of first joint of third finger. Little finger remains idle.

   c) Turn the back of the hand away from you and bend the wrist slightly downward. Then raise the elbow so that you can move the arm freely. This is the position used for back hand stroke with arm movement.

   (Note: Some barbers prefer to use the wrist movement, in which case the arm is not held as high as for the arm movement.)

The position of the left hand is as follows:

a) Keep the fingers of the left hand dry in order to prevent them from slipping.

b) Hold hand as if stretching the skin tightly under razor.

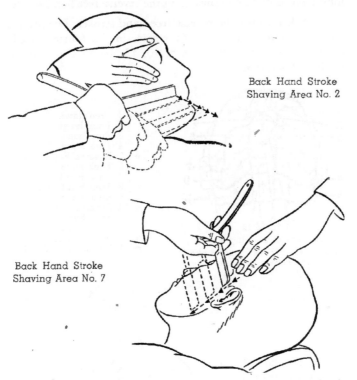

Back Hand Stroke
Shaving Area No. 2

Back Hand Stroke
Shaving Area No. 7

3. **How to stroke the razor.** The back hand stroke is performed in the following manner:

a) Use a gliding stroke away from you.

b) Direct stroke towards the point of the razor in a back and forth sawing movement.

c) Keep the length of the stroke from one inch to three inches, depending upon the location of the part of the face being shaved.

Exercise No. 3
Reverse Free Hand Position and Stroke

The reverse free hand stroke and the free hand stroke are similar in some respects, the main difference being that the movement is directed upwards in the reverse free hand stroke.

1. **When to use the reverse free hand stroke.** The reverse free hand stroke comprises four steps in the fourteen basic shaving areas. See Numbers 5, 10, 13, 14 on the accompanying illustration.

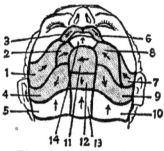

Diagram of Shaving Areas
The Reverse Free Hand strokes
are shown in white.

1. Free hand.
2. Back hand.
3. Free hand.
4. Free hand.
● 5. Reverse free hand.
6. Back hand.
7. Back hand.
8. Free hand.
9. Back hand.
● 10. Reverse free hand.
11. Free hand.
12. Free hand.
● 13. Reverse free hand.
● 14. Reverse free hand.

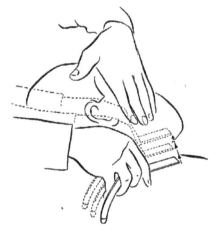

Reverse Free Hand Stroke
Shaving Area No. 5

Note: Left hand is used to stretch skin.

2. **How to hold the razor.** The position of the right hand is as follows:

    a) Hold the razor firmly as in a free hand position, turn hand slightly toward you so that the razor edge is turned upward.

The position of the left hand is as follows:

    a) Keep the hand dry and use it to pull the skin tightly under the razor.

3. **How to stroke the razor.** The reverse free hand stroke is performed in the following manner:

    a) Use small upward semi-arc stroke towards you.

    b) The movement is from the elbow to the hand with a slight twist of the wrist.

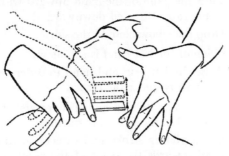

Reverse Free Hand Stroke
Shaving Area No. 10

Note: Left hand stretching skin between thumb and middle finger.

Exercise No. 4

Reverse Back Hand Position and Stroke

• The reverse back hand position and stroke, although not frequently used, must be practiced diligently in order to master this shaving technique.

1. **When to use the reverse back hand stroke.** The reverse back hand stroke is used for making left sideburn outline and for shaving the left side behind the ear when the customer is sitting in an upright position.

2. **How to hold the razor.** The position of the right hand is as follows:

    a) Hold the razor firmly as in the back hand position.

    b) Turn the palm of the hand upward with the point of the razor directed downward.

    c) Drop the elbow close to the side.

The position of the left hand is as follows:

    a) Raise the left arm and hand in order to draw the skin tightly under the razor.

3. **How to stroke the razor.** The reverse back hand stroke is performed in the following manner:

    a) Use a gliding stroke and direct the stroke downward towards the point of the razor in a sawing movement.

Reverse Back Hand
Stroke
Shaving Left Side of
Neck below Ear

Note the position of the razor.

The razor is stroked with the point of the razor in the lead.

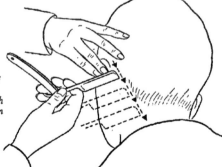

Exercise No. 5

Fourteen Shaving Areas

Before proceeding with the next lesson, review the correct way to handle the razor as for:

1. Free Hand Position and Stroke (Exercise No. 1).
2. Back Hand Position and Stroke (Exercise No. 2).
3. Reverse Free Hand Position and Stroke (Exercise No. 3).

There are fourteen shaving areas in giving a shave the first time over. The right side is shaved first, using the free hand stroke. The shaving areas and strokes used are indicated in numerical order, as follows:

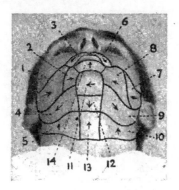

Diagram of Shaving Areas

1. Free hand.	8. Free hand.
2. Back hand.	9. Back hand.
3. Free hand.	10. Reverse free hand.
4. Free hand.	11. Free hand.
5. Reverse free hand.	12. Free hand.
6. Back hand.	13. Reverse free hand.
7. Back hand.	14. Reverse free hand.

To give a face shave with skill and ease, it is necessary to learn the fourteen basic shaving areas in the order named and practice them regularly.

Exercise No. 6

How To Prepare
A Customer For Shaving

As the customer enters the shop, you are to arise and stand at attention on the right side of the chair, facing the prospective customer with an attitude of willingness to serve.

Smile as you greet the customer by name. If the customer is known casually refer to him as Mister with his last name. Only when well acquainted should a customer be called by his first name.

1. Seat customer comfortably in barber chair.

2. Wash hands with soap and warm water, and dry them thoroughly.*

3. Grasp neck-pieces of chair cloth and bring it over front of customer, as in Fig. 1.

4. Change paper cover on headrest and adjust the headrest to the proper height.

5. Lower, adjust and lock barber chair to the proper height and level.

6. Unfold a clean face towel, and lay it diagonally across the customer's chest.

7. Tuck in the left corner of the towel along the right side of the customer's neck, the edge tucked inside the neckband with a sliding movement of the forefinger of the left hand, as in Fig. 2. The lower left end of the towel is crossed over to the other side of the customer's neck and tucked under the neck-band with a sliding movement of the forefinger of the right hand, as in Fig. 3.

*Some barbers prefer to wash hands after Step 5.

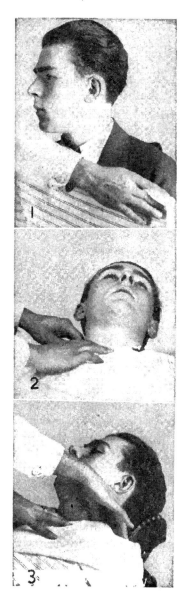

Exercise No. 7

How To Prepare The Face For Shaving.

Lathering and steaming the face are very important steps before shaving the face, for the following reasons:

Lathering the face serves the following purposes:

1. Cleans the face by dislodging dirt and foreign matter.
2. Fills spaces between hairs and keeps them in an erect position.
3. Affords a smooth, flat surface for the razor to glide over.

Steaming the face is helpful for the following reasons:

1. Softens the cuticle or outer layer of the hair.
2. Provides lubrication by stimulating the action of the oil glands.
3. Soothes and relaxes the customer.

Do not use steam towel if the face is sensitive, irritated, chapped or blistered.

The face is prepared for shaving as follows:

1. Prepare lather and spread it evenly over bearded parts of face and neck. To prepare shaving lather, use any of the following:

    a) Electric latherizer.　　c) Tube of shaving cream.

    b) Atomizer latherizer.　　d) Shaving soap or powder.*

2. Rub lather well in-to bearded area, us-ing rotary move-ments with the cu-shion tips of the right hand. Rub la-ther on right side of face, then gently turn the head with the left hand, by gently grasping the back of the head

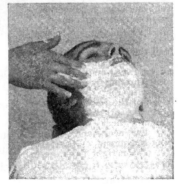

Rubbing Lather
in a Rotary Movement

*Requires the use of a shaving mug and brush. See Exercise 3.

near the crown, and rub lather on the other side of face. Rubbing time from one to two minutes, depending upon the stiffness and density of the beard.

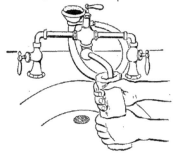

Saturating and Heating the Towel

3. Take a clean Turkish towel, fold it once lengthwise. Then fold it again the short way by bringing together both ends of the towel.

4. Place folded towel under stream of hot water, allowing it to become thoroughly saturated and heated.

5. Wring out towel until fairly dry.

6. Bring the steam towel behind the barber's chair. Unfold it and hold each end. Place center of towel under customer's chin and lower part of neck. Carefully wrap towel around face and forehead, leaving the nose

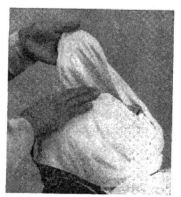

Applying Heated Towel Over Face

exposed. Finally, fold the ends over each other on the forehead.

7. While the steam towel is on the customer's face, strop the razor and immerse it into disinfectant solution.* Then wipe the razor dry on the corner of the face towel, and place it in a dry sterilizer until ready for use.

8. In removing steam towel, wipe lather off in one operation.

*Some barbers prefer to disinfect the razor before stropping or honing.

9. Re-lather the beard a second time, then wipe the hands free of soap.
10. Now pick up the razor, take a position on the right side of the customer, and place sanitary tissue or paper on customer's chest for wiping lather off razor.

Exercise No. 8

How to Use Shaving Mug and Brush

In the absence or breakdown of a mechanical latherizer, extra supplies are needed for producing shaving lather. For this purpose, the barber shop should have on hand shaving mugs, disposable paper linings, shaving brushes and shaving soap or powder in sufficient quantity to meet its needs.

Preparing Lather with Shaving Powder

1. Rinse the brush and mug thoroughly in warm water, insert paper lining, and retain a little water at bottom of mug.
2. Sprinkle shaving powder on brush and mix in mug to form a creamy lather.
3. To apply lather to face, grasp handle of brush in palm of right hand, with the fingertips at base of bristles.

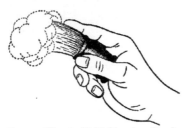

Proper Way to Hold Shaving Brush

4. Starting at right side of neck just below jaw bone, rub lather well, using rotary movements with brush.
5. Gently turn face and rub lather with brush into left side of face.

6. Place brush in mug and work lather into bearded area, using cushion tips of right hand.
7. Continue with steps 3-10 as outlined in Exercise 7.

Preparing Lather with Cake Soap

Pick up the shaving cup with cake soap and brush with the left hand, holding the thumb on the brush so that it will not overbalance and fall. Rinse the brush and mug thoroughly with warm water, leaving some water in the mug. Mix up a lather with the brush until it forms a creamy consistency. Avoid making noise by rattling the handle of the brush on the sides of the mug. Apply lather to the face as explained in steps 3 to 7.

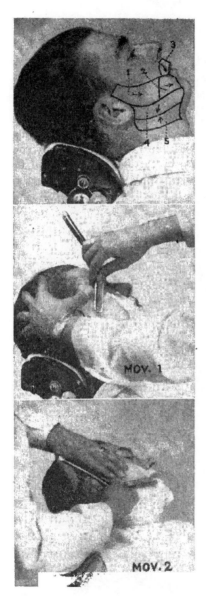

Exercise No. 9
Positions
and Strokes
in Shaving

The barber is now ready to begin shaving. Proper coordination of both hands makes for better and safer shaving. While the right hand holds and strokes the razor, the fingers of the left hand assist in stretching the skin tightly around the part being shaved. A tight skin has the advantage that it allows the beard to be cut more easily. To prevent slipping, the fingers of the left hand must be kept dry at all times.

Shaving Area No. 1

Free Hand Stroke. Barber stands on right side of chair. Gently turn customer's face to the left. With second finger of left hand, remove lather from hairline. Hold razor as for a free hand stroke. Use long gliding diagonal strokes with the point of the razor in the lead. Beginning at hairline on right side, shave downward towards the jawbone. Shave right side of face to the corner of the mouth.

Shaving Area No. 2

Back Hand Stroke. Remaining in the same position, wipe razor clean on lather paper. Hold the razor as for a back hand stroke; use a diagonal stroke with the point of the razor in the lead. Shave all of the beard on the right side of the face up to the point of the chin.

Shaving Area No. 3

Free Hand Stroke. Keeping the same position, wipe razor clean. Hold razor as for a free hand stroke. Shave underneath the nostril and over the right side of upper lip, using the fingers of the left hand to stretch the underlying skin. When shaving underneath the nostril, slightly lift the tip of the nose without interfering with the breathing. To stretch the upper lip, place fingers of left hand against nose while holding the thumb below the lower corner of the lip.

Shaving Area No. 4

Free Hand Stroke. Without wiping the razor, start at point of chin and shave all that portion below the jawbone down to the change in the grain of the beard. While shaving, hold the skin tightly between thumb and fingers of left hand.

Shaving Area No. 5

Reverse Free Hand Stroke. Step to back of chair. Hold the razor as for a reverse free hand stroke. Shave the remainder of the beard upward with the grain. This movement completes shaving the right side of the face.

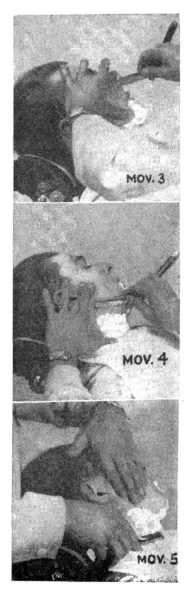

MOV. 3

MOV. 4

MOV. 5

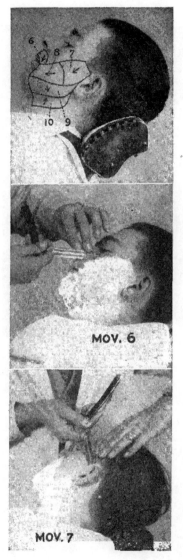

MOV. 6

MOV. 7

Diagram of shaving areas for left side of face.

Shaving Area No. 6

Back Hand Stroke. Wipe razor clean and strop it. Stand on right side of customer and turn customer's face upward so that you can shave the left upper lip. Hold razor as for a back hand stroke. While gently pushing the tip of the nose to the right with thumb and fingers of left hand, shave the left side of upper lip.

Note: Some barbers prefer to shave the upper lip after Step No. 8.

Shaving Area No. 7

Back Hand Stroke. Stand slightly back of customer. Gently turn his face to the right. Re-lather left side of face. Clean lather from hairline. Stretching the skin with the fingers of the left hand, shave downward to the lower part of the ear and slightly forward, on the face. Caution: Be careful to stretch the skin well with the left hand as the razor may dig in along the ear.

Shaving Area No. 8

Free Hand Stroke. Wipe off razor. Step to right side of customer. Hold razor as for free hand stroke. Shave downward on left side of face towards jawbone and point of chin.

Note: Some barbers prefer to shave the upper lip (See Step No. 6) at this time.

Shaving Area No. 9

Back Hand Stroke. Wipe off razor. Keeping the same position, hold razor as for back hand stroke. With the fingers of the left hand tightly stretching the skin, shave downward from point of chin to where the grain of the beard changes on the neck. Complete shaving upper part of neck.

Shaving Area No. 10

Reverse Free Hand Stroke. Wipe off razor. Stand slightly back of customer. Hold razor as for reverse free hand stroke. Stretching the skin tightly with the left hand, shave the left side of the neck in an upward direction.

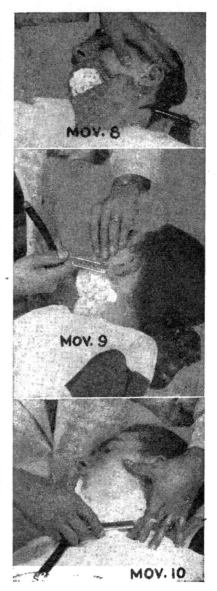

MOV. 8

MOV. 9

MOV. 10

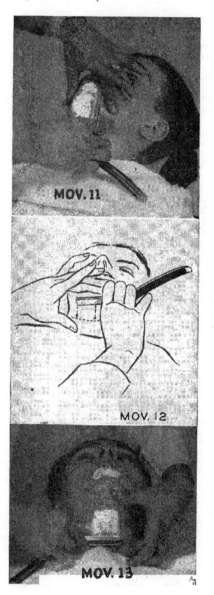

MOV. 11

MOV. 12

MOV. 13

Shaving Area No. 11

Free Hand Stroke. Take your position at the side of the customer and turn his head so the face is pointing upward. Hold razor as for free hand stroke, shave across upper part of the chin. Continue shaving across the chin until it has been shaved to a point below the jawbone. The skin is stretched with the left hand.

Shaving Area No. 12

Free Hand Stroke. Stretch the skin with the left hand and shave the area just below the chin until the change in the grain of the beard is reached.

Shaving Area No. 13

Reverse Free Hand Stroke. Change position to back of chair. Hold the razor as for a reverse free hand stroke. Stretch the skin tightly and shave upward on the lower part of the neck.

Shaving Area No. 14

Reverse Free Hand Stroke. Remain back of chair. Shave upwards on lower lip with a few short reverse free hand strokes.

Wipe off razor again, and in so doing, fold the lather paper in half.

During Steps 13 and 14 the barber should avoid breathing into the customer's face as this is annoying and unhealthy to the customer.

Second Time Over

The second time over is for the purpose of removing any rough spots or unshaved parts.

While the face is steaming, strop the razor and place it on work bench. Remove steam towel, pick up water bottle, and sprinkle a little water in the cupped palm of the left hand. Moisten the bearded part of the face, place bottle on work stand, and proceed with the second time over. Use the free hand and reverse free hand strokes in shaving the second time over.

Stand a little in back of customer. With a free hand stroke (see illustration), start to shave right side of face. Stroking the grain of the beard sideways, shave the upper lip and work downward to the lower jawbone. Shave lower part of neck with a reverse free hand stroke and follow the grain of the beard.

Now, turn the customer's face towards you. With a free hand stroke, start to shave left side of face. Stroking the grain of the beard sideways, shave from ear towards eye. When finished, wipe off razor on lather paper and discard it into container.

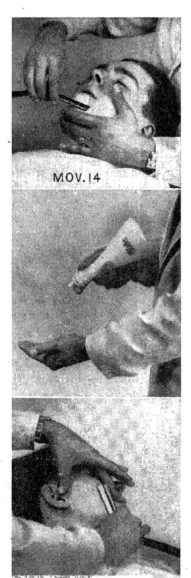

MOV. 14

Once Over Shave

If the customer requests a "once over" shave, the barber should be able to comply with his wishes. The "once over" shave has the advantage that it takes less time to give a complete and even shave. For a "once over" shave, give a few more strokes at different angles when each shaving movement is completed.

Close Shaving

Close shaving is the practice of shaving the beard against the grain of the hair during the second time over. This shaving practice is undesirable because it irritates the skin and may cause an infection or ingrown hairs. For this reason, the barber should avoid close shaving.

Accidental Cuts in Shaving

The barber should know what to do in case the face is cut or scratched in shaving. For a minor cut, apply a little styptic powder with a piece of sterilized cotton. When the bleeding stops, carefully wipe off the powder with clean cotton.

For a deeper cut, apply an antiseptic solution with a piece of sterilized cotton. Then cover cut with a small band-aid.

Exercise No. 10

WRAPPING A TOWEL AROUND THE HAND

A properly trained barber knows how to wrap a towel around the hand with ease and skill for the purpose of:

1. Cleansing and drying the face.
2. Applying powder to the face.
3. Removing all traces of powder, lather and any loose hair from face, neck and forehead.

The student should practice the following exercise until he is able to wrap the towel around the hand with ease and skill.

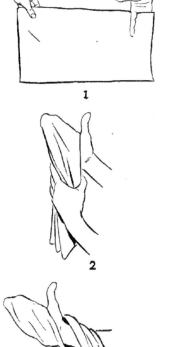

1

1. Hold the towel the long way and grasp both ends as in Fig. 1.

2. Hold the right hand in front of you, draw the upper edge of the towel across the palm of the right hand.

3. Then grasp the towel and draw it towards the right arm as in Fig. 2.

2

4. Holding the towel in this position twist it around the outside of wrist and hold ends of towel from flapping on the face, as in Fig. 3.

3

Exercise No. 11

FINAL STEPS IN FACE SHAVING

The final steps in face shaving require attention to a number of important details.

1. Apply face cream with massage movements.
2. Prepare steam towel and apply it over face.
   Suggest facial treatment at this time.
3. Remove steam towel from face.
4. Apply finishing lotion with several facial manipulations.
5. Pick up towel from customer's chest.
6. Take your position behind the barber chair.
7. Spread towel over customer's face and first dry the lower part and then the upper part of the face.
8. Take your position on the right side of the chair.
9. Wrap towel around hand as described in Exercise 10.
10. Thoroughly dry the face.
11. Select a dry spot of towel and fold it around the hand.

Drying Customer's Face

12. Sprinkle talcum powder over dry towel.
13. Apply powder evenly to face.
14. Raise barber chair to an upright position.
15. Shave the neckline, if necessary, as described in Exercise 12.
16. Comb the hair neatly.
17. With neck towel, wipe off loose hair, lather or powder on face and clothing.
18. Trim mustache, if desired.
19. Remove neck-band and linens.
20. Release customer.

Exercise No. 12

NECK SHAVE

The neck shave, as part of the regular shave, involves shaving the neckline on both sides of the neck below the ears.

Raise the chair slowly in an upright position, tuck the face towel around the back of the neck, and apply lather. Shave neckline, first at the right side using a free hand stroke and then at the left side using a reverse free hand stroke, as described in Exercise No. 4.

Wipe shaved part of the neck with warm damp towel. Remove face towel from around the neck, and dry thoroughly. (This is the time to suggest scalp treatment, or hair tonic.)

Take your position behind the chair, and comb the hair as desired by the customer.

Take towel from the back of neck, and fold it around the right hand. Remove all traces of powder and any loose hair.

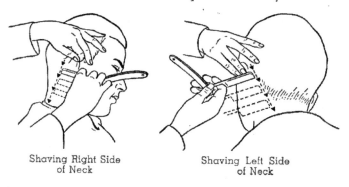

Shaving Right Side   Shaving Left Side
of Neck   of Neck

Points to Remember in Shaving

1. The experienced barber will observe the hair slope and shave with, never against it.

2. A heavy growth of beard requires care in the lathering process and special technique in the use of the razor.

3. The lather should not be scattered carelessly all over the face.

4. The fingers of the left hand should be kept dry in order to grasp and stretch the skin and hold it firmly.

5. Hot towels should not be used on excessively sensitive skin, nor should they be used when the skin is chapped or blistered from cold or heat.

6. Take precaution in shaving: beneath lower lip, lower part of neck, and around the Adam's apple, as these parts of the face and neck are usually the most tender and sensitive, and are easily irritated by very close shaving.

Eleven Reasons Why A Customer May Find Fault With A Shave

1. Dull or rough razors.
2. Unclean hands, towels and shaving cloth.
3. Cold fingers.
4. Heavy touch of hand.
5 Poorly heated towels
6. Lather which is either too cold or too hot.
7. Offensive body odor, foul breath or tobacco odor.
8. Sticking your fingers in customer's mouth.
9. Glaring lights over head.
10. Unshaved hair patches.
11. Scraping the skin and close shaving.

THE MUSTACHE

A shave is not completed unless the barber gives attention to the care of the mustache.

The man who possesses a mustache likes to have it shaped, trimmed, and possibly waxed, because it tends to improve his appearance. If the color of the mustache does not match that of the hair, dyeing or bleaching may be advisable. The barber who is prepared to render such additional services is the one whom the customer will prefer and appreciate.

STYLES OF MUSTACHES

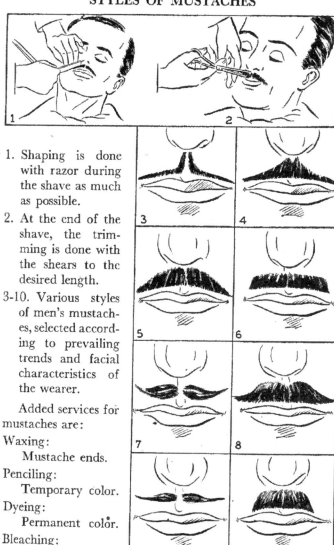

1. Shaping is done with razor during the shave as much as possible.

2. At the end of the shave, the trimming is done with the shears to the desired length.

3-10. Various styles of men's mustaches, selected according to prevailing trends and facial characteristics of the wearer.

Added services for mustaches are:

Waxing:
   Mustache ends.

Penciling:
   Temporary color.

Dyeing:
   Permanent color.

Bleaching:
   Removing color.

SPECIAL PROBLEMS
EYEBROW SHAPING

Eyebrows may be re-shaped either by plucking with tweezers or shaving. The service generally rendered in a barber shop is the shaving or plucking of hair that grows too thick between the brows or of the hair that grows too high above the eyebrows.

TWEEZING

The skin should be softened with cream, and cotton pads dipped in hot water and applied to the brows. Extract the hair by pulling quickly in the direction in which the hair grows, at the same time stretching the skin to reduce pain. Finish with an application of astringent lotion.

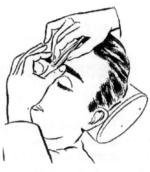

Tweezing Eyebrows

TRIMMING EYEBROWS

If the eyebrows are too thick or bushy they may be trimmed to a uniform shape with the comb and scissors.

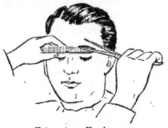

Trimming Eyebrows

STYPTIC POWDER

Whenever a slight cut or scratch drawing blood has occurred, apply styptic powder sparingly to the cut on a small pledget of cotton, and wipe off carefully.

Never use a styptic pencil or any other astringent that will come in contact with more than one face, as there is great danger of infection.

BLACKHEADS OR COMEDONES

Blackheads, which make their appearance on the face and more particularly around the nose, may be removed by means of a comedone extractor, and by steaming.

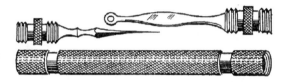

Comedone Extractor

It is not well to attempt to remove all the blackheads appearing on the surface at one time; they should be removed by a series of treatments extending over a period of time.

Facial massage helps to dislodge and remove a number of blackheads.

WHITEHEADS

To remove whiteheads, the skin must first be cleansed with soap and water, followed by the application of steam towels. Then, each whitehead is pierced with the sharp end of a sterilized needle, tweezer or comedone extractor. Gently press out each whitehead with a pledget of sterilized cotton. Finally, apply antiseptic solution over the treated area.

INGROWN OR WILD HAIR

An ingrown hair is one that has grown underneath the skin, causing a lump in which pus forms. Usually caused by very close shaving or the rubbing of a shirt collar.

To remove a wild hair or dead hair, open the affected part with a sterilized needle, pull out the hair with a sterilized tweezer, then apply an antiseptic solution.

NOTES

REVIEW QUESTIONS ON SHAVING

1. What three points should the barber know about the customer's skin and hair?	1. Condition of the skin. 2. Texture of the hair. 3. Slope and grain of beard.
2. What are nine requirements of a good shave?	1. Hands, razor and towels should be properly sterilized. 2. Razor properly honed and stropped. 3. Beard well lathered. 4. Towels properly heated and applied. 5 Beard cut smoothly. 6. Lather completely removed. 7. Astringent or face lotion properly applied. 8. Face dried thoroughly. 9. Powder evenly applied.
3. How should the customer be prepared for shaving?	1. Barber washes hands. 2. Arrange shaving cloth. 3. Adjust headrest paper and adjust headrest to proper level. 4. Recline chair to comfortable position. 5. Tuck in towel.
4. How should the beard be prepared for shaving?	Apply lather to face; apply steam towel over lather; remove lather with steam towel; re-lather beard.
5. What sanitary precautions should be observed by the barber?	1. Use clean hands. 2. Use sterilized razor. 3. Use sanitary receptacle for shaving soap. 4. Use sanitary tissue to wipe lather from razor.
6. What is the most effective way to rub lather into the beard?	To rub lather into the beard use the cushion parts of finger tips with a circular movement.
7. What action does the lather have on the beard?	The lather softens and lubricates the skin and beard.
8. What is the purpose of steaming the face?	The heat softens the outer layer of the hair and stimulates the flow of oil from the skin glands, the added lubrication helps the razor to glide over the face.
9. When should a hot towel not be applied to the face?	If the face is very sensitive, irritated, chapped or blistered.
10. Name the four standard positions and strokes used in shaving.	Free hand; back hand; reverse free hand; reverse back hand.
11. How should the razor be used to accomplish the free hand stroke?	Hold the razor in a free hand position. Use a gliding stroke towards the point of the razor in a sawing movement.

12. How should the razor be used to accomplish the back hand stroke?	Hold the razor in a back hand position and stroke it in a sawing movement away from you towards the point of the razor.
13. How should the razor be used to accomplish the reverse free hand stroke?	The razor is held similarly to the free hand position and the stroke is performed with a slight rotation of the wrist, forming a small upward arc.
14. What should be the direction of the shaving strokes in respect to the grain of the hair?	The shaving strokes are made with the grain of the hair.
15. When is the reverse back hand position and stroke usually used?	As the customer sits in an upright position, the barber evens the sideburn at left temple and outlines the haircut on the left side of the neck behind the ear.
16. How many shaving areas are there in shaving the first time over?	14 shaving areas.
17. Which side of the face is shaved first and which stroke is used first?	The right side is shaved first. The free hand stroke is the first stroke.
18. How is a once-over shave given?	A few more strokes at different angles to the beard may be taken at the completion of each movement, thereby assuring a complete and even shave.
19. What part of the neck is shaved with the standard or regular shave?	The sides of the neck below the ears.
20. What are the final steps after shaving?	Comb the hair neatly, wipe off excessive powder, and any loose hair.
21. When should a facial be suggested to the customer?	As the last steam towel is being removed.
22. When should a hair tonic or scalp treatment be suggested to the customer?	Just before combing the hair.
23. Give eleven reasons why a customer may find fault with a shave.	1. Dull or rough razors. 2. Unclean hands, towels and shaving cloth. 3. Cold fingers. 4. Heavy touch of hand. 5. Poorly heated towels. 6. Lather which is either too cold or too hot. 7. Offensive body odor, foul breath or tobacco odor. 8. Sticking your fingers in customer's mouth. 9. Glaring lights over head. 10. Unshaved hair patches. 11. Scraping the skin and close shaving.

24. **What is an ingrown hair?**	An ingrown hair is one which has grown underneath the skin and causes an infection to develop.
25. **What is the cause of an ingrown hair?**	Usually caused by very close shaving and the wearing of shirt collars which rub against the neck.
26. **What is the proper treatment for an ingrown hair?**	To remove an ingrown hair, open the affected part with a sterilized needle or tweezer and then pull out the hair with the tweezer. Finally, apply an antiseptic such as peroxide or tincture of iodine.
27. **How is a close shave produced?**	Shaving the beard against the grain of the hair during the second time over.
28. **Why is a close shave undesirable?**	A close shave irritates the skin and may cause ingrown hairs or infection.

MEN'S HAIRCUTTING

The art of haircutting involves a distinctive cut and arrangement of the hair to suit the individual requirements of the customer. Each customer presents a new problem which the shop owner cannot afford to neglect by careless or indifferent workmanship. Mistakes should be prevented rather than covered up or changed. Expert workmanship in haircutting can best be acquired by competent instruction and by patient practice on living models.

Fundamentals in Haircutting

It is essential that the barber acquire an easy, graceful position when cutting the hair. Avoid stooping, bending the knees, or twisting the body into awkward positions. In haircutting, work to the right of you, as this will give you a better view of your work. Learning correct habits in haircutting will relieve fatigue and make your work more efficient.

Implements

The principal implements used in haircutting are: clippers, shears and combs.

Important Steps For A Complete Haircut

The important steps in giving a complete haircut are:
1. Preparation.
2. Clipper technique.
3. Shears and comb technique.
4. Arching technique.
5. Finger and shears technique.
6. Front outline.
7. Shaving outlined areas.
8. Final checkup.
9. Combing the hair.

Exercise No. 1

How To Prepare A Customer For A Haircut

Before starting a haircut, the following preparation is required:

1. Have on hand all necessary linens, sterilized implements and supplies.
2. Seat customer comfortably in barber chair, facing mirror.
3. Remove headrest from barber chair.
4. Wash and dry hands.
5. Grasp neck-pieces of chair cloth and bring it over the front of customer, as in Fig. 1.

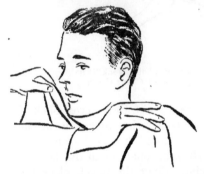

Fig. 1—Placing Chair Cloth Over in Front of Customer

6. Use tissue neck-strip or towel protector under neck-pieces of chair cloth.

   a) If a tissue neck-strip is used, bring it completely around the customer's neck with the ends overlapping in the back, as in Fig. 2.

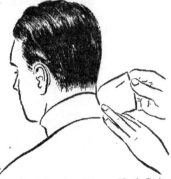

Fig. 2—Adjusting Tissue Neck-Strip Around Neck of Customer

Over the tissue neck-strip, place the neck-pieces of
the chair cloth and fasten it securely in the back.
Extending portion of the tissue neck-strip is folded
neatly over the neck-pieces of the chair cloth, as
in Fig. 3.

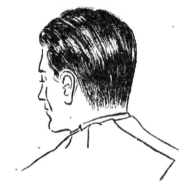

Fig. 3—The extended portion of the Neck-Strip
is folded over Neck-pieces of Chair Cloth

b) If a towel is used, spread it straight across back of
customer, the upper edge being tucked in at the
neckline. Bring both ends of the towel around the
customer's neck, allowing one end to overlap the
other under the chin. Over the towel, place the
neck-pieces of the chair cloth and fasten it securely
in the back.
7. Sprinkle talcum powder on a tissue and apply it over
the back of the customer's neck.

Exercise No. 2

Clipper Technique

For the beginner, it is best to learn how to use the hand clipper before trying the electric clipper. Since the hand clipper is slow cutting, it is easier to control in removing the proper amount of hair from the head.

To learn the proper handling of the clipper the student should practice the following exercises diligently.

1. **How to Hold Clipper and Comb.**
   The position of the right hand is as follows:
   a) Pick up the clipper with the right hand.
   b) Place thumb along still handle attached to lower blade and hold movable handle in the first joint of the fingers, placing the index finger in front of the projecting guide and the rest of the fingers in back of it.

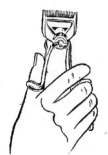

Fig. 1—Holding the Hand Clipper

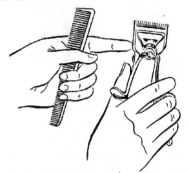

Fig. 2—Using the Index Finger as a Guide

The position of the left hand is as follows:
a) Place the index finger of the left hand on the set

screw and use it as a guide to steady the clipper. See Fig. 2.

b) Hold comb between thumb and index finger, ready to use the comb whenever necessary.

2. **How to Use Clipper and Comb.**

a) Use clipper blade which gives longer cut before using clipper blade which gives shorter cut.

b) For a gradual even taper, tilt the blade as you clip so that the clipper rides on the heel of the bottom blade. See Fig. 3 for correct and incorrect tapering.

c) In order to cut the hair with ease, use the full span of the movable handle with the aid of the fingers. Do not move the clipper up into the hair too fast as it will have a tendency to jam the clipper blades and pull the hair.

d) After tapering one strip of hair, comb hair down smooth and start tapering the unclipped hair to the right.*

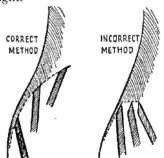

Fig. 3—Correct and Incorrect Methods of Tapering the Hair

Haircut styles that require clipper tapering all around the head should begin at the left temple and continue around the head, finishing at the right temple. Haircut styles that require clipper tapering at the back of the neck only should begin at the left side of the neck, finishing at the right side of the neck.*

*Some barbers prefer to work from right side to left side, in which case the routine of clipping the hair is reversed.

Exercise No. 3

Shears and Comb Technique

Shears and comb technique is used to cut the ends of the hair and even up the clipper taper. It is usually employed after the clipper work is completed.

To learn shears and comb technique the student should practice the following exercises:

1. **How to Hold Shears and Comb.** See Fig. 1.

   The position of the right hand is as follows.

   a) Pick up shears firmly and insert thumb into thumb grip, place third finger into finger grip and leave little finger on finger brace of shears.

   The position of the left hand is as follows:

   a) Hold comb with tips of the first two fingers at the end of teeth and place thumb at the back of the comb.

   b) To comb hair downward turn comb towards customer's head, as in turning a key. See Fig. 2.

   The position of both the right hand and left hand is as follows:

   a) Hold shears and comb slightly to the right front of you.

   b) Hold comb parallel with the still blade of the shears, as in Fig. 1.

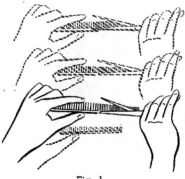

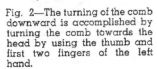

Fig. 2—The turning of the comb downward is accomplished by turning the comb towards the head by using the thumb and first two fingers of the left hand.

Fig. 1

2. **How to Use Shears and Comb.** See Fig. 1.

a) Keep one blade still while moving the other blade with the thumb.

b) While manipulating the shears move both shears and comb upward slowly at the same time.

c) Turn teeth of comb downward when combing the hair downward.

d) Finish one vertical strip at a time before proceeding with the next strip to the left. Working from right to left gives a better view of the work.

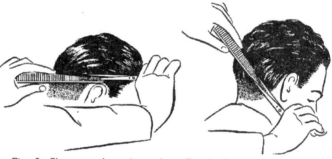

Fig. 3—Shears and comb work over the ear, using the fine teeth of the comb. Start at right side of head, work around the head and finish at left temple.

Fig. 4—Shears and comb work behind the ear. Note the angle in which the shears and comb are held so that they will not interfere with the ear. The fine teeth of the comb are used.

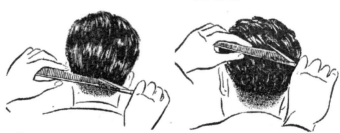

Fig. 5—Using shears and comb to even up the clipper taper at the nape of the neck. The fine teeth of the comb are used in this operation.

Fig. 6—Shears and comb work at the crown, using the coarse teeth of the comb.

Exercise No. 4

Arching Technique

Arching technique means marking the outer border of the haircut in front and over the ears and side of the neck. This outlining is accomplished with the points of the shears and is usually performed while doing the shears and comb work as described in Exercise No. 3.

To learn arching technique the student should practice the following exercise diligently.

1. **How to Hold Shears with Right Hand.**

    a) Pick up shears and insert thumb into thumb grip, place third finger into finger grip and leave the little finger on brace of shears.

    b) Place point of shear blade against scalp. The

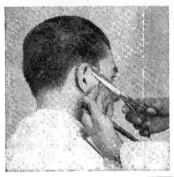

Fig. 1—Outlining the hair in front of and over the ear.

Fig. 2—Outlining the hair on side of neck and back of ear.

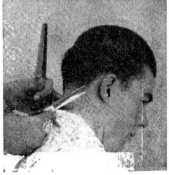

fingers holding the shears are on the bottom and the thumb on top. See Fig 1.

c) Use the most convenient finger-tip of left hand to steady point of shears.

2. **How to Use Shears.**

The proper way to use shears is as follows·

a) Always make outline around ear as close to the edge as possible.

b) Start in front of ear and make a continuous outline around the ear and down the side of neck, as in Fig. 1.

c) Reverse the direction of arching back to the starting point. See Fig. 2.

d) Continue arching around ear until a definite outline is formed.

e) Mark outline for length of sideburns.

Exercise No. 5

Finger and Shears Technique

In order to finish the haircut properly, any noticeable un-evenness remaining after shears and comb work should be removed by means of finger and shears technique. If the top hair needs shortening it may be accomplished during the finger and shears operation.

To perform finger technique on left side of head, stand on left front side of customer.

1. Hold shears and comb as follows:

   a) Hold shears by inserting third finger into finger grip and place little finger on brace.

   b) Grasp comb with left hand.

2. Start just above the left temple, palm shears in right hand, transfer comb from left hand to fingers of right hand and comb a strand of hair two or three inches from you towards the back of the head.

3. Raise the comb sufficiently to permit first and second fingers of the left hand to grasp the hair underneath the comb. The fingers holding the hair should bend to conform with the shape of the head.

4. Place comb between thumb and index finger of left hand.

5. Cut the hair the proper length to blend well with the shorter hair on side of head. See Fig. 1.

6. Hold on to the cut hair, palm the shears, transfer comb from left to right hand and comb through the hair contained in the fingers of the left hand.

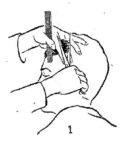

1

7. Release the fingers, sliding the comb and picking up underneath hair beyond the cut just made, and cut the hair.

8. Comb the hair at that point again and repeat the same cutting movements until the back of the head is reached.

9. Start again at the front of the head going a little higher, continue to comb and cut until the back of the head is reached again.

10. Continue to comb and cut, going a little higher each time until the top of the head is reached. See Figs. 2 and 3.

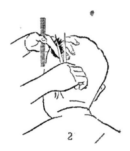

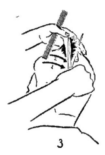

To perform finger technique on right side of head stand in back of the customer.

1. The finger technique for the right side of the head is done in the same manner as on the left side, with the exception that the barber stands in back of the customer and the hair is combed towards the barber. See Figs. 4 and 5.

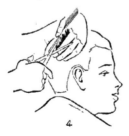

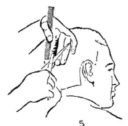

Exercise No. 6

Front Outline

The front outline is shaped soon after completing the finger and shears technique.

The length to which the front outline is cut depends principally on the choice of haircut, whether short, medium or long, and the way the hair is to be parted.

To learn to make the front outline the student should follow these suggestions.

1. Comb all hair to right side bringing the hair straight down over the right temple, as in Fig. 1.

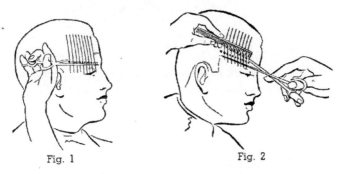

Fig. 1   Fig. 2

2. Hold shears, as in Fig. 1, and cut straight across to the proper length. If necessary, use comb to hold hair in place and cut hair, as in Fig. 2.

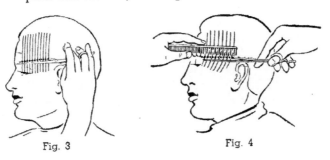

Fig. 3   Fig. 4

3. Comb all hair to left side, bringing the hair straight down over left temple, as in Fig. 3.
4. Hold shears, as in Fig. 3 and cut hair straight across to the proper length. If necessary, use comb to hold hair in place and cut hair, as shown in Fig. 4.

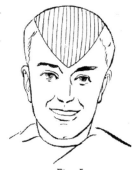

Fig. 5

When the work is properly done the front appearance of the hair as it is combed forward should form to a "V".

Exercise No. 7
Preparation For A Neck Shave

The neck shave contributes to the appearance of the finished haircut. Shaving the outlined areas of the sideburns, around the ears and the sides of the neck below the ears gives the customer a clean cut appearance. If the haircut requires a round or square outline at the nape of the neck, the free hand stroke should be used at the back of the neck.

To prepare for a neck shave follow these steps:

1. Remove all cut hair around the head and neck with clean towel or tissues.
2. Loosen the chair cloth and neck-band carefully, so that no cut hair will go down the neck.
3. Empty the cut hair at the base of the chair in the following manner:
   Pick up the chair cloth at the lower edge and bring it up to the upper edge. Remove chair cloth carefully so that no cut hair will fall on the customer. Drop upper edge of chair cloth, giving a slight shake to dislodge all cut hair.
4. Replace chair cloth as before. It should be left a few inches away from the neck so that it does not come in contact with the customer's skin.
5. Spread a face towel straight across the shoulders, then tuck it in the neck-band

Applying Lather For Neck Shave

1. Prepare lather same as for the beard.
2. Lather both sides of the head and the back of the neck as follows:
   Give a light coat of lather at the hairline around and over the ears, to the temples and down the sides of the neck If round neck shave is to be given, apply lather to the back of the neck up to the hairline.
3. Rub the lather in lightly with the ball part of the finger-tips.

Exercise No. 8

Shaving Outlined Areas

This exercise is a follow-up of Exercise No. 4, on Arching Technique. The purpose of this exercise is to shave over outlined areas of the ears, neck and sideburns.

Before starting this exercise, prepare and apply lather over outlined areas, as explained in Exercise No. 7. Strop razor, then proceed as follows:

1. **Shaving Right Side.**

   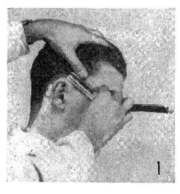

   The proper way to shave outlined area is as follows:

   a) Hold razor as in free hand stroke.

   b) Place thumb of left hand on the scalp above the point of razor, and stretch scalp under razor.

   c) Shave sideburn to the proper length.

   d) Shave around ear at hairline and down side of neck, using a free hand stroke with the point of razor. See Figs. 1, 2 and 3.

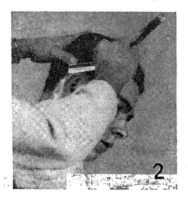

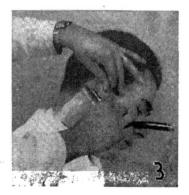

2. Shaving Left Side.

The proper way to shave outlined area is as follows:

a) Hold razor as in reverse back hand stroke.

b) Place thumb of left hand on scalp above point of razor and stretch scalp under razor.

c) Shave sideburn to the proper length.

d) Shave around ear at hairline using a free hand stroke.

e) Shave neck below ear, using the reverse back hand stroke with point of razor. See Fig. 4. Hold ear away with fingers of left hand.

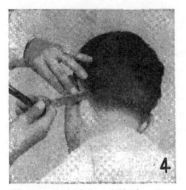 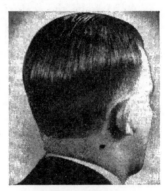

| Shaving Left Side of Neck using Reverse Back Hand Stroke | Medium Haircut with Round Neck Shave |

3. Depending on the customer's preference, shave the neck outline to form a round or square back.

After the neck shave has been completed, remove the excess soap with a warm damp towel. Dry the neck thoroughly. Replace the towel across the customer's shoulder and tuck it in neatly in the neck band.

Exercise No. 9
Final Checkup and Combing of the Hair

A checkup of the haircut and combing of the hair are the steps to complete a haircut. Here is a suggested routine to follow:

1. Replace the face towel across the customer's shoulders and tuck it neatly in neck-band.
2. Retouch parts of the haircut wherever necessary with shears and comb.
3. Trim hair in ears, in nose, and on eyebrows. (Ask the customer before trimming the eyebrows.)
4. Massage the scalp for a few seconds. This is the time to suggest a shampoo, hair tonic or any other hair and scalp service.

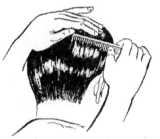

Combing the Hair

5. If the customer's answer is negative, then ask him if he wants his hair combed dry or damp.
6. Comb the hair into its customary style or ask the customer's wishes.

If a hair brush is allowed in your state, be sure that it is properly cleaned and sterilized before using it on the customer.

Final Checkup

1. Go over the finished haircut to correct any uneven parts.
2. Allow customer to see back view of haircut with the aid of a mirror.
3. Make corrections as requested by the customer.
4. Remove all traces of loose hairs around the neck, forehead or nose with a clean towel wrapped around the right hand, or with tissues.
5. Remove chair cloth.
6. Adjust barber chair to level position.
7. Release customer from barber chair.
8. Make out check and thank customer when giving it to him.

REMINDERS
Sanitary Measures

After releasing the customer, take care of the following sanitary measures:

1. Discard used towel and neck-strip,
2. Shake hair cloth at the base of chair, fold and place it on arm of chair.
3. Clean and sterilize used barber implements.
4. Place barber implements into dry (cabinet) sterilizer.
5 Sweep hair from floor and place it into a closed container.
6. Have needed supplies in readiness for next customer.

Ten Reasons Why A Customer May Find Fault With A Haircut

1. Improper hairstyle.
2. Poor workmanship.
3. Cutting off too much or too little hair.
4. Irregular hairlines.
5. Unsanitary practices such as unsterilized implements, unclean towels or chair cloths.
6. Allowing cut hairs to fall down customer's neck.
7. Pulling the hair with dull shears or clippers.
8. Offensive body odor, bad breath or tobacco odor.
9. Blowing loose hair off the customer's neck.
10. Scratching the customer's scalp in combing the hair.

BASIC STEPS OF A STANDARD HAIRCUT

Preparation.

1. Arrange necessary implements and supplies.
2. Wash and dry hands.
3. Adjust chair cloth over customer.
4. Adjust neck-strip or towel around neck and fasten neck-pieces of chair cloth around it.
5. Comb hair just enough to keep it in place.
6. Ask customer how hair is to be cut and styled.

Procedure.

A. **Clipper Work.**

1. Taper hair evenly with hand clipper, working from left side to right side of head. (Some barbers prefer to work from the right side to the left side of the head.)

B. **Shears and Comb Work.**

1. Even up hair taper at right side of head.
2. Trim sideburns, if necessary.
3. Outline right arch, if necessary.
4. Blend in edge of hair with rest, working from right side to left side of the head.
5. Outline left arch, if necessary.

C. **Finger and Shears Work.**

1. Shorten or reduce any pronounced unevenness in the hair, on left top side of head.
2. Shorten or reduce any pronounced unevenness in the hair, on right top side of head.
3. Trim front outline, if necessary.
4. Comb hair and note where further trimming is needed.
5. Drum out loose hair with finger-tips of both hands.
6. Comb hair casually.
7. Brush off loose hair from forehead, ears and neck with towel or tissue.
8. Loosen chair cloth, remove neck-strip and finish dusting off any loose hair.

D. Neck Shave.

1. Place towel around neck.
2. Apply lather over outlined areas of sideburns, around ears and sides of neck.
3. Shave outlined areas. Shave right side of head first and then the left side.
4. Wipe off remaining lather with warm damp towel and dry thoroughly.
5. Place towel around neck to protect clothing.
6. Retouch haircut wherever necessary, with shears and comb.
7. Trim extra hairs from ears, nose and eyebrows, if necessary.
8. Give a few scalp manipulations and suggest a suitable hair tonic or scalp treatment.
9. If no hair tonic is to be used, ask customer if he wishes the hair to remain dry or dampened with water.
10. Comb hair neatly.

E. Final Steps.

1. Wipe off loose hair with towel or tissue.
2. Remove towel and chair cloth from customer.
3. Make out price check for customer.
4. Thank customer as he is handed the price check.

THE ART OF BASIC HAIRCUTTING

To be successful the barber must perfect his skill in hair-cutting. Each haircut should represent a work of art. Try to give the type of haircut that will emphasize the proper contour lines of the head.

From experience the barber has found out that most hair-cuts fall into the following patterns:

1. The short cut.
2. The medium cut. ·
3. Trims (medium or long).
4. Pompadours (short, medium or long).

Each haircut requires the personal touch of the barber. Always keep in mind the customer's needs and wishes and what type of haircut is most becoming to his personality.

Before giving a haircut make sure to ask the customer which type of haircut he desires. If the customer asks for the barber's advice then recommend the type of haircut which best improves his appearance.

THE SHORT CUT

The short cut or full crown haircut is popular in summer time for both young and old.

When giving this cut the barber should keep in mind the following important points.

1. Be guided by the customer's wishes as to any variations in the short cut. The shape of the head should be considered also.
2. Begin clipper work at the left temple, continue around the head, finishing at the right temple* Go up as high as the hat band, tilting the clipper teeth outward at the point where the gradual taper begins.
3. Begin shear and comb work at right temple, continue around the head, finishing at the left temple.

---

*Some barbers prefer to do clipper work from right temple to left temple, in which case the routine is reversed.

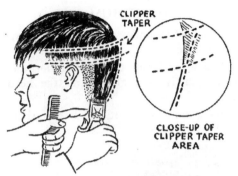

Clipper Taper for Short Cut

4. Use shears and fine teeth of comb for removing traces of the clipper line.
5. Always turn the teeth of the comb out when tapering the hair.
6. Use shears and coarse teeth of comb when removing longer part of hair.
7. Finger work is performed to the top of the head only if necessary.

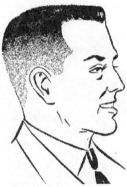

Short Cut with
Pompadour Effect

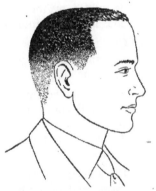

Short Cut with Hair
following the natural shape of
the head

THE MEDIUM CUT

The medium cut is similar to the short cut except for the following differences:

1. The hair is left longer than in the short cut.
2. The clipper is used all around the head, but not so high.

When giving a medium cut, the barber should keep in mind the following points:

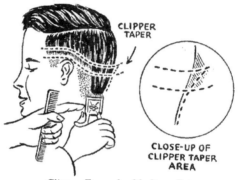

Clipper Taper for Medium Cut

1. Be guided by the customer's wishes as to any variations in the medium cut.

2. Clip the hair about as high as half way up to the crown.

3. Always tilt the clipper teeth outward at the point where the gradual taper begins.

4. Use shears and the coarse teeth of comb for removing longer hair above clipper line.

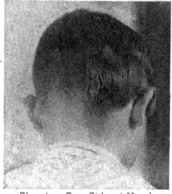

Showing One Side of Head
Properly Tapered with Clippers

5. Always turn the teeth of the comb out when tapering the hair.
6. Use shears and the fine teeth of comb for removing traces of clipper line.

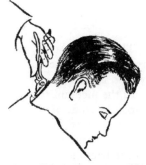

Using Hand Clippers to Clean
Neck of Protruding Hairs

MEDIUM CUT

Left—Front View

Lower Left—Side View

Lower Right—Back View

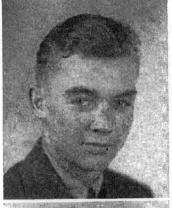

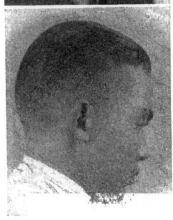

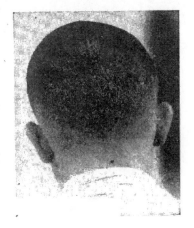

TRIMS

Medium Trim

The medium trim, usually worn by business men, is different from the medium cut, not only in length of the hair, but also in outline.

In the medium trim the No. 1 clipper may be used at the temples in front of the ears. The No. 00 or No. 000 clipper is recommended for the lower part of the neck.

The shears and comb work is started at the right sideburn and the trimming is continued towards the left sideburn.

Caution should be taken not to trim the hair too short.

The finger work is used to reduce the bulk of the top hair and to blend in with the rest of the hair.

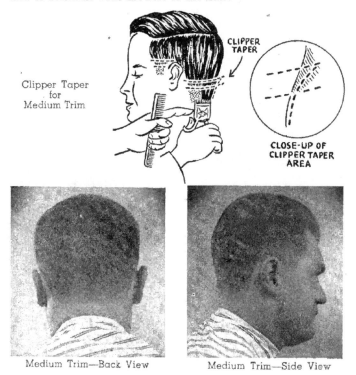

Clipper Taper
for
Medium Trim

CLIPPER TAPER

CLOSE-UP OF
CLIPPER TAPER
AREA

Medium Trim—Back View   Medium Trim—Side View

Long Trim

The long trim is similar to the medium trim with the exception that the hair is left a trifle longer.

In the long trim, clipper work is done at the back of the neck with the taper evident near the lower tip of the ears. With the point of the shears, outline the right sideburn to the desired length and mark off the hairline in front of and around the ears. Trim right sideburn with shears and comb, continue around the head and finish at the left sideburn.

In doing finger work, be careful to cut off the proper amount of hair. (For different lengths of sideburns, see page 144.)

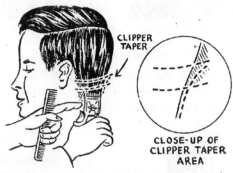

CLIPPER TAPER

CLOSE-UP OF
CLIPPER TAPER
AREA

Clipper Taper for Long Trim

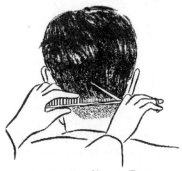

Evening the Clipper Taper
at the Nape of the Neck

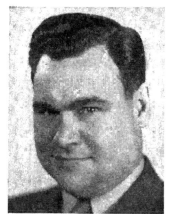

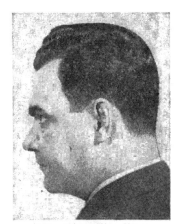

Long Trim—Front View   Long Trim—Side View

Electric Clipper

Experience with the hand clipper makes it easier to use the electric clipper. Because of its rapid cutting action, the electric clipper must be handled skillfully, as follows:

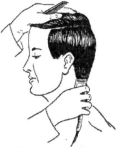

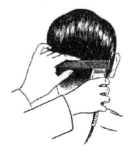

Tapering the Hair
at the Nape of the Neck
with the Electric Clipper

Tapering the Hair
Held through the Teeth
of the Comb
with the Electric Clipper

1. Select the proper size of clipper blade.
2. Feed the clipper slowly into the hair held with the teeth of the comb.
3. In making the taper, gradually tilt the clipper.

THE POMPADOUR

Short Pompadour

For the short pompadour, use the clipper high all around the head, as in the short cut, leaving the top of the head unclipped.

Before using the shears, comb the hair straight back to the crown. Stand to the front, left side of the customer when cutting the hair on top of the head, and start cutting at the forehead, shortening the hair gradually until you reach the crown. Trim and taper the sides and back of the head to blend with the top of the head.

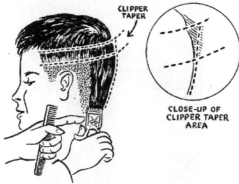

Clipper Taper for Short Pompadour

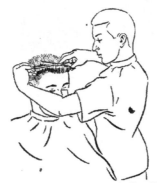

Cutting the Hair in a Brush Top Effect

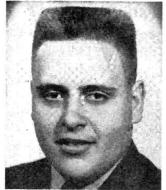

Short Pompadour
(Brush Top)

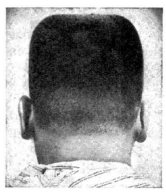

Short Pompadour
(Brush Top) Back View

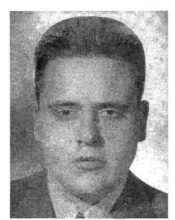

Short Pompadour
(Round Top)

MEDIUM POMPADOUR

The medium pompadour follows the same pattern as the medium trim with the exception that the hair on top of the head is left somewhat longer.

The clipper technique used is similar to the medium cut. (See page 135.)

In doing the finger work, part the hair in the center, then follow the technique as explained in Lesson 5, page 122-123.

Care must be taken that too much hair is not removed.

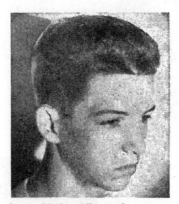

Medium Pompadour

Mark off outline and shave sideburns, around ears and back of neck. Retouch any uneven spots with shears and comb. Finally, the hair is combed straight back.

LONG POMPADOUR

The long pompadour follows the same pattern as the long trim (see pages 138-139) with the exception that the hair is left a little longer on top of the head.

The finger technique is the same as the medium pompadour, but the hair is left a little longer.

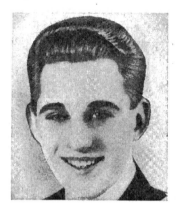

Long Pompadour
with Medium Sideburns,
Dressed with Wide Wave

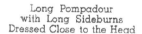
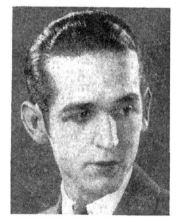

Long Pompadour
with Long Sideburns
Dressed Close to the Head

SIDEBURNS

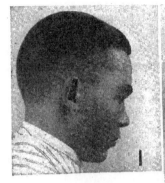

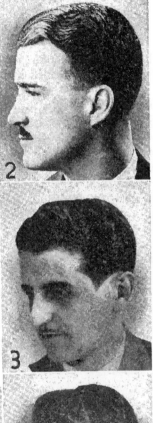

Sideburns should be made according to the desire of the customer, style of the haircut, and the customer's features.

Fig. 1—None.
Fig. 2—Short.
Fig. 3—Pointed (Slant).
Fig. 4—Medium.
Fig. 5—Long.

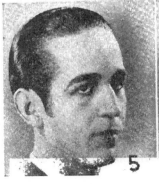

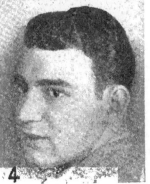

SPECIAL PROBLEMS
HAIR THINNING

Hair thinning is required to reduce the bulk of the hair wherever necessary. Any of the following implements and methods can be used for this purpose.

1. **Thinning (serrated) shears.** The hair strand is combed, and the spread hair held between the index and middle fingers, as in Fig. 1. Then the hair is cut about one inch from the scalp. If another cut is necessary it should be made about one inch from the first cut. To shorten the hair the regular shears is used.

Plan of cutting the hair. The barber stands in back of the customer, combs away the front hair which does not require thinning, as in Fig. 2. The hair is then thinned on both sides of the head, strand by strand as required, and the loose cut hair is combed out. The top part is usually done last.

Caution: Do not cut the hair too close to the scalp nor thin out too much hair.

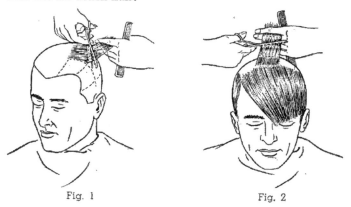

Fig. 1   Fig. 2

2. **Thinning (serrated) shears and comb.** Instead of the index and middle fingers, the comb may be used in holding the hair, as in Fig. 3. The thinning is done in the usual manner.

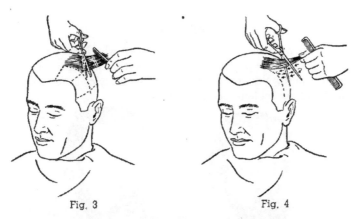

Fig. 3   Fig. 4

3. **Regular shears.** Hold a small strand of hair between the thumb and index finger, insert the strand in the shears, as in Fig. 4. Slide the shears up and down the strand, closing them slightly each time the shears is moved towards the scalp. Slither enough to allow the hair to lie close to the scalp wherever needed.

SHEAR POINT TAPERING

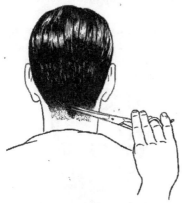

Shear point tapering is a useful technique for thinning out difficult heads of hair occasioned by hollows, wrinkles and creases in the scalp and by whorls of hair on the scalp. Dark and ragged hair patches on the scalp can be minimized by this special technique.

The shear point taper is performed with the cutting points of the shears. Only a few hairs are cut at a time and then combed out. Continue cutting around the objectionable spot until it be-becomes less noticeable and blends in with the surrounding outline of the haircut.

BEARDS

There are still a few professional men who insist on wearing beards, made popular during the sixteenth century by the great painter Van Dyke. However, such styles as shown on this page are seldom seen nowadays.

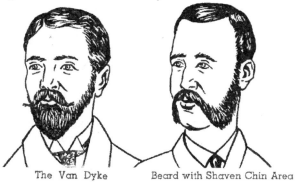

The Van Dyke   Beard with Shaven Chin Area

The cutting of the full beard is done with the shears over the comb, usually starting near the ear and working toward the chin. The length and shape depend upon the customer's wishes.

For the goatee beard, it is customary to first shave the sides of the face and then trim the beard to the desired shape and length. The mustache is trimmed and dressed last in accordance with the customer's wishes.

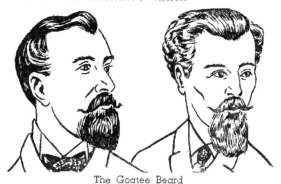

The Goatee Beard

SINGEING

Before commencing to singe, it is necessary to brush and comb the hair thoroughly in order to remove the short hairs which inevitably remain after haircutting.

Singeing by means of the wax taper is done in the following manner. The hair is first combed into position, approxi-

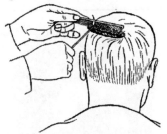

Singeing with the Teeth of the
Comb Pointing Downward

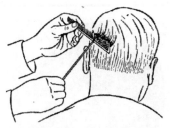

Singeing with the Teeth of the
Comb Pointing Upward

mately as usually worn. Then commence the singeing by placing the comb in the hair at a point just below the crown. The comb is moved slowly down the hair in the direction from the crown toward the nape of the neck. As the comb moves through the hair, the lighted taper is passed along the ends of the hair which protrude through the teeth of the comb, thus singeing off the extreme points. After the back and sides have been treated in this manner, the edges of the short hair in the nape of the neck and sides are singed, using the comb in an upward direction.

VALUE OF SINGEING—Present day authorities claim that singeing is not beneficial to the hair, and classify it as a quack treatment; however, it does provide temporary relief for split hair ends, and some customers desire a finishing touch to their hair that cannot be acquired otherwise. Since there are some customers who desire singeing, and there is an added financial return for the work, it is advisable to learn the technique of singeing thoroughly.

POPULAR HAIR STYLES FOR MEN

The skilled barber should be able to advise his customers as to which type of haircut is best fitted to their age, personality, shape of head and facial features. Study the following hair styles for suggestions as to how to bring out the best qualities in each customer.

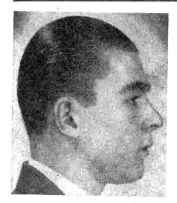
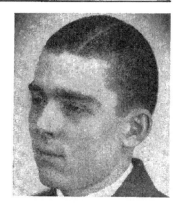

Medium Pompadour with Off-Center Part
The Hair Dressed Close to the Head

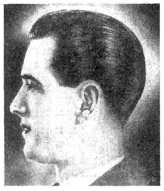
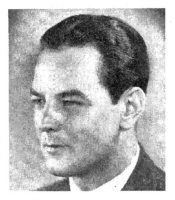

Medium Pompadour
with Side Part

Medium Pompadour
with Center Part

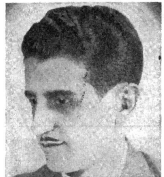

Medium Pompadour, Pointed Sideburns

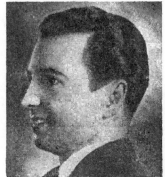

Medium Pompadour, Pointed Sideburns

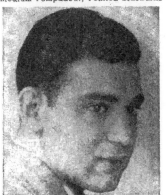

Medium Pompadour
with Side Part

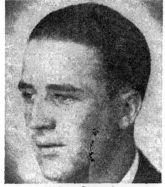

Medium Pompadour
Hair Dressed Close to the Head

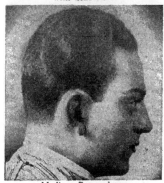

Medium Pompadour

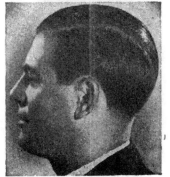

Medium Haircut with Side Part

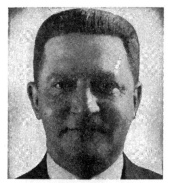
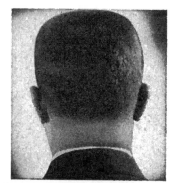

Short Haircut with Brush Top Effect

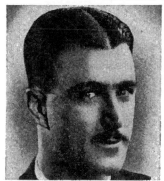
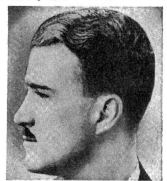

Medium Haircut with Center Part

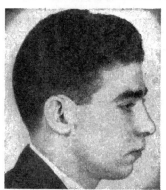
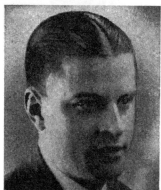

Medium Pompadour

Medium Haircut with Center Part
Hair Dressed Close to the Head

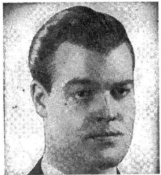
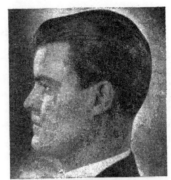

Long Pompadour with Part and Pointed Sideburns

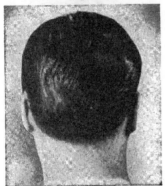

Back View of Long Pompadour

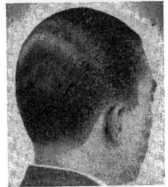

Three-Quarter Back View
of Medium Haircut

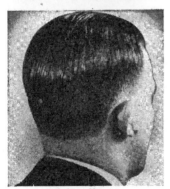

Medium Haircut
with Round Neck Shave

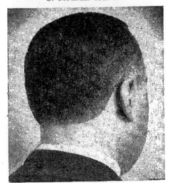

Medium Haircut
with Round Neck Shave

POPULAR HAIR STYLES FOR BOYS

Just as with men's haircuts, it is good business to give flattering haircuts to boys. The barber who caters to boys is likely to win over their fathers as regular customers. For suggestive guidance, study the following individualized types of haircuts for boys.

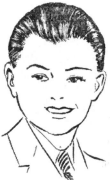

As a general rule, boys' and children's hair should be cut shorter than the men's hair, depending on the age and desire of the customer.

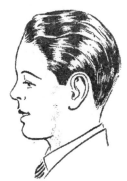

Medium Pompadour
Front View

Medium Pompadour
Side View

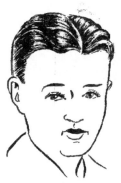

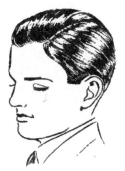

Medium Trim
Center Part

Medium Trim
Side Part

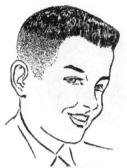

POPULAR HAIR STYLES FOR BOYS

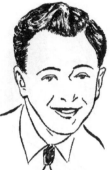

Brush Top Haircut
Cut Close All Around
the Head

Medium Haircut
with Side Part

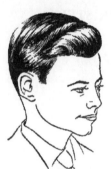

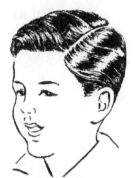

Medium Haircut
with Side Part

Medium Haircut
with Side Part

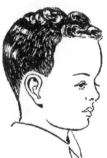

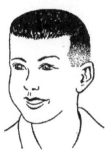

Medium Haircut
with Natural Curls

Short Haircut
Combed Forward

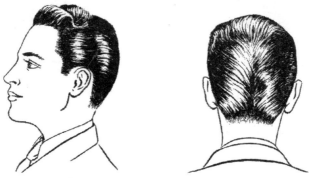

Popular Hair Style During 1950-1951

PASTE HERE — LATEST HAIR STYLES

PRINCIPLES OF MEN'S HAIR STYLING

To render the best service to his customers, the barber should know the principal styles of haircuts and be able to select the one best suited for a particular customer. The barber who knows the fundamentals of artistic hair styling can emphasize the best features of his customers and make them look more attractive for their age, weight and height.

In determining the best way to cut and style the customer's hair, the barber should take into account his preferences, as well as his:

1. Facial contour and features.
2. Head contour.
3. Hairline.

Other factors which influence the choice of haircut are the amount and length of hair on the head, partial baldness and the presence of such characteristics as a high or low forehead, high cheekbones, prominent chin, heavy jowls, small or large ears, and a thin or thick neck.

Although there are numerous variations in facial characteristics, the barber deals most frequently with three basic facial types:

1. Face with regular features.
2. The short, round face.
3. The long, thin face.

Face with Regular Features

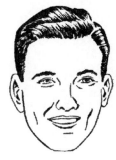

Most customers have regular features, that is, their face is neither fat nor thin, neither long nor short. With the customer's consent, the hair may be cut shorter or left longer. In either event, the hair should be evenly graduated all the way, while the neck is feather edged. The sideburns are left short.

The Short, Round Face

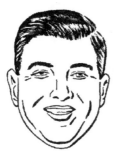

For this facial type, the hair is cut shorter all around and also graduated all the way. The sideburns are kept high.

Should the customer have a full face with hollow temples, allow the hair to grow fuller at the sides and keep the sideburns at medium length.

The Long, Thin Face

Recessed temples are typical of this facial type. In cutting the hair, keep it both long and full at the sides. The rest of the hair is cut medium length. In the back, the hair is kept long, being feather-cut and graduated from the neck up. Long sideburns are recommended.

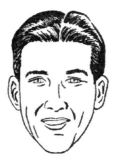

HAIRCUTTING

1. What is meant by the art of haircutting?	The process of cutting, tapering, trimming, moulding, styling and dressing men's hair.
2. What is meant by a hair trim?	Cutting the hair lightly.
3. How can the art of haircutting be acquired?	By obtaining good instruction and by gaining experience and practice on customers.
4. Name four basic styles of haircuts.	1. The short cut or full crown. 2. The medium cut. 3. Trims (medium or long). 4. Pompadours (short, medium or long).
5. Which sanitary precautions should be observed by the barber?	Wash hands and use only sterilized implements, sterile towels and clean linens on customers.
6. How should the customer be prepared for a haircut?	Seat customer comfortably in chair, place neck-strip or towel around neck and then adjust chair cloth over neck-strip or towel.
7. Where is clipper work generally started and finished on the customer's head?	Generally started on the left side of the head and carried around to the right side.
8. Why should the barber first learn to use hand clippers before attempting to use electric clippers?	Hand clippers are slow cutting, and there is less likelihood of making mistakes.
9. How should the clipper be used in tapering the hair?	Gradually tilt the blades in using the clipper so that it rides on the heel of the bottom blade.
10. What is the proper position of the shears and comb in haircutting?	The comb is held parallel to the shears.
11. What is the purpose of finger work in haircutting?	It shortens the hair evenly and helps to reduce any ridges that may appear in the haircut.
12. What plan is followed in shaving the neck outline?	Depending on the desired hair style, shave around the top and back of the ears and the sides and back of the neck.
13. Name the shaving strokes used: 1) over the right side of the neck, 2) Left side of the neck.	1. For the right side of the neck, use a free hand stroke. 2. For the left side of the neck, use a reverse back hand stroke.
14. When should hair singeing be recommended?	To prevent further splitting of hair ends.

15. **How is hair singeing accomplished?**	Run the flame of a wax taper over the hair ends, held straight through the teeth of a comb.
16. **Give ten reasons why a customer may find fault with a haircut.**	1. Improper hairstyle. 2. Poor workmanship. 3. Cutting off too much or too little hair. 4. Irregular hairlines. 5. Unsanitary practices such as unsterilized implements, unclean towels or chair cloths. 6. Allowing cut hairs to fall on the customer's neck. 7. Pulling the hair with dull shears or clippers. 8. Offensive body odor, bad breath or tobacco odor. 9. Blowing loose hair off the customer's neck. 10. Scratching the customer's scalp in combing the hair.

SHAMPOOING

The chief purpose of shampooing the scalp and hair is to maintain a clean and healthy condition of the scalp and hair. The hair should be shampooed on the average of once a week or as frequently as is required to keep the hair and scalp clean.

Preparation

Adequate preparation is the first step in giving a good shampoo. Before starting, the barber should have on hand all necessary supplies and equipment, and should wash his hands with soap and water. Following a definite procedure not only saves time, but makes for greater efficiency.

The essential supplies needed for a shampoo are:

1. Pure liquid soap having a low alkaline content.
2. Soft, warm water capable of producing an abundance of lather with the shampoo. Hard water will not produce lather unless softened by boiling or chemical treatment.
3. Shampoo bowl or tray, chair cloth, and towels.

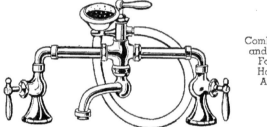

Combination Hot and Cold Water Faucet with Hand Spray Attachment

How To Prepare Customer For Shampoo

1. Seat customer in a comfortable and relaxed position.
2. Arrange chair cloth as follows:
   a) With each hand, grasp each end of the neck of the chair cloth.
   b) Place the chair cloth over the front of the customer.
   c) Place towel around neck.

    d) Secure chair cloth at the back of the neck over
the towel.

  3. Unfold one face towel lengthwise and tuck it around
the customer's left side of neck from center of back
to center of front, allowing remainder of towel to fall
over left shoulder.

  4. Unfold another face towel lengthwise and repeat on
right side of neck.

Depending on available facilities, the barber can use
either the **inclined position** or the **reclined position** for the
customer while giving the shampoo.

How To Prepare Customer For Inclined Position

**The inclined position of sham-
pooing** is used in barber shops having limited facilities. The shampoo
bowl is generally placed at a distance away from the barber chair.
While giving the shampoo, the customer's head is bent forward over
the shampoo bowl.

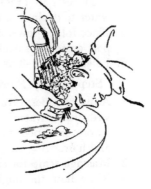

The following procedure is
necessary for the inclined position
in shampooing.

  1. Place clean towel over edge
of shampoo bowl.

  2. Have customer sit on a stool close to shampoo bowl.

  3. Massage scalp to loosen dandruff and to increase the
blood circulation.

  4. Follow steps 1-8 as for a
plain shampoo.

How To Prepare Customer
For Reclined Position

**The reclined position of
shampooing** is generally used if
there is a shampoo bowl next
to the barber's chair. While

giving the shampoo the barber chair is reclined so that the customer's head rests on a shampoo board. This method of shampooing is most comfortable for the customer, while it allows the barber to work rapidly.

The following procedure is necessary for the reclined position in shampooing.

1. Remove the headrest and adjust the shampoo board on shampoo bowl.
2. Massage scalp to loosen dandruff and to increase the blood circulation.
3. Turn the barber chair around with its back facing the shampoo bowl.
4. Tilt the barber chair at an angle so that customer's head rests in groove of shampoo board and allows water to drain into the shampoo bowl.
5. Place folded towel in groove of shampoo board to support customer's neck.
6. Follow steps 1-8 as for a plain shampoo.

Step-by-Step Procedure For Plain Shampoo

1. Adjust temperature of water and wet hair thoroughly with warm water.
2. Apply shampoo to form a thick lather over scalp and hair.
3. Massage scalp for several minutes as described below.
4. Rinse hair thoroughly with warm water and repeat lathering if necessary.
5. Rinse hair thoroughly with cool water.
6. Wipe face and ears thoroughly.
7. Dry the hair completely.
   Suggest hair tonic or hair dressing at this time.
8. Comb hair neatly.

Massage Manipulations During Shampoo

The proper way to massage the scalp during a shampoo is as follows:

1. Stand behind the customer, after the lathering is done.
2. Place the finger-tips at the back of the head just below the ears.

3. Apply rotary movements from the ears to the temples up to the forehead, then over the top of the head down to the neck.
4. Repeat these movements for several minutes.

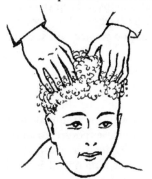

Lathering the Head

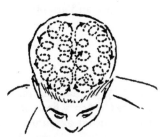

Scalp Massage Movements

Common Faults In Shampooing

A good barber makes every effort to please his customers. A dissatisfied customer may find fault with a shampoo for any of the following reasons:

1. Improper selection of shampoo.
2. Insufficient scalp massage.
3. Insufficient rinsing of hair.
4. Water too cold or too hot.
5. Allowing soapy water to run down the customer's forehead, eyes, or ears.
6. Wetting or soiling the customer's clothing.
7. Scraping the scalp with finger nails.
8. Improper drying of the hair.

Superior Shampoo Service

If the barber is to develop a superior type of shampoo service, he must give individual attention to his customer's needs. First of all, the barber should be able to select the kind of shampoo best suited to the condition of the scalp and hair. The effectiveness of the shampoo will depend in a large measure on:

1. The way the shampoo is applied.
2. The way the scalp is massaged.
3. The way the shampoo is rinsed from the hair.

A good shampoo service, not only removes dirt and dandruff from the scalp and hair, but also helps to keep the scalp and hair in a healthy condition. The barber who gives the utmost care and attention to his shampoo service will succeed in pleasing his customers.

HOT OIL SHAMPOO

A hot oil shampoo is indicated where a dry condition of the scalp is present. The dry scalp may be caused either by a deficiency of natural oil or its removal by frequent hair washings. Men whose occupation require exposure to more than the usual amount of dust and dirt tend to wash their hair frequently. Fresh olive oil or sweet almond oil is used both for its soothing effect as well as for overcoming the dry scalp.

Step-by-Step Procedure For A Hot Oil Shampoo

1. Prepare the customer as for a plain shampoo.
2. Give regular scalp manipulations.
3. Apply cotton swab, dipped into oil, over scalp by parting hair at about every inch.
4. Expose scalp to heat of red dermal lamp or infra-red lamp for five to ten minutes as required.
5. Apply a good shampoo and massage it well into the hair and scalp.

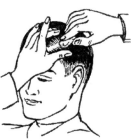

Applying Oil to the Scalp
with a Swab

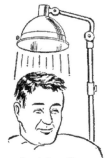

Applying Heat
with Infra-Red Lamp

6. Rinse hair thoroughly with warm water, and repeat lathering if necessary.
7. Dry the hair thoroughly with a clean towel.
8. Heat the oil in a double boiler to the desired temperature.
9. Apply cotton swab, dipped into warm oil, over scalp by parting hair at about every inch.
10. Comb hair neatly.

EGG SHAMPOO

An egg shampoo is a mild cleansing agent for an irritated scalp. None of the natural oil is removed while using an egg shampoo and it is therefore, best for a dry, brittle condition of the hair, and tender scalp.

The egg shampoo is prepared with the following ingredients: One whole egg (or an equivalent amount of prepared egg powder), one tablespoon of witch hazel and one teaspoon of salt.

Step-by-Step Procedure For An Egg Shampoo

1. Prepare the egg mixture.
2. Prepare customer as for a plain shampoo.
3. Apply regular scalp manipulations.
4. Apply one-half of the egg mixture and work it well into the scalp.
5. Rinse the hair with warm or tepid water.
6. Reapply egg mixture as often as necessary to insure a clean scalp.
7. Rinse the hair thoroughly with tepid or warm water.
8. Comb hair neatly.

Only tepid water should be used for rinsing the hair. If the rinse water is too hot, the white of the egg tends to harden and stick to the hair.

SPECIAL SHAMPOOS

There are various shampoo mixtures available for the barber's use on customers. At times, the barber is uncertain as to which particular shampoo to use. To find out for himself, the barber should carefully read the label and literature accompanying the shampoo. Such information will reveal the principal ingredients of the shampoo and the advantages claimed for the product.

One way to test a particular brand of shampoo is to give it a fair trial for a period of time. Make sure to follow the manufacturer's instructions. Keeping a written record of the shampoo used and the results obtained on customers will eliminate guesswork. In this way, the actual merits of the shampoo can be demonstrated to the barber's satisfaction. In addition, the customer will benefit from the barber's experience.

PLAIN SHAMPOO

1. What is the purpose of a plain shampoo?	To keep the hair and scalp in a clean and healthy condition.
2. How often should the hair be shampooed?	At least once a week or as often as necessary.
3. Outline the important steps in giving a shampoo.	1. Proper preparation of customer. 2. Selection of a good shampoo. 3. Proper application of shampoo and water. 4. Sufficient scalp massage to stimulate the scalp. 5. Thorough rinsing to remove dirt and lather. 6. Drying and combing the hair.
4. What kind of soap should be used in a shampoo?	Pure liquid soap having a low alkaline content.
5. What kind of water should be used to shampoo the hair; why?	Soft, warm water. Hard water will not produce any lather unless softened by boiling or chemical treatment.
6. Which supplies are needed to give a shampoo?	Shampoo, shampoo bowl or tray, warm and cold water, chair cloth, and towels.
7. How should the barber prepare himself for a shampoo?	Arrange necessary supplies and wash hands with soap and warm water.
8. How should the customer be prepared for a shampoo?	Seat customer in a comfortable position and properly adjust the towels and chair cloth.
9. Why should the scalp be massaged before giving a shampoo?	To loosen the dandruff and stimulate the circulation of the blood to the scalp.
10. Briefly outline the procedure for giving a plain shampoo.	1. Adjust temperature of water and wet hair with warm water. 2. Apply shampoo to form thick lather over scalp and hair. 3. Massage scalp for several minutes. 4. Rinse hair with warm water and repeat lathering if necessary. 5. Rinse hair thoroughly with cool water. 6. Wipe face and ears thoroughly. 7. Dry and comb hair.
11. Briefly outline the massage manipulations applied to the scalp during a shampoo.	1. After the lathering is done, stand behind the customer. 2. Place the finger-tips at the back of the head just below the ears. 3. Apply rotary movements from the ears to the temples up to the forehead, then over the top of the head down to the neck. 4. Repeat these movements for several minutes.

12. Give eight reasons why a customer may find fault with a shampoo.	1. Improper selection of shampoo. 2. Insufficient scalp massage. 3. Insufficient rinsing of hair. 4. Water too cold or too hot. 5. Allowing soapy water to run down the customer's forehead, eyes, or ears. 6. Wetting or soiling the customer's clothing. 7. Scraping the scalp with finger nails. 8. Improper drying of the hair.
13. For what purpose is a hot oil shampoo indicated?	To correct a dry condition of the scalp.
14. What kind of oil is best for a hot oil shampoo?	Either fresh olive oil or almond oil.
15. When is it advisable to recommend an egg shampoo?	If the customer has a dry, brittle condition of the hair, and a tender scalp.

HAIR TONICS

The barber should be familiar with the different types of hair tonics so that he will be able to advise the correct tonic for a particular condition (dry or oily scalp).

A hair tonic is a solution containing alcohol, water, oil, and an antiseptic or irritant (a chemical agent which has a stimulating action). The liquids cleanse the scalp and help to remove dandruff. Whereas the antiseptic prevents the growth of bacteria on the scalp, the irritant, together with the alcohol, stimulates the circulation. The small amount of oil dresses the hair.

If the label or advertising literature of the hair tonic does not reveal the amount of alcohol, antiseptic or irritant it contains, it is advisable to get this information direct from the manufacturer. To note if there is any improvement in the condition of the scalp over a period of time, the barber should keep a written record of the kind of tonic used and the number of applications. This information will be helpful in judging the relative merits of different hair tonics.

Hair tonics have an important place in the barber shop. They can be used to advantage with many scalp and hair treatments, or when the hair is to be dressed. The barber who knows his work is in a position to discover scalp troubles and recommend suitable hair tonics for their correction. Customers appreciate the friendly interest shown by barbers and generally follow their advice. The most appropriate time to start such a conversation and explain the reason for the tonic is just before the hair is to be combed. Once a customer starts to use a hair tonic, he will probably continue its use if reminded at the proper time.

Scalp Steam

The effectiveness of a hair tonic is increased by means of either:

1. Steaming towels.
2. Scalp steamer.

To increase the effectiveness of a hair tonic application, the steaming of the scalp is recommended. The steam relaxes the pores, softens scalp and hair, increases circulation, making the hair and scalp more receptive to hair tonics.

The scalp steamer is a helpful piece of equipment. It assures a constant and controlled source of steam. When ready to be used, fill the container with water, fit the hood over the customer's head and turn on the electricity. Many hoods have openings on the side for the hands to be inserted in order to give a scalp massage together with the scalp steam.

Steaming towels are used in the absence of a scalp steamer. They are prepared, one at a time, by soaking the towel in steaming water. The excess water is wrung out and the steaming towel is wrapped around the customer's head. As the towel cools, another one is applied in its place.

Step-by-Step Procedure in Giving A Scalp Steam

1. Apply regular scalp manipulations to increase the circulation of the blood.
2. Steam the scalp with two hot towels or scalp steamer.
3. Apply the hair tonic carefully and massage it well into the scalp.
4. Comb the hair neatly.

HAIR TONICS

1. What are hair tonics and what are their benefits?	Hair tonics are lotions or cosmetics applied to the hair or scalp for the purpose of preventing or removing dandruff and for dressing the hair.
2. Why should the barber know the various kinds of hair tonics?	In order to be able to recommend the correct hair tonic for the required condition of the hair or scalp.
3. Where can the barber obtain reliable information about hair tonics?	Read advertising literature, read labels on bottles carefully and consult with the manufacturer of each hair tonic.
4. Why should the barber keep a record of the customer's hair tonic treatments?	To note the progress of the treatment and for future references in similar conditions.
5. What is a scalp steam?	The steaming of the scalp by means of steaming towels or a scalp steamer, followed by the application of a hair tonic.
6. Give the four steps for applying a scalp steam.	1. Apply regular scalp manipulations to stimulate the circulation of the blood. 2. Steam the scalp with two hot towels or scalp steamer. 3. Apply the hair tonic carefully and massage it well into the scalp. 4. Comb the hair neatly.

SCALP TREATMENTS
Scalp Massage

Scalp massage as used in barbering is given either as a separate treatment or in connection with other hair and scalp treatments. To become competent in scalp massage, barbers require sound training as well as continued practice.

The purpose of a scalp massage is to preserve the health of the scalp and hair, and combat such disorders as dandruff and excessive hair loss.

A thorough scalp massage is beneficial in the following ways:

1. The blood and lymph flow is increased.
2. Nerves are rested and soothed.
3. Scalp muscles are stimulated.
4. Sweat and oil glands become more active.
5. Scalp is made more flexible.
6. Promotes hair growth and makes the hair lustrous.

Step-by-Step Procedure For A Scalp Massage

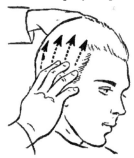

Position: Place the finger-tips of each hand at the hair-line on each side of the customer's head, hands pointing upward. (Fig. 1).

Movement: Slide the fingers firmly upward, spreading the finger-tips. Continue until the fingers meet at the center or top of the scalp. Repeat three or four times.

Fig. 1

Position: Place the fingers of each hand on the sides of the head. (Fig. 2.)

Movement: Use the thumbs to massage from behind the ears towards the crown. Repeat four or five times. Move the fingers so that both thumbs meet at the hair-line at the back of the neck. Rotate the thumbs upwards towards the crown.

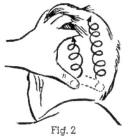

Fig. 2

Position: Step to the right side of the customer. Place the left hand back of the head.
Stretch the thumb and fingers of the right
hand against and over the forehead, just
above the eyebrows. (Fig. 3.)

Movement: Massage the right hand slowly
and firmly in an upward direction towards
the crown; while keeping the left hand
in a fixed position at the back of the head.
Repeat four or five times.

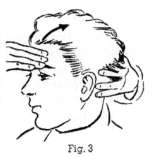

Fig. 3

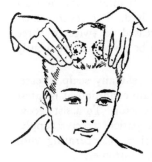

Position: Step to the back of the customer.
Place the hands on each side of the head,
just in front of the hair-line. (Fig. 4.)

Movement: Rotate the finger-tips three
times. On the fourth rotation, apply a
quick, upward twist, firm enough to move
the scalp. Continue this movement on the
sides and top of the scalp. Repeat three
or four times.

Fig. 4

Position: Place the fingers of each hand on
the side of the head.

Movement: Rotate the thumbs behind the
ears. Repeat three or four times. Move
the thumb to the back of the neck at the
hair-line. Apply rotary movements in an
upward direction towards the crown.

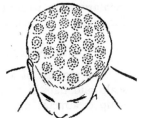

Fig. 5—Diagram of Rotary
Movements of the Scalp

Rotary movements are used in scalp massage because
they loosen the scalp tissue as well as improve the health of
hair and scalp. When giving a scalp massage, care should
be taken to give the manipulations slowly without pulling the
hair in any way.

To derive the greatest benefit from scalp massages, they
should be given at least once a week for normal scalps. In
cases of hair loss or other hair or scalp troubles, give three or
four treatments each week. A series of scalp treatments
yields better results than if given occasionally or irregularly.

When To Recommend Scalp Treatments

The barber employs scalp treatments in his work for any of the following reasons:

1. To keep the scalp clean and healthy.
2. To promote the growth of hair.
3. To prevent the excessive loss of hair.

When advising customers to take scalp treatments, always explain that regular, systematic treatments are necessary to assure lasting improvement. In mild cases, at least one scalp treatment a week is required. For severe cases, the frequency of treatment is increased to twice or three times a week. Scalp treatments can be given less frequently if any improvement is noted.

No barber should undertake to treat any scalp disease. If the customer has any abnormal scalp condition, it is safest and best to refer him to his private doctor. To assist recovery, the doctor may suggest that the patient receive supplementary scalp treatment by the barber. Cooperating with the doctor is in the best interests of the customer.

GENERAL SCALP TREATMENT

The purpose of a general scalp treatment is to keep the scalp and hair in a clean and healthy condition. Regular scalp treatments are also beneficial in preventing baldness.

Step-by-Step Procedure After A Shampoo

1. Dry the hair and scalp thoroughly.
2. Part the hair and apply a scalp ointment directly to the scalp.
3. Place both thumbs about ¾ of an inch apart on each side of the parted hair.
4. Rotate the thumbs in a circular manner, pressing firmly against the scalp.
5. Make another hair part about an inch away from the first one. Apply ointment and massage.
6. Repeat steps 2-5 and continue until the entire scalp has been treated.

7. Expose scalp to red dermal light or infra-red lamp for four to eight minutes, parting the hair to permit maximum exposure.

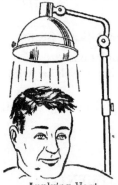

Applying Heat
with Infra-Red Lamp

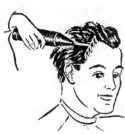

Applying High-Frequency
Current

8. Stimulate the scalp with high-frequency current for three to five minutes.

9. Apply hair tonic and work it well into the scalp.

10. Comb hair neatly.

Scalp Treatment with Vibrator

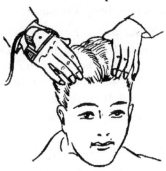

Massaging the Scalp
with Vibrator

A vibrator is an effective mechanical aid in giving a stimulating scalp massage.

Before using the vibrator, it is adjusted on the back of the hand, leaving the thumb and fingers free. Then, turn on the current. The vibrations are transmitted through the cushions of the finger-tips. The same movements are followed as for a regular hand scalp massage.

When using the vibrator on the scalp, be careful to regulate the intensity and duration of the vibrations as well as the pressure used.

SCALP STEAM

A scalp steam is used to stimulate the blood supply going to and from the scalp.

Step-by-Step Procedure For A Scalp Steam

1. Apply regular scalp manipulations.

2. Steam the scalp with two hot towels or with scalp steamer.

3. Apply hair tonic carefully and massage it well into the scalp.

4. Comb hair neatly.

DRY SCALP TREATMENT

Inactivity of the oil glands or the excessive removal of natural oil from the hair and scalp may produce a dry condition of the scalp. Among the contributory causes of a dry scalp are leading an indoor life, frequent washing of the hair with strong soaps or alcoholic shampoos and the continued use of drying tonics or lotions on the hair and scalp.

Step-by-Step Procedure For A Dry Scalp Treatment

1 Massage and stimulate the scalp.

2. Apply prepared egg shampoo and work it into the hair and scalp. If scalp is exceedingly dry, hot oil should be applied and massaged into the scalp before the egg shampoo.

3. Rinse hair with tepid water and dry scalp thoroughly.

4. Apply tissue cream into the scalp with rotary frictional movements.

5. Apply a red dermal light or infra-red lamp over the scalp for a period of five minutes.

6. Apply high-frequency current over the scalp for five to six minutes.

7. Comb hair neatly.

OILY SCALP TREATMENT

The main causes of an oily scalp are excessive intake of fatty foods in the diet and the resultant over-activity of the oil glands.

Step-by-Step Procedure For An Oily Scalp Treatment

1. Gently massage the scalp to relax the nerves and muscles.

2. Wash the scalp with tar shampoo.

3. Dry excessive moisture from the hair, leaving the hair in a damp condition.

4. Apply a mild astringent lotion to the scalp by parting the hair, and steam it well with several steam towels.

5. Dry excessive moisture with a towel.

6. Barber and customer wear eye goggles.

7. Expose scalp to ultra-violet rays for six to eight minutes.

8. Apply an astringent or alcoholic scalp lotion to the scalp.

9. Expose the scalp to the red dermal lamp for five minutes.

10. Dress the hair, without brushing, using comb only.

DANDRUFF TREATMENT

The principal signs of dandruff are the appearance of white scales on the hair and scalp and the accompanying itching of the scalp. Dandruff may be associated with either a dry or oily condition of the scalp. The more common causes of dandruff are poor circulation of blood to the scalp; improper diet, neglect of cleanliness and infection. To prevent the spread of dandruff in the barber shop, the barber must sterilize all barber implements and avoid the use in common of combs, brushes and scalp applicators.

Step-by-Step Procedure For A Dandruff Treatment

1. Shampoo according to the condition of the scalp (dry or oily dandruff).

2. Dry the hair thoroughly.

3. Apply a dandruff lotion or antiseptic lotion to the scalp with a cotton pledget.

4. Apply four or five steam towels or use scalp steamer over the lotion.

5. Dry the hair thoroughly.

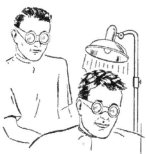

Applying Ultra-Violet Rays

6. Barber and customer put on goggles.

7. Expose scalp to ultra-violet rays for six to ten minutes, parting the hair every half-inch across the head from temple to temple.

8. Apply regular scalp manipulations for five minutes.

9. Apply dandruff ointment to the scalp and retain it until the next treatment.

10. Expose scalp to red dermal light for five minutes.

11. Apply high-frequency current for 6 to 8 minutes.

12. Comb hair neatly.

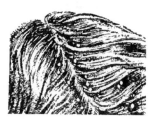

Simple Dandruff

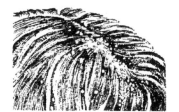

Excessive Dandruff

TREATMENT FOR ALOPECIA

Alopecia refers to a condition of premature baldness or excessive hair loss. The chief causes responsible for alopecia are poor circulation, lack of proper stimulation, improper nourishment and certain infectious skin diseases such as tinea, erysipelas and syphilis. The treatment for alopecia is directed at stimulating the blood supply and reviving the hair papillae involved in hair growth.

Step-by-Step Procedure For Treating Alopecia

1. Apply regular scalp manipulations.

2. Shampoo the scalp as required. For a dry scalp, use an oil shampoo; for an oily scalp, use a tar shampoo.

3. Dry the scalp thoroughly.

4. Cover the eyes with goggles.

5. Expose the scalp to ultra-violet rays for about five minutes.

6. Apply scalp ointment or lotion.

7. Apply high-frequency current with glass rake electrode for about five minutes, without sparking.

8. Comb hair neatly.

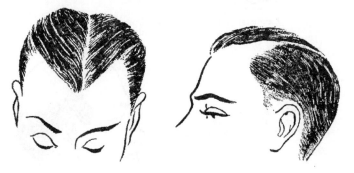

Beginning baldness in men from 30 to 40
Scalp treatments are most beneficial at this stage

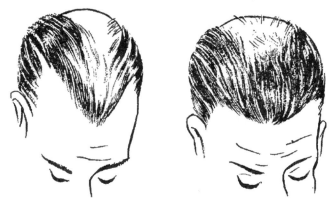

Partial baldness in men from 40 to 50
Scalp treatments are worth trying at this stage

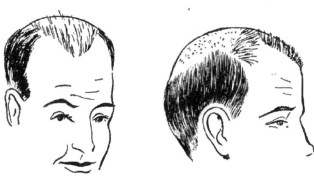

Extensive baldness in men from 50 to 60
Too late for scalp treatments

Extensive baldness in men
from 61 and over
Too late for scalp treatments

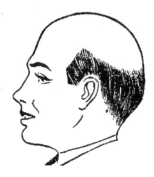

SCALP TREATMENTS

1. What is the purpose of scalp massage?	To maintain a healthy scalp and hair, and to combat such disorders as dandruff and excessive hair loss.
2. In what ways does scalp massage benefit the blood and nerves?	The blood flow is increased, while the nerves are rested and soothed.
3. What is the purpose of general scalp treatment?	To keep the scalp and hair in a healthy condition, and to prevent baldness.
4. What is accomplished by using a scalp steam?	A scalp steam stimulates the blood supply to the scalp.
5. When is a dry scalp treatment recommended?	If there is a deficiency of natural oil in the scalp and hair.
6. What are some of the common causes of a dry scalp?	Leading an indoor life, frequent washing of the hair and the continued use of alcoholic lotions, tonics and shampoos on the scalp and hair, and inactivity of the oil glands in the scalp.
7. What are the main causes of an oily scalp?	Excessive intake of fatty foods in the diet, and the resultant over-activity of the oil glands in the scalp.
8. What are the principal signs of dandruff?	The appearance of white scales on the scalp and hair and the accompanying itching of the scalp.
9. What are the common causes of dandruff?	Poor circulation of blood to the scalp, improper diet, uncleanliness and infection.
10. What are the chief causes of alopecia?	Poor blood circulation, lack of proper stimulation, improper nourishment and certain infectious skin diseases such as tinea, erysipelas and syphilis.
11. What is the aim in treating alopecia?	Stimulating the blood supply to the hair papillae encourages the growth and replacement of hairs.
12. Give the four steps for applying a scalp steam.	1. Apply regular scalp manipulations. 2. Steam the scalp with either 2 hot towels or a scalp steamer. 3. Apply hair tonic carefully and massage it well into the scalp. 4. Comb hair neatly.

THEORY OF MASSAGE

Most customers enjoy a facial or scalp massage for its stimulating and relaxing effects. It produces a glow in the cheeks and a sparkling feeling in the scalp, besides removing that tired look. The barber who has acquired a skillful touch in applying massage movements is the one whose services will be in greatest demand.

Massage involves the application of external manipulations to the face or any other part of the body. This is accomplished by means of the hands or with the aid of mechanical or electrical appliances. Each massage movement is applied in a definite way to accomplish a particular purpose.

Parts of the body usually massaged by the barber are the head, face and neck.

The **basic manipulations** used in massage are as follows:

1. **Effleurage** (stroking movement): This is a light, continuous movement applied in a slow and rhythmic manner over the skin. No pressure is employed. Over large surfaces, the palm is used; while over small surfaces, the finger-tips are employed. Effleurage is frequently applied to the forehead, face and scalp, for its soothing and relaxing effects.

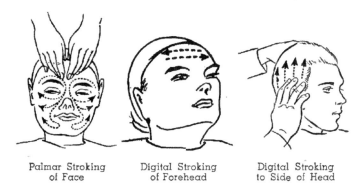

Palmar Stroking
of Face

Digital Stroking
of Forehead

Digital Stroking
to Side of Head

2. **Petrissage** (kneading movement): In this movement, the skin and flesh are grasped between the thumb and fingers. As the tissues are lifted from their underlying structures, they are squeezed, rolled or pinched with a light, firm pressure. This movement exerts an invigorating effect on the part being treated.

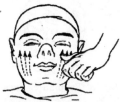

Digital Kneading of Cheeks

3. **Friction** (deep rubbing movement): This movement requires pressure on the skin while it is being moved over the underlying structures. The fingers or palm are employed in this movement. Friction has a marked influence on the circulation and glandular activity of the skin.

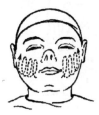 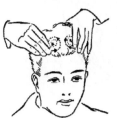 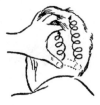

Palmar Circular   Circular Friction   Circular Friction
Friction of Face   with Finger-Tips   with Thumb

4. **Percussion** or **tapotement** (tapping, slapping and hacking movement): This form of massage is the most stimulating. It should be applied with care and discretion. Tapping is more gentle than slapping movements. Percussion movements tone the muscles and impart a healthy glow to the part being massaged.

In tapping, the finger-tips are brought down against the skin in rapid succession; whereas *in slapping*, the whole palm is used to strike the skin. *Hacking movement* employs the outer ulnar borders of the hands which are struck against the skin in alternate succession.

In facial massage, **light** digital tapping only is used.

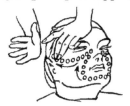

Digital Tapping of Face

5. **Vibration** (shaking movement): The hands or vibrator are used to transmit a trembling movement to the skin and its underlying structures. To prevent over-stimulation, this movement should be used sparingly and should never exceed a few seconds duration on any one spot.

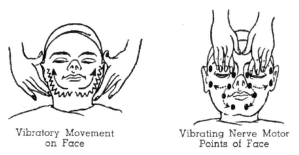

Vibratory Movement   Vibrating Nerve Motor
on Face   Points of Face

Physiological Effects of Massage

Skillfully applied massage influences the structures and functions of the body, either directly or indirectly. The immediate effects of massage are first noticed on the skin. The part being massaged responds by increasing its functional activities, as noticed by a more active circulation, secretion, nutrition and excretion. There is scarcely an organ of the body which is not favorably affected by scientific massage treatments.

Beneficial results may be obtained by proper facial and scalp massage, as follows:

1. The skin and all its structures are nourished.
2. The muscle fiber is stimulated and strengthened.
3. Fat cells are reduced.
4. The circulation of the blood is increased.
5. The activity of the glands is stimulated.
6. The skin is rendered soft and pliable.
7. The nerves are soothed and rested.
8. Pain is sometimes relieved.'

Rest and relaxation are brought about by giving soft, light, slow rhythmical movements, or very slow, light vibrations for a very short time.

The tissues are stimulated by movements of moderate pressure, speed and time, or by light vibrations of moderate speed and time.

Contours or fatty tissues are reduced by firm kneading or fast slapping movements, producing a sensation of heat or warmth over a fairly long period of time. Moderately fast vibrations with firm pressure will also accomplish this reduction.

Electrical appliances most commonly used in giving facial and scalp massage are as follows:

1. Vibrators.
2. High-frequency applicators.
3. Therapeutic lamps.
    a) Infra-red lamp
    b) Ultra-violet lamp.
    c) White or colored bulbs.

THEORY OF MASSAGE

1. What is massage?	A system of manipulation applied with the hands or with the aid of mechanical or electrical devices.
2. Which parts of the body are usually massaged by the barber?	The head, face and neck.
3. Name five basic movements used in massage.	1. Effleurage or stroking movements. 2. Petrissage or kneading movements. 3. Friction or deep rubbing movements. 4. Percussion movements (tapping, slapping or hacking). 5. Vibration or shaking movements.
4. What are the effects of massage on the skin?	The skin is nourished, stimulated and rendered soft and flexible.
5. What is the effect of massage on the blood?	The blood circulation is improved.
6. What are the effects of massage on the nerves?	The nerves are rested and soothed.
7. What are the effects of massage on the muscles?	The muscles are stimulated and strengthened.
8. What is the effect of massage on fatty deposits?	Fat cells are reduced.
9. Which massage movements produce a relaxing effect on the customer?	Soft, light, slow movements, either with the hands or vibrator.
10. Which massage movements produce a stimulating effect on the customer?	Moderate pressure and speed, either with the hands or vibrator.
11. Which massage movements reduce fatty tissue?	Firm kneading movements.

FACIAL TREATMENTS

Facial treatments can be developed into profitable services which will keep customers satisfied. Discriminating men seek facials for their soothing and refreshing benefits. Special facials are available for particular conditions of the skin A tactfully directed sales talk can materially help to stimulate revenue from facial business.

To be competent with facials, the barber should know how to analyze the condition of the customer's skin and recommend the most effective treatment. To accomplish this scientifically requires a knowledge of the anatomy of the head, face and neck in connection with facial massage.

Quiet, orderly surroundings are essential for giving facials. A quiet manner on the part of the barber is conducive to the customer's relaxation. Customers appreciate a clean, comfortable facial service.

Facial treatments are beneficial for the following reasons.

1. To cleanse, nourish and stimulate the skin.
2. To rest tired nerves and eyes.
3. To strengthen weak or sagging muscles.
4. To preserve the youthful texture and complexion of the skin.
5. To prevent the formation of wrinkles, ageing lines or double chin.

To give various facial treatments, the following supplies and equipment should be available:

Hot and cold water, towels, vibrator, therapeutic lamp, and various preparations such as facial creams, ointments, lotions, oils, packs, masks and powders.

Plain Facial

The plain facial is a general treatment beneficial for its cleansing and stimulating action on the skin. It also exercises as well as relaxes the facial muscles, thereby preserving a youthful appearance and preventing the formation of wrinkles.

The five causes of wrinkles are:

1. Loosening of the elastic skin fibers because of abnormal tension or relaxation of the facial muscles.

2. Shrinking of the skin tissue because of advancing years.

3. Excessive dryness or oiliness of the skin.

4. Facial expressions which continually crease and fold the skin.

5. Improper hygienic care of the skin.

Preparation For Plain Facial

In preparing the customer for a plain facial, the barber should pay attention to the following points:

1 Arrange all necessary supplies in their proper place.

2. Adjust chair, linens and towels.

3. Protect customer's hair by fastening a towel around his head.

4. Recline the barber chair.

5. Wash hands with soap and warm water.

All creams and other products should be removed from their containers with a spatula; never, under any circumstances, should the fingers be dipped into any of the products used.

Step-by-Step Procedure For A Plain Facial

The following steps are employed in giving a plain facial:

1. Apply cleansing cream over the face, using stroking and rotary movements.

2. Remove cleansing cream with a smooth warm towel.

3. Steam face mildly with three towels.

4. Apply tissue cream with finger tips into the skin.

5. Gently massage the face, using continuous and rhythmic movements. (See facial movements on page 192.)

6. Wipe off excess cream with a hot towel.

7. Steam the face with hot towels.

8. Remove hot towel and follow with a cool towel.

9. Pat an astringent or face lotion over the face and dry.

10. Apply powder over the face and remove excess powder.

11. Raise the barber chair.

12. Comb hair neatly.

ROLLING CREAM MASSAGE

The purpose of a rolling cream massage is to cleanse and massage the skin of the face.

Step-by-Step Procedure For A Rolling Cream Massage

1. Prepare the customer and steam the face with warm towels.

2. Apply the soft rolling cream.

3 Manipulate the face with rhythmic, rotary, stroking, rubbing movements, performed with the tips of the fingers, until most of the cream has been rolled off.

4. Apply a little cold cream, and cleanse the skin with a few lighter manipulations.

5. Remove all the cream with a warm towel, and follow with a mild witch-hazel steam.

6. Apply one or two cool towels and apply a toilet lotion.

7. Dry thoroughly and powder.

Points To Remember In Facial Massage

1. Have customer thoroughly relaxed.
2. Provide quiet atmosphere.
3. Maintain a clean, orderly arrangement of supplies.
4. Follow systematic procedure.
5. Give facial massage properly.

Seven Reasons Why A Customer May Find Fault With A Facial Massage

1. Not being careful or sanitary
2. Harming or scratching the skin.
3. Excessive or rough massage.
4. Getting facial creams into eyes.
5. Using towels that are too hot.
6. Breathing into the customer's face.
7. Offensive body odor, foul breath or tobacco odor.

FACIAL MASSAGE MOVEMENTS USING HANDS

Facial Massage Movements

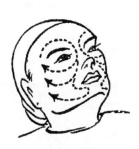

Fig. 1

1. Apply cleansing cream lightly over the face with stroking, spreading and circular movements. (Fig. 1).

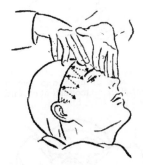

Fig. 2

2. Stroke fingers across forehead with up and down movements. (Fig. 2).

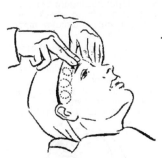

Fig. 3

3. Manipulate fingers across forehead with a circular movement. (Fig. 3).

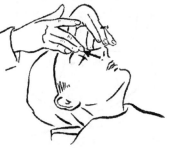

Fig. 4

4. Stroke fingers upward along side of nose (Fig. 4).

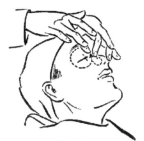

Fig. 5

5. Apply a circular movement over side of nose and use a light, stroking movement around the eyes. (Fig. 5).

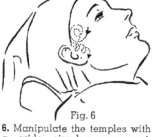

Fig. 6

6. Manipulate the temples with a wide circular movement. (Fig. 6).

7. Manipulate the front and back of the ears with a circular movement. (Fig. 6).

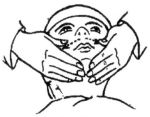

Fig. 7

8. Gently stroke both thumbs across upper lip. (Fig. 7).

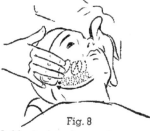

Fig. 8

9. Manipulate fingers from corners of mouth to cheeks and temples with a circular movement. (Fig. 8).

10. Manipulate fingers along lower jaw bone from tip of chin to ear with a circular movement. (Fig. 8).

11. Stroke fingers above and below along lower jaw bone from tip of chin to ear (Fig. 8).

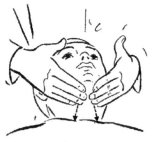

Fig. 9

12. Manipulate fingers from under chin and neck to back of ears, and up to temples. (Fig. 9, 10).

Repeat all massage movements **three to six times.**

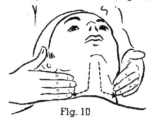

Fig. 10

FACIAL MASSAGE MOVEMENTS USING VIBRATOR

1. Adjust the vibrator on right hand and place finger-tips on left nostril. Vibrate left side of face as follows:

2. Vibrate a few light up and down movements on the left side of nose.

3. Gently slide fingers around eyes and then direct them toward center of forehead.

4. Vibrate rotary movement towards the left temple. Pause for a moment.

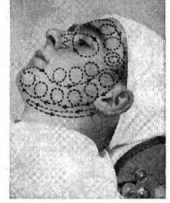

Facial Massage Movements
Using Vibrator

5. Continue the rotary movements down along the jaw line toward the tip of chin.

6. Vibrate from the chin towards the cheek, using wider, firmer movements.

7. Continue with a slow, light stroke at the temple, around the left ear, over the jaw bone, towards the center of the neck and then below the chin.

8. Vibrate rotary movements over the neck, behind the ear, up to the temple and then towards the center of the forehead.

9. Repeat steps 2-8 on the right side of the face.

10. Repeat steps 2-8 on the left side and then over on the right side of face.

Rules to Follow in Using Vibrator

1. Regulate the number of vibrations to avoid over-stimulation.

2. Do not use the vibrator too long in any one spot.

3. Vary the amount of pressure in accordance with the results desired.

4. Do not use vibrator over the upper lip as the vibrations may cause discomfort.

5. For soothing and relaxation effects, give very slow, light vibrations for a very short time.

6. For stimulating effects, give light vibrations of moderate speed and time.

7. For reducing fatty tissues, give moderate, fast vibrations with firm pressure.

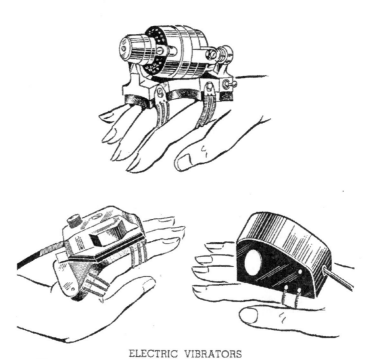

ELECTRIC VIBRATORS
Illustrations of three different types of electric hand vibrators
popular with barbers which are used for
facial and scalp massage.

FACIAL TREATMENTS

1. What are five benefits of facial treatments?	1. To cleanse, nourish and stimulate the skin. 2. To rest tired nerves and eyes. 3. To strengthen weak or sagging muscles. 4. To preserve the youthful texture and complexion of the skin. 5. To prevent the formation of wrinkles, ageing lines or double chin.
2. Name five causes of wrinkles.	1 Loosening of the elastic skin fibers because of abnormal tension or relaxation of the facial muscles. 2. Shrinking of the skin tissue because of advancing years. 3. Excessive dryness or oiliness of the skin. 4. Facial expressions which continually crease and fold the skin. 5. Improper hygienic care of the skin.
3. Which supplies and equipment are required for facial treatments?	Hot and cold water, towels, vibrator, therapeutic lamp and various preparations such as facial creams, ointments, lotions, oils, packs, masks and powders.
4. Why should the barber know the histology of the skin and the anatomy of the head, face and neck in giving facial massage?	In order to select the proper cream for each type of skin and be able to apply the proper massage manipulations as required by the customer.
5. Why should the barber know the composition and action of various creams applied to the skin?	In order to select and recommend the proper preparation for the particular condition of the skin being treated.

PLAIN FACIAL

1. In giving a plain facial, what attention should the barber show toward his customer?	Make customer comfortable and make a facial as restful and refreshing as possible.
2. Why should the barber never lean over the customer's face?	To avoid inhaling each other's breath or smelling each other's body odor.
3. How should the customer be protected from offensive tobacco odor?	The barber should never use tobacco while working on a customer. If tobacco was used, rinse mouth before starting to work.
4. What preparation should be made before giving a plain facial?	Arrange all necessary supplies in their proper place; wash hands; adjust linens and towels; protect the customer's hair by fastening a towel around his head; recline the customer.

5. **Briefly outline the procedure for giving a plain facial.**	1. Apply cleansing cream over the face, using stroking and rotary movements. 2. Remove cleansing cream with a smooth, warm towel. 3. Steam face mildly with three towels. 4. Apply tissue cream into the skin with finger-tips. 5. Gently massage the face, using continuous and rhythmic movements. 6. Wipe off excess cream with a hot towel. 7. Steam the face with hot towels. 8. Remove hot towels from face and follow with a cool towel. 9. Pat an astringent or face lotion over the face, and dry. 10. Apply powder over the face and remove excess powder. 11. Raise the barber chair. 12. Comb hair neatly.
6. **What are five important points to remember in giving a plain facial?**	1. Have customer thoroughly relaxed. 2. Provide quiet atmosphere. 3. Maintain clean, orderly arrangement of supplies. 4. Follow systematic procedure. 5. Give facial massage properly.
7. **Give seven reasons why a customer may find fault with a plain facial.**	1. Not being careful and sanitary. 2. Harming or scratching the skin. 3. Excessive or rough massage. 4. Getting facial cream into eyes. 5. Using towels that are too hot. 6. Breathing into customer's face. 7. Offensive body odor, foul breath or tobacco odor.

SPECIAL PROBLEMS

DRY SKIN FACIAL

The purpose of a dry skin facial is to stimulate the activity of the oil glands and to replenish a deficiency of the natural oil on the skin.

Step-by-Step Procedure For A Dry Skin Facial

1. Prepare customer as for a plain facial.
2. Apply cleansing cream over the face.
3. Remove the cream with a soft, dry towel.
4. Swab face with cotton pads dipped in witch hazel.
5. Steam the face moderately with 3 or 4 warm towels.
6. Massage a tissue cream containing lanolin gently into the skin, using stroking, circular and rotary movements.
7. Expose the skin to a red dermal light or infra-red lamp for three to six minutes.

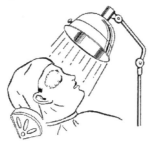 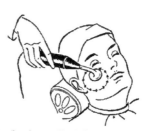

Applying Heat
with Infra-Red Lamp

Applying High-Frequency
Current

8. Knead the skin between the finger-tips and thumb by gently twisting it to the right and then to the left.
9. Apply the high-frequency current with a glass electrode for three to four minutes.
10. Wipe excess cream with three or four warm towels, followed by a cold towel.
11. Dry the face thoroughly with a soft towel.
12. Rub several drops of muscle oil into the skin.
13. Apply powder.

FACIAL FOR OILY SKIN AND BLACKHEADS

An excessively oily skin or any skin showing signs of enlarged pores or blackheads will benefit from this special facial treatment. This condition may be due to excessive use of starchy and oily foods, and also due to faulty hygienic habits.

Step-by-Step Procedure For An Oily Skin Facial

1. Prepare customer as for a plain facial.

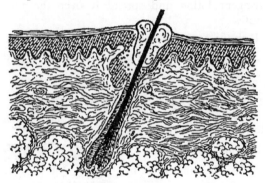

Notice Plug, or "Blackhead" Around Mouth
of Hair Follicle

2. Cleanse the skin either with cleansing cream or soap and warm water.

3. Steam the skin with three hot towels.

4. Press out blackheads with a sterilized comedone extractor.

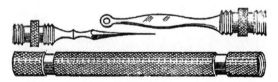

Comedone Extractor

5. Pat the face with an astringent lotion and then apply an astringent cream.

6. Apply regular hand manipulations for about five minutes.

7. Apply the mild high-frequency current for three to four minutes.

8. Apply warm towels to remove astringent cream.

9. Sponge the face with a soda solution (one table-spoonful of baking soda to one quart of water).

10. Dip several layers of cheese cloth or a piece of linen into astringent lotion and spread it over the face for a few minutes.

11. Remove covering and apply one or two cold towels.

12. Apply an astringent lotion, dry and powder the face.

FACIAL FOR WHITEHEADS (MILIA)

Follow routine of **facial for oily skin and blackheads** for steps 1 to 3. The milia must be removed by opening the tiny sacs with the sharp sterilized end of the comedone extractor and expelling the contents. A piece of cotton dipped in an antiseptic solution should then be applied. Continue the treatment from steps 5 to 12.

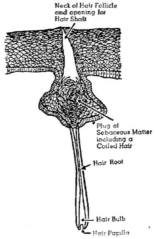

Formation of Milia (Whitehead) and Enlargement of Sebaceous Gland with Horny Plug

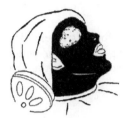

Clay Pack

CLAY PACK

The clay pack is suitable for all types of skin except a dry skin. It has a mild bleaching and tonic effect which prevents undue wrinkling of the skin.

Step-by-Step Procedure For A Clay Pack

1. Prepare a warm clay pack according to the manufacturer's directions.

2. Prepare the customer by arranging the linen and fastening a towel around the head to protect the hair.

3. Steam the skin with three moderately hot towels.

4. Spread the warm clay pack over the warm skin, using continuous stroking and rotary movements.

5. Cover the eyes with cotton pads moistened in witch hazel.

6. Dry the pack on the skin by exposure to a red dermal lamp.

7. Remove the pack with warm, damp steam towels.

8. Expose the face to the soothing blue light for a few minutes.

9. Apply cold cream or tissue cream with a few soothing massage movements.

10. Remove cream, and apply two cold towels,

11. Apply a mild lotion, dry and powder.

HOT OIL MASK

The hot oil mask is recommended for extremely dry, parched and scaly skins, prevalent during dry, hot or windy weather. It is used to soften, smooth and stimulate the skin tissues.

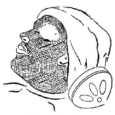

Hot Oil Mask

Step-by-Step Procedure for Hot Oil Mask

1. Prepare customer as for plain facial.
2. Prepare mask. Saturate cotton pads (4x4 inches) or an 18-inch square of gauze, in warm mineral or muscle oil.
3. Follow steps 1 to 5 as in plain facial on page 190.
4. After the manipulations, do not remove cream, but place the cotton pads or gauze over the face.
5. Adjust eye pads.
6. Use red dermal light or infra-red lamp from ten to fifteen minutes.
7. Remove mask and cream.
8. Finish the facial as in plain facial.

BLEACH PACK

The bleach pack is used for the purpose of lightening the shade of any tan or freckles present on the skin. Repeated treatments are necessary before any noticeable improvement can be obtained.

A bleach pack can be prepared by mixing together the following ingredients: One tablespoon of fine almond meal, one tablespoon of starch, two tablespoons of citric acid, ten drops of tincture of benzoin, and two or three tablespoons of peroxide.

Step-by-Step Procedure For A Bleach Pack

1. Prepare bleach pack freshly for each application.

2. Prepare customer by arranging linen and fastening a towel around the head to protect the hair.

3. Cover the eyes with cotton pads and protect the eyebrows and sideburns with cold cream.

4. Steam the skin with three warm towels.

5. Spread the bleach mixture with the finger-tips over the entire face.

6. Retain the bleach mixture on the face for six to eight minutes.

7. Remove the pack gently with warm, moist towels.

8. Apply lemon cream with light, soothing manipulations.

9. Remove excess cream and apply two cool towels.

10. Apply a mild lotion, dry and powder.

ACNE FACIAL

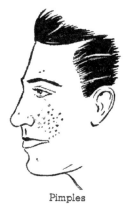

Pimples

Upon the advice of a physician local treatments are helpful in correcting acne and in clearing up the skin. Cleanliness and sterilization must be strictly observed in treating any form of acne.

Step-by-Step Procedure
For An Acne Facial

1. Cleanse the skin with cleansing cream.

2. Steam the face with three moderately hot towels, and remove the cream with the last towel.

3. Press out whiteheads and blackheads with a sterilized comedone extractor.

4. Sponge the skin well with an antiseptic acne lotion.

5. Rub an acne cream gently into the skin.

6. Cover the eyes with cotton pads moistened in witch hazel.

7. Expose the face to the red dermal light or infra-red lamp from five to ten minutes.

8. Apply high-frequency current for five minutes. Do not spark.

9. Wipe off excess cream with two or three warm towels.

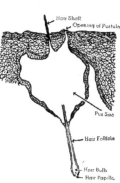

Formation of Acne Pustule and Enlargement of Sebaceous Gland with Pus

10. Sponge the skin with an astringent lotion.

11. Apply one or two cool towels, followed by an application of witch hazel.

12. Dry and powder the face.

ACNE ROSACEA FACIAL
Acne Rosacea is also known as Rosacea

Acne rosacea is a chronic, inflammatory congestion of the cheeks and nose. It is characterized by redness, dilation of the blood vessels, and the formation of papules and pustules.

Acne rosacea is usually caused by bad digestion and over-indulgence in alcoholic liquors. It may also be caused by over-exposure, constipation, faulty elimination and hyper-acidity It is usually aggravated by eating and drinking hot, highly spiced, or highly seasoned foods or drinks.

The treatment of acne rosacea belongs in the hands of a physician, but the barber can improve the condition by giving the following treatment under the guidance of the physician.

Step-by-Step Procedure For Treating Rosacea

No hot towels are used in this facial.

1. Apply cleansing cream.

2. Remove cream gently with a soft towel.

3. Sponge the face with a soda lotion (dissolve one large tablespoon of baking soda in one quart of water).

4. Apply astringent cream.

5. Expose the face to the blue light for five minutes.

6. Apply high-frequency current from ten to fifteen minutes. (The galvanic current may be used with the positive electrode instead of the high-frequency current).

7. Sponge face with witch hazel.

8. Dry and powder the face.

FARADIC FACIAL

Faradic facial is recommended as a general stimulant: It gives the muscles and tissues a mild passive exercise with a soothing relaxation to the nerves. It has no chemical effect.

Step-by-Step Procedure For A Faradic Facial

1. Cleanse the skin with a cleansing cream.
2. Steam the face mildly and apply a cold cream.
3. Apply the faradic current, using the electrode.
4. Give facial manipulations as in facial massage.
5. Wipe the cream with a couple of warm towels, and finish with two cool towels.
6. Apply a good antiseptic astringent.
7. Dry and powder the face.

SPECIAL PROBLEMS—FACIAL TREATMENTS

1. What is the purpose of a dry skin facial?	To stimulate the activity of the oil glands and to replenish a deficiency of natural oil on the skin.
2. What are the principal causes of an oily skin?	Excessive intake of starchy and oily foods, and faulty hygienic habits.
3. When is a bleach pack advised for a customer?	To lighten the shade of tan or freckles.
4. Which instrument is used to press out blackheads and whiteheads?	Sterilized comedone extractor.
5. What is the action of a clay pack on the skin?	It has a mild bleaching and tonic effect which prevents undue wrinkling of the skin.
6. Which facial treatments require the guidance of a physician?	Acne facial and rosacea facial.
7. What are the beneficial effects of a faradic facial?	Affords mild exercises for the facial muscles and relaxes the nerves.
8. In which facial treatments should the eyes be covered with cotton pads?	Clay pack, bleach pack, and acne facial.
9. In which facial treatments should an astringent lotion or cream be applied?	Oily skin facial, acne facial, rosacea facial and faradic facial.
10. In which facial treatment are hot towels omitted?	Rosacea facial.
11. When is a hot oil mask recommended?	For customers whose skin is extremely dry, parched and scaly.

PART III

BARBER SCIENCE

ANATOMY AND PHYSIOLOGY

Anatomy and physiology are sciences dealing with the structure and functions of the body. The body is organized into a complex network of bones, muscles, nerves and blood vessels. What affects one part ultimately influences the welfare of the entire body.

The study of anatomy and physiology will help the barber to adjust his procedures in accordance with bodily conditions.

Physiology is the study of the functions or activities performed by the various organs of the body.

Anatomy is the study of the gross structure of the body, which can be seen with the naked eye, such as muscles, bones and arteries.

Histology is the study of the minute structure of the body which can be seen only with the aid of a microscope such as the layers of the skin or hair.

To practice barbering it is necessary for the barber to shave with the grain of the beard and to know the reaction of the skin to shaving. It is equally important that he know the reaction of the skin, scalp and hair to the applications of hot and cold towels, soaps, hair tonics, creams, massage and electricity. For these reasons, the barber should study histology of the skin, scalp and hair as well as the anatomy of the underlying structures of the head, face and neck.

CELLS

In order to understand anatomy and physiology it is necessary to study the structure and activities of cells. The human body is composed of millions of specialized cells which perform the functions required for living.

Cells are the basic units of all living matter—animals, plants and bacteria. Living cells differ from each other in respect to their size, shape, structure and function. In the human body, the cells are **highly specialized,** and perform such vital functions as movement, absorption, reproduction, growth and elimination.

The cell consists of protoplasm and contains the following essential parts:

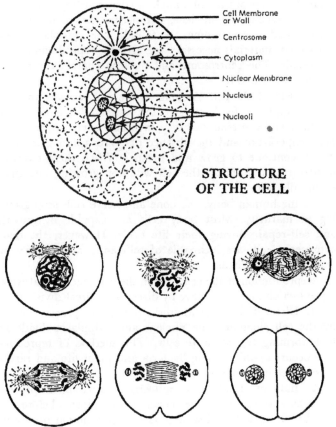

Diagram illustrating Indirect Division or Mitosis of the Cell

Composition. Most cells consist of the following parts:
1. Protoplasm:
    a) Cytoplasm.   b) Centrosome.   c) Nucleus.
2. Cell membrane or wall.

All living cells contain **protoplasm,** a colorless jelly-like substance in which protein, fat, carbohydrate, water and mineral salts are present. A thin **cell membrane or wall** permits soluble substances to enter and leave the protoplasm. Near the center of the cell a nucleus (dense protoplasm) is located. Outside the nucleus, **cytoplasm** (less dense protoplasm) and a **centrosome** are found. The cytoplasm contains food materials necessary for growth, reproduction and self-repair. The centrosome and nucleus control the reproduction of the cell.

Growth of the cell. As long as the cell receives an adequate supply of food, oxygen and water, eliminates waste products and is surrounded by a favorable environment (proper temperature and the absence of poisons and pressure), it will continue to grow and prosper. When these requirements are not fulfilled, the cell will stop growing and may eventually die.

In the human body, the bone and nerve cells stop growing at maturity. Most body cells are capable of growth and self-repair during their life cycle. However, the delicate nerve cells are incapable of self-repair after injury or destruction by disease.

Reproduction of the cell. When the cell reaches maturity, reproduction may take place by direct or indirect division.

1. **Direct division,** or **amitosis,** is a simple process whereby the cell elongates, the nucleus and cytoplasm divide in half, forming two separate cells. This method of reproduction occurs mainly among bacteria and plant life and rarely takes place in human tissues.

2. **Indirect division,** or **mitosis,** is a complex process whereby a series of changes occur in the nucleus before the cell divides in half. This method of reproduction occurs in human tissues (See illustration on preceding page.)

Metabolism is a complex chemical process whereby the body cells are nourished and supplied with energy to carry on their many activities. In a healthy body, the metabolic rate is kept under control by a secretion from the thyroid gland.

There are two phases to metabolism:
1. **Anabolism,** a constructive process.
2. **Catabolism,** a destructive process.

During anabolism, the cells of the body absorb water, food and oxygen for the purposes of growth, reproduction and repair. In catabolism, the cells consume what they have absorbed in order to perform specialized functions, such as muscular effort, secretion or digestion.

TISSUES

Tissues are composed of groups of cells of the same kind. Each tissue has a specific function and can be recognized by its characteristic appearance. Body tissues are classified as follows:

1. **Connective tissue:** serves to support, protect and bind together other tissues of the body. Bone, cartilage, ligament, tendon, and adipose tissue are examples of connective tissue. Adipose or fatty tissue forms a protective layer underneath the skin, surrounds the vital organs and affords support to blood vessels and nerves in these areas.

2. **Muscular tissue:** serves to contract and move various parts of the body.

   a) **Voluntary muscle tissue** (striated) is under the control of the will and permits the movements of muscles such as those of the face, arms and legs.

   b) **Involuntary muscle tissue** (non-striated) is under the control of special nerve centers which permit the movement of the intestines, stomach, and blood vessels.

   c) **Heart muscle tissue** (cardiac) permits the movement of the heart as the blood is pumped through it.

3. **Nerve tissue:** serves to carry messages, controls and coordinates body functions by means of neurons or nerve cells found in the muscles, skin, vital organs and glands.

4. **Epithelial tissue:** serves as a protective covering of the outer and inner body surfaces such as that found on the skin, mucous membranes, linings of the heart, digestive and respiratory organs and glands.

5. **Liquid tissue:** serves as a carrier of food, waste products, and hormones, by means of the blood and lymph.

ORGANS

Organs are structures containing two or more different tissues which are combined to accomplish a definite function. Each organ is so constructed that in a state of health it will perform its function with ease and efficiency. Among the important organs found in ·the body are the brain, heart, lungs, kidneys, and the various glands.

SYSTEMS

Systems are groups of organs which cooperate for a common purpose. The human body is composed of the following important systems.

Skeletal System   Circulatory System   Respiratory System
Muscular System   Endocrine System   Digestive System
Nervous System   Excretory System   Reproductive System

The **skeletal system** is the physical foundation of the body. It is composed of differently shaped bones united by movable and immovable joints. The function of the skeletal system is to serve as a means of protection, of support or of locomotion.

The **muscular system** covers and shapes the skeleton. Practically every contraction and movement of the body is due to the action of muscles. The obvious movements of the arms and hands, the contraction of the heart and stomach, and the changes in facial expression, are ·the direct result of muscular activity.

The **nervous system** is a highly developed and sensitive organization of nerve tissues. Through it the individual is made aware of his existence and relation to the outside world. Nerves, branching out from the brain and. spinal cord, carry messages to and from all parts of the body.

The **circulatory system** is composed of the heart, blood vessels, blood and lymph. The pumping action of the heart distributes the vital fluids, blood and lymph, through the blood vessels to all parts of the body. The blood acts as

216   ANATOMY AND PHYSIOLOGY

a two-way carrier of supplies, bringing oxygen and food materials to the cells and taking away waste products and secretions from the cells. The lymph reaches all parts of the body not reached by the blood, and assists in the exchange of supplies required by the cells.

The **endocrine system** represents a group of specialized glands which produce secretions called hormones. Among the important endocrine glands are the pituitary and thyroid glands whose hormones regulate the processes of growth and metabolism.

The **excretory system** includes the skin, kidneys, liver, lungs and large intestine, which are engaged in the process of eliminating waste products from the body. The skin gives off perspiration, the lungs exhale carbon dioxide gas, the kidneys excrete urine, and the large intestine discharges refuse from the body. The liver produces bile which contains certain waste products.

The **respiratory system** is confined to the chest cavity where the lungs are located. The blood, as it passes through the lungs, is purified by the removal of carbon dioxide gas and the intake of oxygen gas.

The **digestive system** includes the mouth, stomach and intestines, which are part of a continuous tube about thirty feet in length. The function of digestion is to break down complex food substances into simple materials fit to be absorbed and used by the body cells. Various digestive glands, including the pancreas and liver, form and discharge, at various points along the route, enzymes that act on food in the process of digestion

The **reproductive system**, the function of which is to insure the continuance of the race by the reproduction of other human beings.

ANATOMY AND PHYSIOLOGY

1. Define anatomy.	Anatomy is the study of gross structures of the body, such as muscles, bones or arteries.
2. Define physiology.	Physiology is the study of the functions or activities performed by various organs of the body.
3. Why should the barber study the anatomy of the head, face and neck?	In order to have a knowledge of those parts upon which the barber works.

Cells

1. What is a cell?	A cell is the basic unit of all living matter.
2. Of what are cells composed?	Cells are composed of protoplasm and a cell membrane or wall.
3. Name the principal parts of the cells and their functions.	1. Cytoplasm—contains food materials. 2. Nucleus—necessary for reproduction of the cell. 3. Centrosome—controls reproduction of the cell. 4. Cell membrane or wall—permits soluble substances to enter and leave the protoplasm.
4. What is metabolism?	Complex chemical process whereby body cells are nourished and perform their functions.
5. Name two phases of metabolism.	Anabolism and catabolism.
6. Which activities occur during anabolism?	The cell takes in whatever it needs of food, water and oxygen.
7. Which activities occur during catabolism?	The cell uses up whatever it has taken in.
8. Name two methods of cellular reproduction.	Direct division or amitosis. Indirect division or mitosis.
9. What are tissues? Name 5.	Groups of cells performing the same function. Bone tissue, muscle tissue, nerve tissue, liquid tissue and epithelial tissue.
10. What is an organ? Give five examples.	A structure containing two or more different tissues and performing a vital function of the body. Brain, heart, lungs, kidneys and various glands.
11. What are systems?	A group of organs which work together in performing the various functions of the body.
12. Name nine body systems.	Skeletal, muscular, nervous, circulatory, endocrine, excretory, respiratory, digestive and reproductive systems.

THE SKELETAL SYSTEM

The skeletal system is the framework of the body which supports and protects the other body systems. It is composed of bones, cartilages and ligaments.

The **skeleton** of the adult consists of 206 bones, comprising about 16% of the weight of the body, as follows:

Skull	22	Upper extremities	64
Spinal column	26	Lower extremities	62
Hyoid bone	1	Ear bones	6
Ribs and sternum	25		

Total 206

Bones*

Composition. Bone is the hardest structure, forming the framework of the body. It is composed of about one-third animal matter and two-thirds mineral or earthy matter.

1. The **animal (organic) matter** consists of bone cells, blood vessels, connective tissues and marrow.

2. The **mineral (inorganic) matter** consists mainly of phosphate and carbonate of lime.

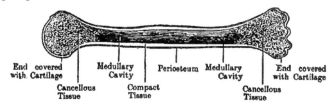

End covered with Cartilage   Medullary Cavity   Periosteum   Medullary Cavity   End covered with Cartilage

Cancellous Tissue   Compact Tissue   Cancellous Tissue

Longitudinal Section of a Long Bone

Appearance. Externally, bone appears to be light pink color; internally, deep red.

Bone tissue. There are two types of bone tissue: cancellous (spongy) and dense (compact).

*Throughout this text the official B.N.A. (Basle Anatomical Nomenclature) system of classifying anatomical terms has been adopted. Old terms are placed in parentheses.

NOTE: Side views of anatomical drawings have identical structures on both sides.

1. The **compact tissue** forms the hard bone found in the shafts of long bones, and outside of flat bones   The compact bony tissue is traversed by small channels called Haversian canals, containing minute blood vessels.

2. The **cancellous tissue** forms the interior of bones, the ends of bone shaft, and the very thin bones. It consists of a meshwork of bony arches through which blood vessels and nerves pass.

Marrow is a soft fatty substance filling the cavities of bones whose function is largely concerned with the formation of red corpuscles (red blood cells).

Covering. The covering of bone is called periosteum, a fibrous membrane whose function is to protect the bone, and serve as an attachment for tendons, ligaments, blood vessels and nerves.

Nutrition. Bone receives its nourishment through blood vessels (capillaries) which make their way through the periosteum into the interior of bones. Bone marrow also aids in the nutrition of bone.

Functions of bones are as follows:

1. To give shape and strength to the body, and keep the various parts and organs in position.

2. To protect organs from injury.

3. To afford a solid place for the attachment of muscles.

4. To act as levers for all bodily movements.

Forms or Shapes. There are several forms or shapes of bones found in the human body, namely:

1. Flat bones, as the skull.

2. Long bones, as the legs and arms.

3. Short bones, as the fingers and toes.

4. Irregular bones, as the vertebrae (spine),

The various bones of which the skeleton consists are connected at different parts of their surfaces, and such connections are called joints, or articulations.

Joints. The various joints come under the following classifications.

1. Movable—as in fingers.

2. Immovable—as in the skull.

3. Slightly movable—as in the spine.

Types of Joints. The various types of joints found in the human body are as follows:

1. Pivot—the neck.

2. Hinge—the elbow and knees.

3. Ball and socket—the hips and shoulders.

4. Gliding—the spine.

5. Condyloid—the wrist and ankle.

Cartilage and Ligaments

Cartilage (also called gristle), is a firm and tough non-vascular, elastic substance, similar to bone but without its mineral content It serves the following purposes:

1. To cushion the bones at the joints.

2. To prevent jarring between bones in motion, as in walking.

3 To give shape to certain external features, such as the nose or ears.

Ligaments are bands or sheets of fibrous tissues, which help to support the bones at the joints, such as the wrist or ankle.

The synovial fluid is a lubricating fluid whose function is to prevent friction at the joints.

The Bones of the Head and Face

The skull is the skeleton of the head. It is an oval bony case which shapes the head, and protects the brain. The skull is divided into two parts: the cranium, consisting of eight bones; and the skeleton of the face, consisting of fourteen bones.

The Eight Bones of the Cranium

Occipital bone—Situated at back and lower part of the cranium.

Two parietal bones—By their union the sides and roof of the cranium are formed.

Frontal bone—This bone is divided into two portions: the vertical portion forming the forehead, and the horizontal or orbital portion, which is a part of the formation of the roof of the orbits (eye sockets) and nasal fossae (depressions).

Two temporal bones—Situated on either side of the skull below the parietal bones.

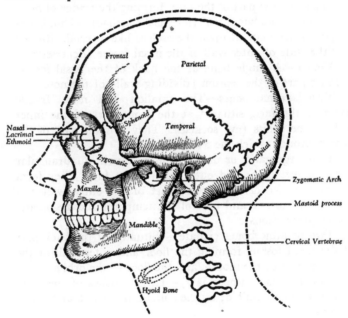

BONES OF THE HEAD, FACE AND NECK

Cranial Bones:
Occipital—Base of skull.
Two parietals—Crown.
Frontal—Forehead.
Two temporals—Ear region.
Ethmoid—Between the orbits.
Sphenoid—Base of cranium and
 back of orbits (eye sockets).

Facial Bones:
Two nasals.
Two turbinals (inferior nasal
Vomer.   conchae)
Two lacrimals.
Two zygomatics (malar).
Two palatines (palate).
Two maxillae (upper jaw).
Mandible (lower jaw).

Cervical Vertebrae—Neck region of the spinal column.
Neck Bone—Hyoid bone—Front of throat.

Ethmoid bone—Light and spongy, situated between the orbits (eye sockets) at the root of nose, forming part of the nasal cavities.

Sphenoid bone—Situated at the base of the cranium and back of orbits, joins together all the bones of the cranium.

The Fourteen Bones of the Face

Two nasal bones—Oblong bones placed side by side in the upper middle part of the face, forming the bridge of nose.

Two turbinal bones (inferior nasal conchae)—Thin layers of spongy bone curled upon themselves like a scroll, situated on either side of outer wall of the nasal fossae (depressions).

Vomer—A single bone at the back of the nasal fossae, forming part of the septum (dividing wall) of the nose.

Two lacrimal bones—The smallest and most fragile bones of the face, situated at the front part of the inner wall of the orbits (eye sockets). They contain part of the canals through which the tear ducts run.

Two zygomatic or malar bones—Small quadrangular bones in the upper and outer part of the face. They form the prominence of the cheeks, part of the outer wall and floor of the orbits, and part of the temporal and zygomatic fossae (depressions).

Two palatine bones (palate)—Situated at the back part of the nasal fossae, forming the floor and outer wall of the nose, the roof of the mouth, and the floor of the orbits.

Two maxillae (upper jaw)—Largest bones of the face, excepting the mandible; by their union the whole upper jaw is formed.

Mandible bone (lower jaw)—The largest and strongest bone of the face.

Bones of the Neck

Hyoid bone—A "U" shaped bone, between the root of the tongue and the laryngeal prominence (Adam's Apple). It supports the tongue.

Cervical vertebrae—Form the top part of the vertebral column located in the neck region.

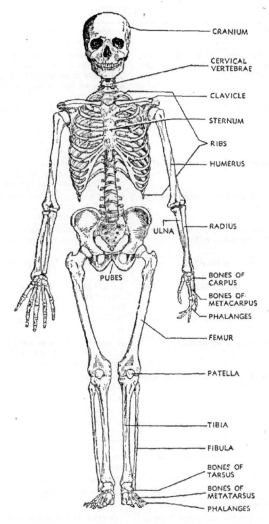

CRANIUM

CERVICAL
VERTEBRAE

CLAVICLE

STERNUM

RIBS

HUMERUS

RADIUS

ULNA

BONES OF
CARPUS

PUBES

BONES OF
METACARPUS

PHALANGES

FEMUR

PATELLA

TIBIA

FIBULA

BONES OF
TARSUS

BONES OF
METATARSUS

PHALANGES

Diagram illustrating the Human Skeleton

Front view, showing the principal bones, their size and shape.

BONES

1. What is bone?	Bone is the hard tissue forming the framework of the body.
2. What are four important functions of bones in the body?	1. Gives shape and strength to the body. 2. Protects organs from injury. 3. Serves as an attachment for muscles. 4. Acts as levers for all bodily movements.
3. Of what is bone composed?	About one-third organic matter (bone cells, blood vessels, connective tissue and marrow) and about two-thirds inorganic matter (mainly phosphate and carbonate of lime).
4. Describe the external part of bones.	It has a light pink color and consists of hard tissue protected by an outer covering known as the periosteum.
5. Describe the internal part of bones.	It has a deep red color and consists of a spongy tissue containing cavities filled with marrow.
6. How does the bone receive its nourishment?	Through blood vessels which enter the interior of the bone by way of the periosteum.
7. What is a joint?	A connection between the surfaces of bones.
8. What is cartilage or gristle?	Cartilage is a firm, elastic substance resembling bone but lacking its mineral content, making it softer than bone.
9. What is the main purpose of cartilage?	It serves to cushion the bones at the joints.
10. What is a ligament?	A band of fibrous tissue which helps to support the bones at the joints as in the wrist or ankle.
11. What is the function of synovial fluid?	To lubricate the joints to prevent friction.
12. What is the skull?	An oval, bony case which shapes the head and protects the brain.
13. How many bones are found in the skull?	22 bones.
14. How many bones are found in the cranium? Name them.	8 bones. One occipital, two parietals, one frontal, two temporals, one ethmoid and one sphenoid.
15. Locate the occipital bone.	Back and lower part of the skull.
16. Locate the parietal bones.	The sides and top of head.
17. Locate the frontal bone.	Forehead.
18. Locate the temporal bones.	Located in the ear region.
19. Locate the ethmoid bone.	Placed between the eye sockets.
20. Locate the sphenoid bone.	Situated at the base of the cranium and back of the eye sockets.

21. How many bones are found in the face? Name them.	14 bones. Two nasals, two turbinals, two lacrimals, one vomer, two zygomatics, two palatines, two maxillae (upper jaw), and one mandible (lower jaw).
22. Locate the nasal bones.	Placed side by side in the upper middle part of the face.
23. Locate the vomer bone.	Located back of nasal depressions.
24. Locate the turbinal bones.	Situated on the side wall of the nose.
• 25. Locate the lacrimal bones.	Situated at the front part of inner wall of eye sockets.
26. Locate the zygomatic bones.	Form the cheek bones at the upper and outer part of the face.
27. Locate the palatine bones. What does it form?	Situated at back part of nasal dedepressions. Forms roof of mouth.
28. Which bony structure is formed by the maxillae?	Upper jaw.
29. Which bony structure is formed by the mandible?	Lower jaw.

THE MUSCULAR SYSTEM

The muscular system covers, shapes and supports the skeleton, and its function is to effect all movements of the body. The muscular system relies upon the skeletal and nervous systems for its activities.

The muscular system consists of over 500 muscles, large and small, comprising approximately 40% to 50% of the weight of the body.

Muscles

Muscle is fibrous contractile and elastic tissue by which movements of every part of the body are accomplished. Muscles do not cover and surround the body in continuous sheets, but consist of separate bundles made up of elastic fibers varying in size and length, according to the function of each muscle.

Muscles are attached to bones, cartilage, ligaments, tendons, skin, and sometimes to each other.

Usually muscles are not directly connected to bones, but are joined by means of glistening cords, called **tendons,** or sinews. Where one muscle connects with another, each muscle ends in a flat expanded tendon or fibrous sheet, called an **aponeurosis.** A delicate membrane of connective tissue called **fascia** covers the muscles and separates their numerous layers.

Origin of muscle is the term applied to the more fixed attachments, such as muscles attached to bones (referred to as skeletal muscles) or to some other muscle. **Insertion** of muscle is the term applied to the more movable attachments, such as muscles attached to the skin, or movable muscles.

Nutrition. Each muscle has its own set of blood vessels, nerves and lymphatics, from which it receives nourishment.

Types of muscles. There are three kinds of muscular tissue, namely: voluntary, involuntary and cardiac.

1. **Voluntary** or **striated** muscles, which are controlled by the will. These muscles are attached to the skeleton and are in turn fastened to the bones, skin, and other muscles,

by tendons. They are composed of cells which appear striated or striped under the microscope.

MUSCLE CELLS

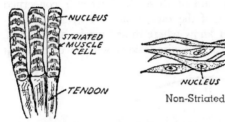

Striated   Non-Striated   Cardiac

2. **Involuntary** or **non-striated muscles,** which function without the action of the will. These muscles are found in the walls of the stomach, intestines and blood vessels. They consist of smooth spindle-shaped cells which overlap at the ends.

3. **Cardiac** or **heart muscles** are found in the substance of the heart. They are composed of cells which are not as distinctly striated as the cells of skeletal muscle. They are quadrangular in shape, joined end to end, and are grouped in bundles supported by a framework of connective tissue.

Stimulation. Muscular tissue may be stimulated by any of the following agencies: chemical (acid or salt), mechanical (massage), electrical agents (vibrator and faradic current), thermal agents (heat and therapeutic lamps) and nerve impulses.

Several characteristics that enable muscular tissue to perform the **functions of motion** are:

1. Excitability or irritability—the power of responding to stimulation.

2. Contractibility—the thickening of a muscle when in action and its thinning when at rest.

3. Extensibility—the ability to stretch.

4. Elasticity—the ability to recover the original form.

5. Muscle tone—normal degree of tension and the quickness with which the muscle responds to stimulation.

MUSCLES OF THE HEAD, FACE AND NECK

The voluntary muscles are the only ones affected by external manipulations, and of these the barber is concerned only with the muscles of the face, head and neck. It is essential that the barber know where these muscles are located, so that facial and scalp manipulations will be directed at the muscles.

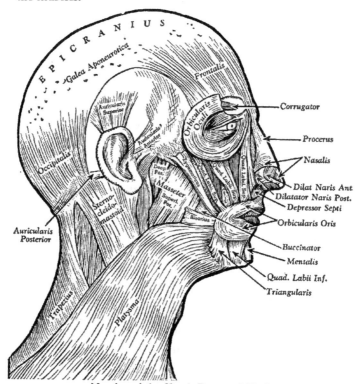

Muscles of the Head, Face and Neck

Muscle of the Scalp

Epicranius (occipito-frontalis)—A broad muscle covering the top of the skull. It consists of two parts: the **occipitalis,** or posterior part, and the **frontalis,** or anterior part, which are connected by an aponeurosis called **galea aponeurotica.** The two muscles act independently. The frontalis raises the eyebrow, draws the scalp forward and causes transverse wrinkles across the forehead. The occipitalis draws the scalp backward.

Muscles of the Ear

Muscles of the ear are practically functionless.

Auricularis superior—Raises the ear slightly.

Auricularis posterior—Draws the ear backward slightly.

Auricularis anterior—Draws the ear forward slightly.

Muscles of the Eyebrow and Eyelid

Orbicularis oculi (orbicularis palpebrarum)—Surrounds the margin of the orbit, and closes the eyelid. It has an external or orbital section, which is controlled by the will; and an internal or palpebral portion, whose action is involuntary, as in blinking.

Corrugator (corrugator supercilii)—Extends along the line of the brow. It draws the eyebrow downward and inward, forming vertical wrinkles above the nose, as in frowning.

Levator palpebrae superioris—Opens the eye by raising the upper eyelid. (An internal eye muscle not affected by massage treatment.)

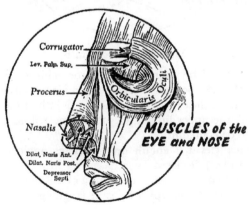

Muscles of the Nose

Procerus (pyramidalis nasi)—Covers the bridge of the nose. Draws down eyebrow and puckers up the skin over bridge of nose, causing transverse wrinkles over bridge of nose.

Nasalis (compressor nasi)—Compresses the nostril.

Depressor septi (depressor alae nasi)—Contracts the opening of the nostril.

Dilatator (dilator) **naris posterior and anterior**—Expands the opening of the nostrils.

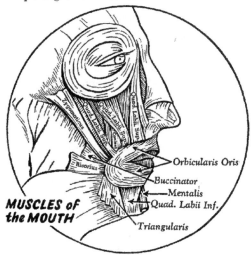

Muscles of the Mouth

Quadratus labii superioris (levator labii superioris)—Consists of three portions (angular head, infra-orbital head and zygomatic head) which function jointly to raise and draw back the upper lip and elevate the nostril, as expressed in distaste or contempt.

Caninus (levator anguli oris)—Raises angle of mouth and aids to keep it closed.

Zygomaticus (zygomaticus major)—Raises angle of mouth backward and upward, as in laughing or smiling.

Mentalis (levator menti)—Raises and pushes up lower lip, causing wrinkling of the chin.

Quadratus labii inferioris (depressor labii inferioris)— Depresses the lower lip down and a little to one side, as in the expression of sarcasm.

Triangularis (depressor anguli oris)—Pulls down the corner of the mouth.

Buccinator—Contracts and compresses the cheek, as in blowing; accessory muscle of mastication.

Orbicularis oris—Forms a flat band around the upper and lower lips. Holds mouth closed when contracted; puckers and wrinkles lips as in kissing or whistling.

Risorius—Draws corner of mouth out and back, as in a broad grin.

Facial Expressions

Most of the changes in the expression of the face are caused by the action of the mouth and eye muscles and of those which are attached to them. For example, the lifting of the eyelids by the frontalis expresses surprise. The wrinkling of the brows by the corrugator speaks disapproval or bewilderment. The risorius, or grinning muscle, draws the corners of the mouth outward and backward. The quadratus labii superioris lifts the nostrils and upper lip together, expressing distaste or contempt. Pleasure is expressed by the lifting of the angles of the lips upward and outward, while grief depresses them. (There are but three of the depressors, or grieving muscles, on each side, and six for the manifestation of happier feelings.)

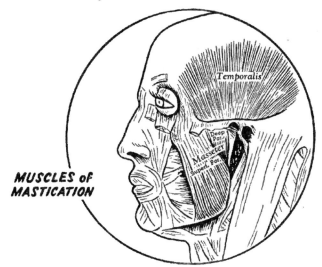

*Superficial muscles have been removed to show
the underlying muscles of mastication.*

Muscles of Mastication

Masseter—This muscle is made up of two layers, deep portion and superficial portion. Closes jaws, as in chewing.

Temporalis (temporal muscle)—Closes the jaws.

Pterygoideus internus and externus (not shown on illustration)—Between mandible and cheek bone. Draw lower jaw (mandible) forward. (Not affected by massage treatment:)

Muscles of the Neck and Back

Platysma (platysma myoides)—Depresses the lower jaw and draws down the lower lip.

Sterno-cleido-mastoideus (sterno-cleido-mastoid muscle) —Turns head obliquely to one side; pulls head downward and forward.

Trapezius—Covers the back of the neck and upper region of the back. Draws the head to one side or backward; rotates shoulder blade.

NOTE: *BNA terms for various muscles are recorded in heavy type.*

MUSCLES OF THE SCALP

NAME	ORIGIN	INSERTION	FUNCTION
Epicranius Occipitalis Occipito-frontalis Frontalis	Occipital bone Aponeurosis	Aponeurosis Skin of forehead on the line of eyebrows	Draws scalp backward. Raises eyebrow, draws scalp forward, causes transverse wrinkles across the forehead.

NERVES. *The frontalis is supplied by the temporal branches, and the occipitalis by the posterior auricular branch of the facial nerve.*

MUSCLES OF THE NECK

NAME	ORIGIN	INSERTION	FUNCTION
Platysma Platysma myoides	Deep skin of neck and shoulder region	Lower border of mandible & skin & muscles of mouth.	Depresses lower jaw and draws down lower lip.

NERVES. *The platysma is supplied by the cervical branch of the facial nerve.*

Trapezius	Middle of occipital bone, and the vertebrae of neck and chest	All around the shoulder, the clavicle in front and spine of the scapula in back	Draws head to one side or backward; rotates the shoulder blade.

Sterno-cleido-mastoideus Sterno-cleido-mastoid muscle	Sternum and clavicle, by two heads	Mastoid process of temporal bone, and occipital bone.	Turns head obliquely to one side; draws head downward and forward.

NERVES. *Trapezius and sterno-cleido-mastoideus are supplied by the spinal part of the accessory nerve and branches from the second and third cervical nerves.*

MUSCLES OF THE EYELIDS AND EYEBROWS

NAME	ORIGIN	INSERTION	FUNCTION
Orbicularis oculi Orbicularis palpebrarum *This muscle consists of palpebral (internal) or orbital (external) parts.*	Palpebral—Upper part of nasal bone Orbital—Frontal process of maxilla and frontal bones	Palpebral—Skin at outer corner of eye Orbital—Near its own origin	Palpebral—Closes the eye involuntarily as in blinking. Orbital—Closes the eye forcibly, wrinkling the surrounding skin.
Corrugator Corrugator supercilii	Nasal prominence at inner end of eyebrow	Skin about half way across the orbital arch	Draws eyebrow downward & inward, causing vertical lines above nose, as in frowning.

NERVES. *The orbicularis oculi and corrugator are supplied by the temporal and zygomatic branches of the facial nerve.*

Levator palpebrae superioris raises the upper eyelid. This muscle, being an internal eye muscle, is not affected by massage treatment. It is supplied by the oculomotor nerve.

MUSCLES OF THE NOSE

NAME	ORIGIN	INSERTION	FUNCTION
Procerus Pyramidalis nasi	Skin covering bridge of nose.	Skin over lower part of forehead between eyebrows	Draws down the eyebrow and produces transverse wrinkles over bridge of nose.
Nasalis Compressor nasi	Maxilla near wing of nose	Skin at lower bridge of nose	Compresses the nostril.
Depressor septi Depressor alae nasi	A depression in front of maxilla	Septum and back part of wing of nose	Contracts the opening of the nostril.
Dilatator (dilator) naris anterior and posterior	Nasal notch of maxilla and cartilage of nose	Skin near margin of nostril	Expands the opening of the nostril.

NERVES. *Muscles of the nose are supplied by the buccal branches of the facial nerve.*

MUSCLES OF THE MOUTH

NAME	ORIGIN	INSERTION	FUNCTION
Quadratus labii superioris Levator labii superioris	Maxilla next to nose, lower margin of orbit and zygomatic bone	Cartilage wing and skin of nose, orbicularis oris and upper lip	Raises and draws back upper lip and elevates nostril to express distaste or contempt.
This muscle consists of three portions: angular head, infraorbital head, and zygomatic head.			
Caninus Levator anguli oris	Canine depression of maxilla	Skin at angle of mouth	Raises angle of mouth, & aids to keep it closed.
Zygomaticus Zygomaticus major	Outer arch of zygomatic bone	Skin at angle of mouth	Draws angle of mouth backward and upward, as in laughing or smiling.
Orbicularis oris	Other muscles of the mouth surrounding orbicularis oris.	Acts as insertion for other muscles of the mouth	Holds mouth closed when contracted; puckers & wrinkles lips as in kissing or whistling.

NERVES. *The above muscles of the mouth are supplied by the buccal branches of the facial nerves.*

NAME	ORIGIN	INSERTION	FUNCTION
Mentalis Levator menti	Incisive depression of mandible	Skin of chin	Raises and pushes up lower lip, causing wrinkling of chin.
Quadratus labii inferioris Depressor labii inferioris	Oblique line of mandible	Skin of lower lip	Depresses lower lip down and a little to one side, as in expression of sarcasm.
Triangularis Depressor anguli oris	Oblique line of mandible	Skin at angle of mouth	Pulls down corner of mouth.
Risorius	Fascia near ear over the masseter	Skin at angle of mouth	Draws corner of mouth out and back, as in a broad grin.

NERVES. *The above four muscles of the mouth are supplied by the mandibular and buccal branches of the facial nerve.*

NAME	ORIGIN	INSERTION	FUNCTION
Buccinator	Alveolar portions of upper and lower jaw bones	Orbicularis oris	Contracts and compresses cheek, as in blowing; accessory muscle of mastication.

NERVES. *The buccinator is supplied by the buccal branches of the facial nerve. Buccinator nerve from the trigeminal is sensory only in this area.*

MUSCLES OF MASTICATION

NAME	ORIGIN	INSERTION	FUNCTION
Masseter	Arch of zygomatic bone	Lower border and around the corner of mandible	Closes jaws, as in chewing.
Temporalis Temporal muscle	Temporal fossa and fascia	Anterior border of crown-shaped process of mandible	Closes the jaws.

Pterygoideus externus and internus are two muscles which draw the lower jaw forward. These muscles are not affected by massage treatments.

NERVES. *Muscles of mastication are supplied by branches from the mandibular division of the trigeminal nerve.*

MUSCLES OF THE EAR

NAME	ORIGIN	INSERTION	FUNCTION	
Auricularis anterior Attrahens aurem	Frontalis and aponeurosis	Front of ear	Draws the ear forward slightly.	*Ear muscles are practically functionless.*
Auricularis superior Attollens aurem	Aponeurosis	Upper part of ear	Raises the ear slightly.	
Auricularis posterior Retrahens aurem	Mastoid portion of temporal bone	Back of ear	Draws ear backward slightly.	

NERVES. *The auriculares anterior and superior are supplied by the temporal branches; the auricularis posterior is supplied by the posterior auricular branch of the facial nerve.*

THE MUSCULAR SYSTEM

1. What are the important functions of muscles in the body?	Muscles cover, shape and support the skeleton, and effect all bodily movements.
2. Of what is a muscle composed?	Muscle is composed of fibrous contractile and elastic tissue.
3. Name three kinds of muscular tissue.	1. Voluntary or striated muscle. 2. Involuntary or non-striated muscle. 3. Cardiac or heart muscle.
4. Distinguish between voluntary and involuntary muscles.	Voluntary muscles such as those of the face, arms and legs, are controlled by the will. Involuntary muscles such as those of the stomach and intestines, are not controlled by the will.
5. What is a tendon or sinew?	A tendon is a white glistening bundle of fibrous tissue which attaches a muscle to a bone.
6. What is an aponeurosis?	An aponeurosis is an expanded tendon which serves to connect one muscle with another.
7. What is a fascia?	A fascia is a membrane of connective tissue which covers and separates muscular layers.
8. How do the muscles receive their nourishment?	Food elements are brought to the muscles by small blood and lymph vessels.
9. Name five agents capable of stimulating muscular tissue.	1. Chemical agents, such as acids or salts. 2. Mechanical agents, such as massage. 3. Electrical agents, such as the vibrator and faradic current. 4. Thermal agents, such as heat and therapeutic lamps. 5. Nerve impulses.
10. Name the scalp muscle and its two portions.	Epicranius muscle, consists of occipitalis and frontalis.
11. Locate the scalp muscle and its two portions.	The epicranius covers the entire top of the scalp, from the base of the skull to the eyebrows. The occipitalis is the back portion; the frontalis is the front portion.
12. Which structure connects the occipitalis and frontalis?	An aponeurosis called galea aponeurotica.
13. What is the function of the occipitalis?	Occipitalis draws the scalp backward.
14. What is the function of the frontalis?	Raises the eyebrow and draws scalp forward, causing transverse wrinkles across forehead.
15. Name two muscles of the eyes.	Orbicularis oculi and corrugator.

16. Which muscle draws the eyebrow downward and inward?	Corrugator.
17. Which muscle closes the eye?	Orbicularis oculi.
18. Which muscle covers the bridge of the nose?	Procerus.
19. Which muscle depresses the lower lip?	Quadratus labii inferioris.
20. Which muscle raises and draws back the upper lip?	Quadratus labii superioris.
21. Which muscle raises the angle of the mouth backward and upward?	Zygomaticus.
22. Which muscle holds the mouth closed when contracted?	Orbicularis oris.
23. Which muscle pulls down the corner of the mouth?	Triangularis.
24. Which muscle raises and pushes up the lower lip?	Mentalis.
25. Which muscle contracts and compresses the cheek?	Buccinator.
26. What is mastication?	The act of chewing.
27. Name four important muscles of mastication.	Masseter, temporalis, pterygoideus internus and pterygoideus externus.
28. Name three important muscles of the neck and back.	Platysma, trapezius and sterno-cleido-mastoid muscle.
29. Which muscle draws the head downward and forward?	Sterno-cleido-mastoid muscle.
30. Which muscle depresses the lower jaw and draws down the lower lip?	Platysma.
31. Which muscle draws the head backwards or to one side?	Trapezius.

THE NERVOUS SYSTEM

The nervous system is considered to be one of the most important systems of the body because it controls and coordinates the functions of all the other systems and makes them work harmoniously and efficiently.

The nervous system is composed of the brain, spinal cord, cranial nerves and spinal nerves.

The **functions** of the nervous system are:

1. To rule the body by controlling all visible and invisible activities.

2. To control human thoughts and conduct.

3. To govern all internal and external movements of the body.

4. To give the power to see, hear, smell, taste, move, talk, feel, think and remember.

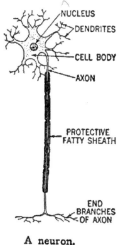

A neuron.

A neuron is the structural unit of the nervous system. It is composed of a nerve cell (cell body) and its outgrowth of long and short fibers, called **cell processes**. The nerve cell (cell body) stores energy and nutriment for the cell processes which convey the nerve impulses throughout the body. Practically all the nerve cells are contained in the brain and spinal cord.

Nerves are long white cords made up of fibers (cell processes) from nerve cells. They have their origin in the brain and spinal cord, and distribute branches to all parts of the body.

Nerves furnish both sensation and motion.

Sensory nerves, termed **afferent nerves,** carry impulses or messages from sense organs to the brain where sensations of touch, cold, heat, sight, hearing, smell, taste and pain are experienced.

Motor nerves, termed **efferent nerves,** carry impulses from the brain to the muscles, the transmitted impulses causing movement

NERVOUS SYSTEM
1. Cerebro-spinal nervous system
 1. Central System
  1. Brain
  2 Spinal cord
 2. Peripheral System
  1. Cranial nerves
  2 Spinal nerves
2. Sympathetic nervous system
 1 Ganglia: issued from spinal cord
 2 Communicating Branches

The **nervous system** is divided into two main divisions, namely: the cerebro-spinal nervous system, and the sympathetic nervous system.

The **cerebro-spinal nervous system,** which consists of both the **brain** and the **spinal cord,** as well as the **spinal nerves** and **cranial nerves,** controls speech, taste, sight, touch and smell, and governs the voluntary muscles. Making up this large system are the central and peripheral systems.

The **central system** consists of the **brain** and **spinal cord.**

The **brain,** the principal nerve center, is the largest and most complex nerve tissue. It controls sensations, voluntary muscles, and the power to think and feel. It includes:

1. **Cerebrum,** large frontal part, presides over such mental activities as reasoning, will, and higher emotions.

2. **Cerebellum,** the smaller, lower part, keeps the body balanced, makes muscular movements smooth and graceful.

3. **Medulla oblongata,** connecting the brain with the spinal cord, regulates the movements of the heart, and organs of respiration and digestion.

4. **Twelve pairs of cranial nerves,** originating in the brain, reach various parts of the head, face and neck.

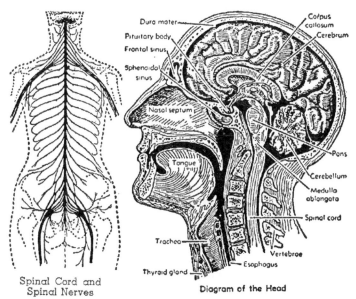

Spinal Cord and
Spinal Nerves

Diagram of the Head

The **spinal cord is** composed of masses of nerve cells with fibers running upward and downward. It originates from the brain and extends down to the lower extremity of the trunk, being enclosed and protected by the spinal column. **Thirty-one pairs of spinal nerves** extending from the spinal cord are distributed to the muscles and skin of trunk and limbs; and connect with the nerves of the sympathetic system.

The **peripheral system** is located in the skin, muscles and sense organs. It consists of the terminal endings of the cranial and spinal nerves. These nerves send sensory impulses to the brain and spinal cord and receive motor impulses from the brain.

The **sympathetic or autonomic nervous system** governs the involuntary muscles controlling the functions of circulation, digestion and respiration, and controls secretion of the glands as well.

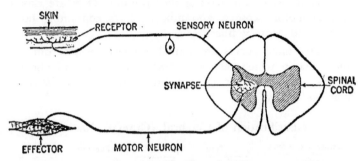

The Path of a Nerve Impulse

A **reflex arc** is the path through which a nervous impulse travels in responding to a stimulus. For example, the quick removal of the hand from a hot object.

Nerve fatigue is caused by excessive mental or muscular work, resulting in an accumulation of waste products. Weariness, poor complexion, and dull eyes may be signs of nerve exhaustion. Rest and relaxation, assisted by massage, help to relieve nerve fatigue.

Nutrition. Nerves are nourished through blood vessels, lymph spaces, and lymphatics found in the connective tissues surronding them.

The nervous system may be **stimulated** by physical agents and chemical agents.

1. Physical agents such as light, heat, electricity or massage.
2. Chemical agents such as acids, bases or salts.

Cerebral (Cranial) Nerves

There are twelve pairs of cranial nerves all connected to some part of the brain surface. They issue through openings on the sides and base of the cranium. They are classified as motor, sensory, and mixed nerves containing both motor and sensory fibers.

The cranial nerves are named numerically according to the order in which they arise from the brain, and also by names which describe their nature, function, or distribution, as follows:

Classification of Cerebral (Cranial) Nerves

Number and Names	Type	Function
1. Olfactory	Sensory	Sense of smell.
2. Optic	Sensory	Sense of sight.
3. Oculomotor	Motor	Motor nerve to eye muscles.
4. Trochlear	Motor	Motor nerve to the superior oblique muscle of the eye.
*5. Trigeminal or Trifacial	Sensory-Motor	Sensory nerve to scalp, forehead and face; motor nerve to muscles of mastication.
6. Abducent	Motor	Motor nerve to lateral rectus muscle of eye.
*7. Facial	Sensory-Motor	Sensory nerve to tongue (taste); motor nerve to muscles of facial expression, part of scalp and muscles of neck.
8. Acoustic or Auditory	Sensory	Sense of hearing and maintenance of equilibrium.
9. Glossopharyngeal	Sensory-Motor	Sensory nerve to tongue (taste); motor nerve to muscles of pharynx.
10. Vagus or Pneumogastric	Sensory-Motor	Sensory nerve to respiratory and digestive organs; motor nerve to heart, respiratory and digestive organs.
*11. Accessory	Motor	Motor nerve to sterno-cleido-mastoid and trapezius muscles of neck.
12. Hypoglossal	Motor	Motor nerve to muscles of tongue and hyoid bone.

*Important nerves for the barber to know in facial and scalp services.

NERVES OF THE HEAD, FACE AND NECK

Of the twelve cerebral nerves, only three are of interest to the barber in giving facial and scalp treatments. These are:

1. Fifth cerebral (trigeminal or trifacial) nerve.
2. Seventh cerebral (facial) nerve.
3. Eleventh cerebral (accessory) nerve.

The cervical nerve, originating from the spinal cord in the neck, is also of interest to the barber.

The proper use of massage or electric current can favorably influence the nerve and muscular functions of the area being treated.

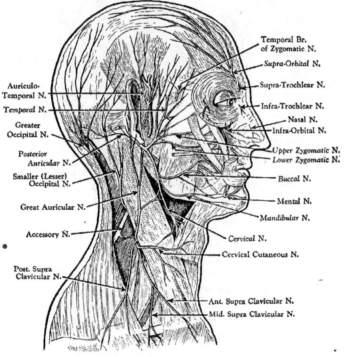

Nerve Supply to Scalp, Face and Side of Neck.
(Facial Nerves are marked in italics)

Fifth Cerebral (Cranial) Nerve

Fifth cerebral (trigeminal or trifacial) nerve is the largest of the cerebral nerves and is the chief sensory nerve of the face and the motor nerve of the muscles of mastication. It emerges from the brain, forms a ganglion just inside of the skull, just forward of the ear. It splits into three main divisions and many branches, all of which are inside of the skull with the exception of a few terminal branches. The three main divisions and their branches are ophthalmic, maxillary, and mandibular.

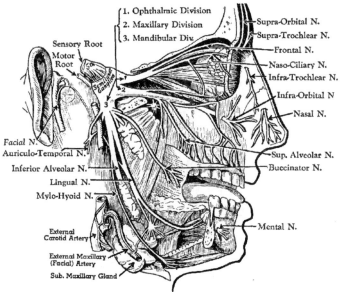

1. Ophthalmic Division
2. Maxillary Division
3. Mandibular Div.

Supra-Orbital N.
Supra-Trochlear N.
Frontal N.
Naso-Ciliary N.
Infra-Trochlear N.
Infra-Orbital N
Nasal N.

Sensory Root
Motor Root

Facial N.
Auriculo-Temporal N.
Inferior Alveolar N.
Lingual N.
Mylo-Hyoid N.

Sup. Alveolar N.
Buccinator N.

External Carotid Artery
External Maxillary (Facial) Artery
Sub. Maxillary Gland

Mental N.

Fifth Cerebral Nerve

Only important anatomical terms are explained in the text. Anatomical terms of lesser importance are not explained in the text.

A. **Ophthalmic Division** (sensory nerve) supplies branches to the skin of the forehead, eyelid, eyebrow and nose. Its principal branches are:

   1. **Frontal nerve** is subdivided to form:

      a) **Supra-orbital nerve;** affects the forehead, scalp, eyebrow, and upper eyelid.

b) **Supra-trochlear nerve**; affects skin between eyes and upper side of nose.

2. **Naso-ciliary** (nasal) nerve is subdivided to form:

a) **Infra-trochlear nerve**; affects membrane and skin of nose.

b) **Nasal nerve**; affects point and lower side of nose.

c) **Lacrimal nerve**; affects upper eyelid and tear glands. (Not shown on illustration.)

B. **Maxillary Division** (sensory nerve) supplies the forehead, lower eyelid, upper lip and skin of cheek and nose. Its principal branches are:

1. **Zygomatic nerve**; affects the temple, side of forehead and skin of upper part of cheek.

2. **Infra-orbital nerve**; affects skin of lower eyelid, side of nose, upper lip, mouth and their corresponding glands.

C. **Mandibular Division** (motor and sensory nerve) supplies the temple, auricle of ear, lower lip, lower part of face and muscles of mastication. Its principal branches are:

1. **The anterior portion** (motor and sensory nerve) which is subdivided to form:

a) **Masseteric nerve**; affects the masseter muscle. (Not shown on illustration.)

b) **Deep temporal nerves**; affect the muscles above the temple. (Not shown on illustration.)

c) **Buccinator nerve** (sensory); affects the buccinator muscle and the skin of the cheek.

2. **The posterior portion** (motor and sensory nerve) of the mandibular division is subdivided to form:

a) **Auriculo-temporal nerve**; affects the external ear and the skin above the temple and up to the top of the skull.

b) **Inferior alveolar nerve**; affects all the teeth along the lower jaw. Its principal branch is:

1. **Mental nerve**; affects the skin of lower lip and chin.

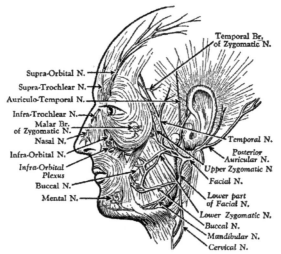

Distribution of the Fifth and Seventh Cerebral (Cranial) Nerves
To Head, Face and Neck.
(Facial nerves are marked in italics.)

Seventh cerebral (facial) nerve is the chief motor nerve of the face. It emerges near the lower part of the ear; its divisions and their branches spread through all the muscles of expression, and down to the muscles of the neck. Of all the branches of the facial nerve, those most important to the barber are:

1. **Posterior auricular nerve**; affects the muscles behind the ear and at the base of skull.

2. **Temporal nerve**; affects the muscles of the forehead, eyelid, temple and upper part of cheek.

3. **Zygomatic nerve (upper and lower)**; affects the muscles of the upper part of cheek.

4. **Buccal nerve**; affects the buccinator and orbicularis oris muscles.

5. **Mandibular nerve**; affects the muscles of chin and lower lip.

6. **Cervical nerve**; affects the side of the neck and the platysma muscle.

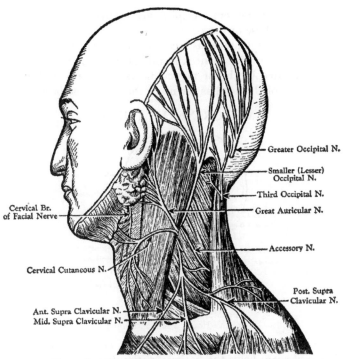

Greater Occipital N.

Smaller (Lesser)
Occipital N.

Third Occipital N.

Great Auricular N.

Accessory N.

Post. Supra
Clavicular N.

Cervical Br.
of Facial Nerve

Cervical Cutaneous N.

Ant. Supra Clavicular N.
Mid. Supra Clavicular N.

Nerve Supply to Side of Neck and Back of Head

Eleventh cerebral (accessory) nerve (motor) extends over the neck and upper part of back by means of two branches.

1. **Accessory portion** is distributed only to internal structures.
2. **The spinal portion** affects the sterno-cleido-mastoid and trapezius muscles of the neck and back.

Cervical nerves originate at the spinal cord and their branches supply the muscles and skin at the back of the head and neck, as follows:

1. **Great Auricular nerve** is subdivided to form:
   a) **Anterior branches** which affect the skin of the face and external ear.
   b) **Posterior branches** affect the skin behind the ear.

2. **Smaller (Lesser) Occipital nerve** affects the scalp area at the base of the skull.
3. **Cervical Cutaneous (cutaneous colli)** extends over front and side of neck as far down as the breast bone.
4. **Greater Occipital nerve** affects the scalp and back part of the head as far up as the top of the head.

MOTOR NERVE POINTS

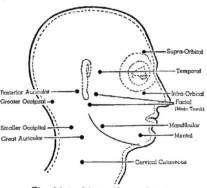

The Main Motor Nerve Points
of the Head, Face and Neck

Knowing the location of important nerve points of the face and scalp helps the barber to stimulate particular muscles with the least outside force. A nerve point represents that part of a nerve which comes closest to the surface of the skin and can, therefore, be reached by direct contact.

Stimulation of the following nerve points has a beneficial effect in facial and scalp massage.

  A. Derived from the **fifth cerebral (cranial)** nerve are:
1. **Supra-orbital nerve point,** located just above the eye socket, affects the forehead, scalp, eyebrow and upper eyelid.
2. **Infra-orbital nerve point,** located just below the eye socket, affects the lower eyelid, side of nose, upper lip and mouth.
3. **Mental nerve point,** located just below the premolar teeth on either side of the lower jaw, affects the lower lip and chin.

B. Derived from the **seventh cerebral (cranial) nerve** are:

1. **Facial nerve point,** located in front of the ear lobe, affects all the muscles of facial expression.
2. **Temporal nerve point,** located on sides of head, affects the muscles of the forehead, eyelid, temple and upper part of cheek.
3. **Posterior auricular nerve point,** located back of the ear, affects the muscles behind the ear and at the base of skull.
4. **Mandibular nerve point,** located slightly above and in front of angle of jaw, affects muscles of chin and lower lip.

C. Derived from the **cervical nerve of the spinal cord** are:

1. **Greater occipital nerve point,** located in back of the head, affects the scalp as far up as the top of the head.
2. **Smaller occipital nerve point,** located at base of scalp, affects the skin and muscles of this region.
3. **Great auricular nerve point,** located at side of neck, affects the external ear and area in front and back of ear.
4. **Cervical cutaneous nerve point,** located at side of neck, affects the front and side of neck as far down as the breast bone.

THE NERVOUS SYSTEM

1. What are the important functions of the nerves in the body?	1. To rule the body by controlling all visible and invisible activities. 2. To control human thoughts and conduct. 3. To govern all internal and external movements of the body. 4. To give the power to see, hear, move, talk, feel, think and remember.
2. What is a neuron?	A neuron is a nerve cell containing a central portion or cell body and short and long fibers called processes
3. What is a nerve?	A nerve is a long white cord consisting of nerve fibers and capable of carrying messages to and from various parts of the body.
4. Name two kinds of nerves found in the body.	1. Sensory or afferent nerves. 2. Motor or efferent nerves.

5. What is the function of sensory nerves?	Sensory nerves carry messages regarding touch, heat, cold, sight, hearing, smell, taste and pain to the nerve centers in the brain.
6. What is the function of motor nerves?	Motor nerves carry messages from the brain to the muscles which produce bodily movements.
7. Name the two main divisions of the nervous system.	1. The cerebro-spinal nervous system. 2. The sympathetic nervous system.
8. Of what is the cerebro-spinal nervous system composed?	Brain, spinal cord, cranial nerves and spinal nerves.
9. What is the function of the cerebro-spinal nervous system?	To control all the voluntary muscles as well as speech, taste, sight, touch and smell.
10. What is the function of the sympathetic nervous system?	To control involuntary muscles and the functions of digestion, circulation, respiration and secretions of the various glands.
11. What is the cause of nerve fatigue?	Excessive mental or muscular work.
12. What are the signs of nerve fatigue?	Weariness, poor complexion and dull eyes.
13. What is the best way to relieve nerve fatigue?	Proper use of rest, relaxation and massage.
14. How many pairs of cerebral (cranial) nerves are there, and how are they known?	There are twelve pairs of cerebral nerves, and they are known by their number or name.
15. How many pairs of nerves issue from the spinal cord, and what are they called?	Thirty-one pairs of nerves issue from the spinal cord, and they are called spinal nerves.
16. Which two cerebral (cranial) nerves are the most important in facial treatment?	1. The Fifth or trigeminal nerve. 2. The Seventh or facial nerve.
17. Which is the largest cerebral (cranial) nerve?	The Fifth or trigeminal nerve.
18. What is the function of the fifth or trigeminal nerve?	It is the chief sensory nerve of the face and the motor nerve of the muscles of mastication.
19. Name three nerve points originating from the fifth cerebral nerve.	The supra-orbital, infra-orbital and mental nerve points.
20. Which cerebral (cranial) nerve controls the muscles of expression?	The Seventh or facial nerve.
21. Name four nerve points originating from the seventh cerebral nerve.	The facial, posterior auricular, temporal, and mandibular nerve points.
22. Name four nerve points originating from the cervical nerve of the spinal cord.	Greater occipital, smaller occipital, great auricular, and cervical cutaneous nerve points.

23. Which cerebral (cranial) nerve controls the sense of sight? — The optic nerve.

24. Which cerebral (cranial) nerve controls the sense of smell. — The olfactory nerve.

25. Which cerebral (cranial) nerve controls the sense of hearing? — The acoustic (auditory) nerve.

26. Which cerebral (cranial) nerves control the motion of the eyes? — The oculomotor nerve, trochlear nerve and abducent nerve.

27. Which region of the head is supplied by the greater occipital nerve? — The scalp of back part of the head as far up as the top of the head.

28. Which cerebral nerve supplies the sterno-cleido-mastoid and trapezius muscles? — The spinal portion of the eleventh or accessory nerve.

29. Which branches of the fifth cerebral (cranial) nerve supply the following regions?
   a) Forehead
   b) Lower side of nose
   c) Skin of upper lip
   d) Skin of lower lip
   e) Skin above temple
   f) Skin of upper part of cheek

   a) Supra-orbital
   b) Nasal
   c) Infra-orbital
   d) Mental
   e) Auriculo-temporal
   f) Zygomatic

30. Which branches of the seventh cerebral nerve supply the following regions or muscles?
   a) Muscle of the forehead
   b) Muscles of chin and lower lip
   c) Platysma muscle
   d) Muscle behind ear
   e) Orbicularis oris
   f) Muscles of upper part of cheek

   a) Temporal
   b) Mandibular

   c) Cervical
   d) Posterior Auricular
   e) Buccal
   f) Zygomatic

THE CIRCULATORY (VASCULAR) SYSTEM

The circulatory (vascular) system controls the circulation of the blood through the body in a steady stream, by means of the heart and blood vessels, and supplies body cells with nutrient materials and carries away waste products.

There are two divisions to the vascular system:

1. The **blood-vascular system**, which comprises the heart and blood vessels (arteries, capillaries and veins) for the circulation of the blood.

2. The **lymph-vascular system**, or **lymphatic system**, consisting of lymph glands and lymphatics through which the lymph circulates.

These two systems are intimately linked with each other. Lymph is derived from the blood and is gradually shifted back into the blood stream.

THE BLOOD-VASCULAR SYSTEM

The Heart

The heart is an efficient pump which keeps the blood moving in a steady stream through a closed system of arteries, capillaries and veins.

The heart is a muscular, conical-shaped organ, about the size of a closed fist, located in the chest cavity, and enclosed in a membrane, the **pericardium**. Two sets of nerves, the **vagus** and **sympathetic**, regulate the heart beat. In a normal adult, the heart beats about 72 to 80 times a minute.

The interior of the heart contains four chambers and four valves. The upper thin-walled cavities are the right **atrium** (auricle) and left **atrium**. The lower thick-walled chambers are the right **ventricle** and left **ventricle**. Valves allow the blood to flow in only one direction. With each contraction and relaxation of the heart, the blood flows in, travels from the auricles (atria) to the ventricles, and is then driven out, to be distributed all over the body. The atrium (pl., atria) is also called the auricle.

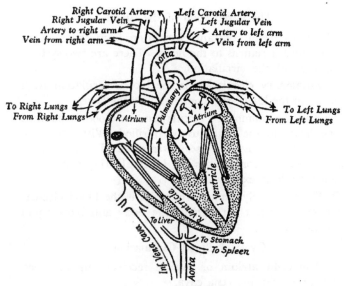

Right Carotid Artery   Left Carotid Artery
Right Jugular Vein   Left Jugular Vein
Artery to right arm   Artery to left arm
Vein from right arm   Vein from left arm

Aorta

To Right Lungs   To Left Lungs
From Right Lungs   From Left Lungs
          R.Atrium   Pulmonary   L.Atrium

                                        L.Ventricle
                            R.Ventricle

              To Liver
                           To Stomach
                           To Spleen
    Inf. Vena Cava   Aorta

Diagram of the Heart

The Blood Vessels

The arteries, capillaries and veins, transport blood to
and from the heart and the various tissues of the body.
The main artery of the body is the **aorta** which starts at
the left ventricle of the heart, and subdivides into smaller
arteries.

Arteries are thick-walled muscular and elastic vessels that
carry pure blood from the heart to the capillaries. They
vary in size from the aorta, which is about an inch in diameter, to others which are but a small fraction of an inch.

Capillaries are minute thin-walled blood vessels whose
network connects the smaller arteries with the veins. Through
their walls, the tissues receive nourishment and eliminate
waste products.

Veins are thin-walled, inelastic blood vessels containing
cup-like valves to prevent backflow, and carrying impure
blood from the various capillaries back to the heart.

The Circulation of the Blood

The blood is in constant circulation from the moment it leaves until it returns to the heart. There are two systems taking care of the circulation.

1. **Pulmonary circulation** is the blood circulation from the heart to the lungs, and back again to the heart.

During the pulmonary circulation the blood is pumped by the heart to the lungs to be purified. With each respiration, an exchange of gases takes place. During inhalation, oxygen is absorbed into the blood. During exhalation, carbon dioxide is expelled.

2 **General or Systemic Circulation** is the blood circulation from the heart throughout the body and back again to the heart.

Cycle of Blood Circulation

1. The **right atrium** or **auricle** receives impure blood from a large vein, the **vena cava**.

2. From the right atrium or auricle, the venous blood passes through a valve into the **right ventricle**.

3. From the right ventricle, the venous blood is carried through the **pulmonary artery** up to the lungs to be oxygenated or purified.

4. The **left atrium** or **auricle** receives the purified blood through the **pulmonary vein**.

5. From the left atrium or auricle, the purified blood passes through a valve into the **left ventricle**.

6. From the left ventricle, the **aorta** sends the arterial blood to all parts of the body, except the lungs.

7. This cycle is repeated when the venous blood is brought back again to the right atrium or auricle.

The Blood

Blood is the nutritive fluid circulating throughout the blood-vascular system. It is salty and sticky, has an alkaline reaction, and maintains a normal temperature of 98 6° Fahrenheit. From 8 to 10 pints of blood fill the blood vessels of an adult and constitute about 1/16th to 1/20th of the body's weight. The skin holds about 1/2 to 2/3 of all the blood in the body.

Color of blood. The blood has a distinct color, varying from bright red to scarlet in the arteries, and possessing a dark-red to crimson tint in the veins. The exceptions to this rule are the pulmonary artery (dark-red to crimson tint) and the pulmonary vein (bright red to scarlet color). This change in color is due to the gain or loss of oxygen as the blood passes through the lungs and other tissues of the body.

Composition of blood. The blood is a liquid tissue consisting of blood plasma, red corpuscles, white corpuscles and blood platelets. Plasma constitutes about two-thirds of the blood and the other bodies about one-third.

Plasma is the fluid part of the blood, straw-like in color, in which the red corpuscles, white corpuscles and blood platelets flow. About nine-tenths of plasma is water. The blood plasma also contains proteins, nutrients, mineral salts, waste products and other substances. Plasma is derived from the food and water taken into the body.

Red corpuscles (red blood cells) or **erythrocytes** are circular bi-concave discs colored with a substance called **hemoglobin.** The function of the red corpuscles is to carry oxygen from the lungs to the body cells and transport carbon dioxide from the cells to the lungs. The red blood cells are formed in the red bone marrow and from cells lining the capillaries. They are far more numerous than the white blood cells.

White corpuscles (white blood cells) or **leucocytes** differ from red blood cells in many respects. They are larger in size, colorless, and can change their form by movements. White corpuscles are produced in the spleen, lymph glands, and the yellow marrow of the long bones. The most important function of these cells is to protect the body against disease by fighting harmful bacteria and their poisons.

Blood platelets or **thrombocytes** are colorless, irregular bodies, much smaller than the red corpuscles. They are formed in the bone marrow. These cells play an important role in the clotting of the blood.

Clotting. When the blood leaves the body and comes in contact with the air, it hardens and clots. This clotting is due to the hardening of the **fibrin** in the blood and the clot thus prevents the further flow of the blood.

Diseases of the blood. Hemophilia is characterized by extremely slow clotting of blood and excessive bleeding from even very slight cuts. This disease is a sex-linked disease affecting only males, but transmitted by the female.

Anemia is a condition in which there are too few red blood cells or too little hemoglobin. **Iron** (furnished by liver, calf-brain, spinach, and oatmeal) is frequently beneficial.

Chief Functions of the Blood

1. It carries water, oxygen, food and secretions to all cells of the body.

2. It carries away carbon dioxide and waste products to be eliminated through the lungs, skin, kidneys and large intestine.

3. It helps to equalize the body temperature, thus protecting the body from extreme heat and cold.

4. It aids in protecting the body from harmful bacteria and infections through the action of the white blood cells.

5. It coagulates or clots, thereby closing injured blood vessels and preventing the loss of blood through hemorrhage.

THE LYMPH-VASCULAR SYSTEM

(Lymphatic System)

The **lymph-vascular system** acts as an aid to the venous system, and consists of lymph spaces, lymphatics and lymph glands.

Lymph spaces are channels found between the walls of the capillaries and the body cells.

Lymphatics are minute vessels that convey lymph.

The smaller lymphatics unite to form two principal vessels (the right lymphatic duct and the thoracic duct), which empty their contents into a vein found below the base of the neck. This, in turn, empties into the vena cava, and also mixes the lymph with the venous blood just before it is returned to the heart.

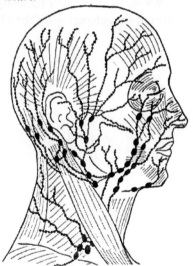

Lymph Nodes of the Head and Face

Lymph glands or **nodes** are ductless organs in the course of lymphatic vessels. They filter the lymph and are a defense against the spread of infection.

Lymph

Composition. Lymph is a slightly viscid, alkaline fluid, circulating through the lymph-vascular system. It is derived from plasma which has been forced through the capillary walls both by the pressure of the blood in the capillaries and by osmosis (an exchange of fluids through a thin membrane).

Dissolved food materials and oxygen pass through the blood vessels by **osmosis** and are conveyed by the lymph to the body cells, which they enter by osmosis. In like manner, water, carbon dioxide and wastes are removed from the body cells. Lymph is well supplied with white blood cells.

The **functions** of lymph are:

1. To reach parts of the body not reached by the blood.
2. To carry nourishment from the blood to the body cells.
3. To remove waste material from the body cells.
4. Carries constant interchange with the blood.

ARTERIES OF THE HEAD, FACE AND NECK

The **common carotid arteries** are the main sources of blood supply to the head, face and neck. They are located on either side of the neck, and each artery subdivides into an internal and external branch. The **internal branch** of the common carotid artery supplies the cranial cavity, while the **external branch** supplies the superficial parts of the head, face and neck.

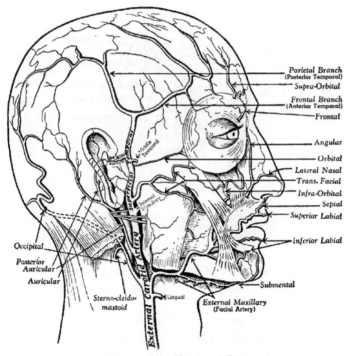

Arteries of the Head and Face

The **external carotid artery** subdivides into a number of branches which supply blood to various regions of the head and face. Of particular interest to the barber are the following arteries:

1. External maxillary (facial artery).
2. Superficial temporal.
3. Occipital.
4. Posterior auricular.

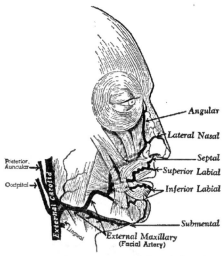

EXTERNAL MAXILLARY (Facial Artery)
AND BRANCHES

The muscular tissue of the lips must be supposed
to have been cut away, in order to show the course
of the labial arteries.

A. **External maxillary** (facial artery) supplies the lower region of the face, and mouth and nose. Some of its branches are.

   1. **Submental artery;** supplies chin and lower lip.

   2. **Inferior labial artery;** supplies the lower lip.

   3. **Angular artery;** supplies side of nose.

   4. **Superior labial;** supplies the upper lip, septum (dividing wall) of nose, and wing of nose.

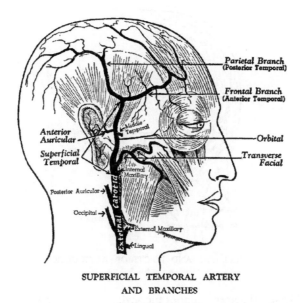

SUPERFICIAL TEMPORAL ARTERY
AND BRANCHES

B. **Superficial temporal artery;** continuation of the external carotid artery supplies muscles, skin and scalp to front, side and top of head. Some of its important branches are:

1. **Frontal artery;** supplies the forehead.

2. **Parietal artery;** supplies crown and side of head.

3. **Transverse facial artery;** supplies the masseter.

4. **Middle temporal artery;** supplies the temporalis.

5. **Anterior auricular artery;** supplies the anterior part of the ear.

6. **Orbital artery;** supplies the orbicularis oculi.

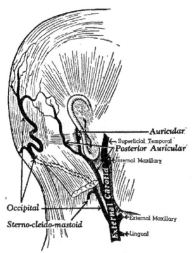

OCCIPITAL AND POSTERIOR AURICULAR
ARTERIES

C. **Occipital artery** supplies the scalp, back of head up to the crown. Its most important branch is the **sterno-cleido-mastoid artery** which supplies muscle of the same name.
D. **Posterior auricular artery** supplies the scalp above and back of the ear. Its most important branch is the **auricular artery** which supplies the skin back of ear.

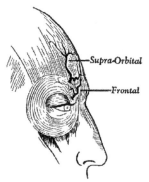

Branches of the **Ophthalmic Artery**
Originating from the
Internal Carotid Artery

The **internal carotid artery** consists of several branches, all of which are inside the skull with the exception of the **ophthalmic artery.** This artery subdivides to form the **supra-orbital artery** which supplies the orbit, eyelid and forehead.

The **frontal artery** is an end branch of the ophthalmic artery; supplies the forehead.

VEINS OF THE HEAD, FACE AND NECK

The blood returning to the heart from the head, face and neck, flows on each side of the neck into two principal veins: the **internal jugular** and **external jugular**. The most important veins of the face are placed almost parallel with the arteries and take the same names as the arteries.

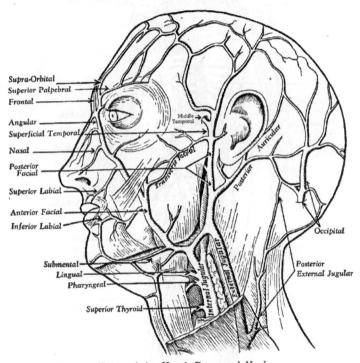

Veins of the Head, Face and Neck

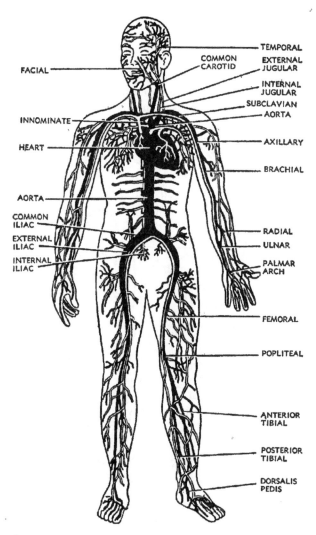

Diagram illustrating the General Circulation of the Blood,
Showing the Important Arteries and Veins of the Body

CIRCULATION

1. Name the two main divisions of the circulatory system.	1. The blood-vascular system. 2. The lymph-vascular system.
2. Name the principal parts of the blood-vascular system.	Heart and blood vessels (arteries, veins and capillaries).
3. What are the important functions of the blood-vascular system?	1. Carries water, food and oxygen to all cells of the body. 2. Removes waste products. 3. Regulates heat. 4. Fights harmful bacteria. 5. Clots to prevent loss of blood.
4. What is the function of the heart?	Pumps blood to all parts of the body by means of blood vessels and receives the blood on its return.
5. Describe the interior of the heart.	The heart consists of four chambers, two upper auricles and two lower ventricles, and four valves which control the flow of blood.
6. Name three kinds of vessels found in the blood-vascular system.	Arteries, veins, capillaries.
7. Which blood vessels are the smallest in size?	The capillaries.
8. Which blood vessels carry blood away from the heart?	The arteries.
9. Which vessels generally carry blood back to the heart?	The veins.
10. What is the normal temperature of the blood?	98.6 degrees Fahrenheit.
11. What is the composition of blood?	The blood is composed of two-thirds plasma and one-third cells (red blood cells, white blood cells and blood platelets).
12. What is the composition of blood plasma?	Blood plasma is composed of about 90% water, and balance consists of proteins, nutrients, mineral salts, waste products and other substances.
13. Which blood cells carry oxygen to the body cells?	The red blood cells.
14. Which blood cells destroy harmful bacteria?	The white blood cells.
15. Which blood cells aid in the clotting of the blood after an injury?	The blood platelets.
16. Which two systems take care of the blood circulation?	1. The general circulation. 2. The pulmonary circulation.
17. Which path is taken by the general circulation?	The blood flows from the heart throughout the body and then back again to the heart.
18. Which path is taken by the pulmonary circulation?	The blood circulates from the heart to the lungs and then back again.

Lymphatic System

1. Name the principal parts of the lymphatic system.	Lymph glands, lymphatic vessels and lymph spaces.
2. What is lymph?	Lymph is a slightly viscid, alkaline fluid originating from the blood plasma and circulating through the lymphatic system.
3. What are the important functions of the lymph?	1. The lymph reaches parts of the body not reached by the blood. 2. The lymph carries nourishment to body cells. 3. The lymph removes waste products from body cells. 4. Carries constant interchange with the blood.
4. In what way is the lymph related to the blood?	Lymph is derived from the blood plasma and contains white blood cells.

Blood Vessels of the Head, Face and Neck

1. Which main arteries supply blood to the entire head, face and neck?	Common carotid arteries.
2. Name two main branches of the common carotid arteries.	Internal branch and external branch.
3. Which branch of the common carotid artery supplies the cranial cavity?	Internal branch of the common carotid artery.
4. Which branch of the common carotid artery supplies blood to the skin and muscles of the head and face?	External branch of the common carotid artery.
5. Name four important branches of the external carotid artery.	External maxillary, superficial temporal, occipital, and posterior auricular.
6. Inferior labial and superior labial arteries branch out from what artery?	External maxillary.
7. The angular artery is the end branch of what artery?	External maxillary.
8. Parietal branch and frontal branch originate from what artery?	Superficial temporal.
9. Name two arteries that branch out from the ophthalmic artery.	Supra-orbital and frontal.

10. What parts of the head do the following arteries supply?

a) Angular — a) Side of nose.
b) Parietal branch — b) Crown and side of head.
c) Superior labial — c) Upper lip.
d) Occipital — d) Back of head up to crown.
e) Posterior auricular — e) Scalp above and back of ear.
f) Supra-orbital — f) Forehead, eyelid and orbit.
g) Frontal artery — g) Forehead.
h) Submental — h) Chin and lower lip.
i) Inferior labial — i) Lower lip.

11. What muscles do the following arteries supply?

a) Middle temporal — a) Temporalis.
b) Orbital — b) Orbicularis oculi.
c) Transverse facial — c) Masseter.

12. Name the principal veins by which the blood from the head, face and neck is returned to the heart. The internal jugular and the external jugular.

THE ENDOCRINE SYSTEM

The **endocrine system** comprises a group of specialized glands which may beneficially or adversely affect the growth, reproduction and health of the body, depending on the quality and quantity of their secretions. The hormones present in the blood stream have a profound influence on external appearance and body processes. The absence or deficiency of certain hormones in the blood may cause certain glandular diseases.

Glands are specialized organs which vary in size and function. The blood and nerves are intimately connected with the glands. The nervous system controls the functional activities of the glands. The glands have the ability to remove certain substances from the blood and to convert them into new compounds. The secretions manufactured by the endocrine glands are known as **hormones.**

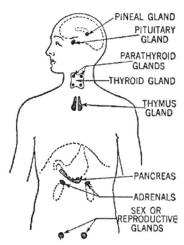

The human endocrine glands.

There are two main sets of glands. One group is called the **duct glands** (possess canals leading from the gland to a particular part of the body). Sweat and oil glands of the skin and intestinal glands belong to this group. The other group, known as **ductless or endocrine glands,** have their secretions thrown directly into the blood stream which in turn influences the welfare of the entire body.

The **endocrine glands** operate as a unit. If there is an under or an over functioning of any ductless gland, it is bound to upset the delicate balance of the entire chain of endocrine glands. Some of the endocrine glands exert a regulatory and restraining influence over the other glands.

Among the important endocrine glands are the following:

The **pituitary gland,** located at the base of the brain, regulates the water balance and the height of the body.

The **thyroid gland,** situated on either side of the trachea (wind pipe) produces a hormone, **thyroxin,** which controls the weight and the metabolic rate of the body.

The **adrenal glands,** found immediately above the kidneys, regulate the blood circulation.

The **sex glands** are both duct and ductless glands. The male and female sex glands manufacture the reproductive cells and the sex hormones which are required for fertility and reproduction.

The **pancreas** is located behind the stomach. Certain cells in the pancreas produce a hormone, known as **insulin.** This hormone is absorbed by the blood, brought to the tissues, and helps in the use of sugars by the body.

THE ENDOCRINE SYSTEM

1. What is the endocrine system?	The endocrine system is composed of glands whose functions are to aid the growth, health and reproduction of the body.
2. How are the glands connected with other parts of the body?	Each gland is linked with other parts of the body by means of nerves and the blood stream.
3. Why are glands dependent upon an adequate nerve and blood supply?	The blood supplies the raw materials which glands utilize to produce secretions. The nerves control the functional activities of the glands.
4. What is the function of duct glands?	Duct glands produce secretions which are carried away through canals to particular parts of the body.
5. Give examples of duct glands and explain their functions.	The skin glands are duct glands. They excrete perspiration and secrete sebum which keeps the skin moist and lubricated.
6. What is the function of a ductless or endocrine gland?	A ductless or endocrine gland has no duct but delivers its secretion directly into the blood or lymph streams, causing actions remote from the regions of their formation.
7. Give 2 examples of ductless or endocrine glands and explain their functions.	The pituitary gland regulates the water balance of the body. The thyroid gland controls the weight and metabolic rate of the body.
8. What is an important difference between a duct and ductless gland?	A duct gland possesses a duct or canal; whereas a ductless gland has no duct.
9. Which glands are both duct and ductless glands?	The pancreas and sex glands.
10. Which type of glands produce hormones?	The ductless or endocrine glands.
11. Why are hormones important to the body?	The hormones in the blood stream have a profound influence on external appearance and body processes.
12. Briefly describe the location and function of the adrenal glands.	Located immediately above the kidneys. They regulate the blood circulation.

THE EXCRETORY SYSTEM

The excretory system, including the kidneys, liver, skin, intestines and lungs, purifies the body by the elimination of waste matter.

1. The **kidneys** excrete urine.

2. The **liver** discharges bile pigments.

3. The **skin** eliminates perspiration.

4. The **large intestine** evacuates decomposed and undigested food.

5. The **lungs** exhale carbon dioxide.

Metabolic activities of body cells form various poisons which if retained would harm the body.

Urinary System

The important organs of the urinary system are the **kidneys** and the **bladder**. The kidneys are two bean-shaped glands located at the lower end of the spinal column and kept in place by the fatty tissues and the ureters. The ureters are tubes leading from the kidneys to the bladder where the urine is stored. The emptying of the bladder is accomplished by the passage of the urine through the urethra. As the blood circulates through the kidneys it gives up a certain amount of water and rejects the various end products of metabolism such as urea and uric acid.

Liver

With the exception of the skin, the liver is the largest organ in the body and is situated on the upper right side of the abdomen, immediately below and in contact with the diaphragm. The liver neutralizes poisonous substances which may have been absorbed from the intestines. The liver salvages a portion of the old red blood cells, the remainder being eliminated in the bile. The main functions of the liver are the production of bile, which aids the digestion of fats, and the storage of glycogen (animal starch) which is a reserve form of energy to be used when the body needs it.

THE EXCRETORY SYSTEM

1. Name the important organs of the excretory system.	The lungs, kidneys, skin, liver and large intestine.
2. What is the function of the excretory system?	The excretory system eliminates waste products formed in the body.
3. What happens if waste products are retained instead of being eliminated?	The body will become poisoned by its own waste products.
4. Enumerate the waste products removed by the various excretory organs.	The kidneys excrete urine. The skin eliminates perspiration. The lungs exhale carbon dioxide. The large intestine evacuates undigested food. The liver discharges bile.

THE RESPIRATORY SYSTEM

The **respiratory system** is situated within the chest cavity which is protected on both sides by the ribs. The diaphragm, a muscular partition which controls breathing, separates the chest from the abdominal regions.

The most **important organs** of the respiratory system are the nose, trachea (wind pipe), the bronchial tubes, and the lungs. When air is inhaled through the nose, it passes down the pharynx, trachea and bronchial tubes, into the lungs. Between the trachea and the base of the tongue, the larynx (voice box) is located.

Nasal breathing is healthier than mouth breathing because the air is warmed by the surface capillaries and the bacteria are caught by the hairs which line the mucous membranes of the nasal passages.

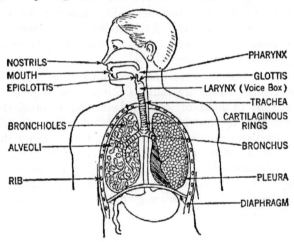

NOSTRILS
MOUTH
EPIGLOTTIS
BRONCHIOLES
ALVEOLI
RIB

PHARYNX
GLOTTIS
LARYNX (Voice Box)
TRACHEA
CARTILAGINOUS RINGS
BRONCHUS
PLEURA
DIAPHRAGM

The human respiratory system.

Lungs

The lungs are spongy tissues composed of microscopic cells into which the inhaled air penetrates. These tiny air cells are enclosed in a skinlike tissue or epithelium. Behind this epithelium, the fine capillaries of the blood vascular system are found.

With each respiration, an exchange of gases takes place. During inhalation, oxygen is absorbed into the blood, while carbon dioxide is expelled during exhalation. As oxygen is brought to the body cells, it reacts chemically with liquid food, previously digested, to form living tissue. As a result, heat, energy and carbon dioxide gas are formed.

Oxygen is more essential than either food or water to the body. Although a man may live more than sixty days without food, and a few days without water, if air is excluded for a few minutes, death ensues.

Breathing

Breathing is instinctive because it is necessary to carry on the life functions. The rate of breathing is conditioned by the activity of the individual. Muscular activity and energy expenditures increase the bodily demands for oxygen. As a result, the rate of breathing is increased. A person requires about three times as much oxygen when walking than when standing at rest.

The cultivation of **abdominal breathing** is of value in building health. **Costal breathing** is common to many people. This type of light or shallow breathing involves the use of the ribs to the exclusion of the diaphragm. Abdominal breathing means deep breathing, which brings the diaphragm into action. The maximum intake of oxygen and expulsion of carbon dioxide is accomplished with abdominal breathing. The rhythmic movements of the diaphragm exert a favorable effect by massaging the liver and other intestinal organs.

THE RESPIRATORY SYSTEM

1. Name the important organs of the respiratory system.	Nose, trachea or wind pipe, bronchial tubes and lungs.
2. What are the functions of the respiratory system?	An exchange of gases takes place through the capillaries in the lung tissue, oxygen gas being inhaled and carbon dioxide gas being exhaled.
3. What is the diaphragm and what function does it perform?	The diaphragm is a muscular sheet separating the chest from the abdominal cavity. It helps in expanding and contracting the lungs.
4. Describe the appearance of the lung tissue.	The lungs are two spongy sacs composed of microscopic cells into which the inhaled air penetrates.
5. Why is abdominal breathing preferred to costal or shallow breathing?	Abdominal breathing utilizes all the lung space, thereby permitting a greater intake of oxygen and a greater expulsion of carbon dioxide.
6. Why is nasal breathing preferable to mouth breathing?	Nasal breathing warms and cleans the air before entering the lungs.

THE DIGESTIVE SYSTEM

The **digestive system** changes food into a form suitable for use by the body. Digestion is started in the mouth and completed in the small intestine. From the mouth, the food passes down the pharynx and the esophagus (food pipe) into the stomach. In the small intestine, the food is completely digested with the aid of the secretions from the liver and the pancreas. The large intestine (colon) stores the refuse before being eliminated through the rectum. The time required for the complete digestion of a meal is about nine hours.

Physical and Chemical Changes in Digestion

Digestion is a process involving physical and chemical changes in the food taken into the body. Physical changes take place when the food is chewed and mixed with the digestive secretions. Responsible for the chemical changes in food are the enzymes present in the digestive secretions.

Digestive enzymes are chemical agents which change certain kinds of food into a form capable of being used by the body. Each enzyme is specific and can act only on a certain food constituent.

The principal chemical constituents found in foods are starches, sugars, fats, proteins, minerals and vitamins.

The Process of Digestion

The mouth prepares the food for entrance into the stomach. Chewing stimulates the flow of saliva and tends to soften the food. The saliva, secreted by the salivary glands, contains an enzyme, **ptyalin,** which can change carbohydrate foods into the sugar stage. The tongue aids in the tasting and swallowing of the food. The chewed food easily passes down the pharynx and esophagus into the stomach.

The **stomach** is a muscular sac, found below the diaphragm, and capable of holding from one to two quarts. The soft, velvety lining of the stomach walls secrete an enzyme, **pepsin,** which partly digests protein in the presence of hydrochloric acid. The churning action of the stomach brings the food in contact with the gastric juice. Protein and fatty foods remain in the stomach for a much longer period of time than do starches and sugars.

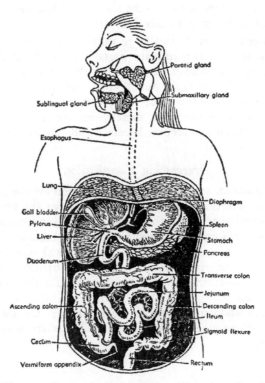

Diagram illustrating the Human Alimentary Canal with its Principal Digestive Glands

As the stomach contents empties into the small intestine, it is acted upon by the pancreatic juice. The pancreatic secretion contains three enzymes capable of completing the digestion of carbohydrate, fat and protein containing foods. The liver secretes bile which aids in the digestion of fats. Besides the bile and the pancreatic secretion, the intestinal secretion also assists in the process of digestion.

The final end products of carbohydrate digestion are the simple sugars; the end products of fat digestion are fatty acids and glycerine; and the end products of protein digestion are the amino salts. In the small intestine, the digested food is absorbed into the blood stream.

Between the small and large intestine is found a valve, which must open to permit the passage of the digested food. The appendix is located on the right side of the large intestine. Although the exact function of the appendix is unknown, it is believed to be of value to the body. In the large intestine, water is absorbed, thereby making the waste matter firm. When the rectum becomes full, bowel movement occurs.

Overcoming Constipation

Constipation and intestinal decomposition are the basis of many skin infections such as acne, acne rosacea and urticaria. The absorption of toxic substances from the intestine, and its subsequent elimination through the skin accounts for the presence of many skin blemishes. The logical remedy is to remove the underlying cause, namely constipation. A balanced diet containing plenty of water to make the intestinal contents soft, enough cellulose to stimulate intestinal movement, and abdominal exercises to strengthen the intestinal muscles—these measures will be helpful in overcoming constipation.

THE DIGESTIVE SYSTEM

1. What is digestion?	Digestion is a process involving physical and chemical changes in the food taken into the body.
2. Name the principal chemical constituents found in foods.	Starches, sugars, fats, proteins, minerals and vitamins.
3. Name the important organs of the digestive system.	Mouth, pharynx, esophagus, stomach, small intestine, liver and pancreas.
4. In which organ is digestion started?	The mouth.
5. In which organ is digestion completed?	The small intestine.
6. How do digestive enzymes aid digestion?	Digestive enzymes are chemical agents which convert certain kinds of food into a form capable of being used by the body.
7. What digestive changes occur in the mouth?	Food is chewed and mixed with salivary juice. Starchy foods are partly digested.
8. What digestive changes occur in the stomach?	The food is combined with gastric juice. Protein foods are digested.
9. What digestive changes occur in the small intestine?	Foods are completely digested and absorbed into the blood.
10. How does the liver aid digestion?	The liver produces bile which enters the small intestine and digests fats in foods.
11. How does the pancreas aid digestion?	The pancreas produces a juice which enters the small intestine and digests starches, proteins and fats in foods.

THE SKIN

The scientific study of the skin forms the basis for an effective program of skin care and barber treatments. The skin is the largest organ in the body and performs many vital functions required for health. The barber who has a thorough understanding of the skin, its structure and functions, will be in a better position to give professional skin treatments.

A healthy skin shows signs of being smooth and flexible, has proper color and is free from any blemish or disease.

The skin varies in thickness, being thinnest on the eyelids and thickest on the palms and soles Continued pressure over any part of the skin will cause it to thicken.

The structure of the skin contains two clearly defined divisions:

1. The **epidermis, cuticle** or **scarf skin** is the outermost protective layer.

2. The **dermis, corium** or **true skin** is the deeper layer of the skin.

Subcutaneous (adipose) **tissue** is a fatty tissue found below the dermis. (See footnote *.)

The **epidermis** or **cuticle** forms the outer protective covering for the body. It contains no blood vessels but has many small nerve endings. The epidermis contains the following layers:

1. The **stratum corneum** (horny layer) consists of tightly packed, scale-like cells which are continually being shed and replaced. As these cells develop, they form keratin which acts as a water-proof covering. This layer of cells plays an important part in determining the character of the complexion.

2. The **stratum lucidum** (clear layer) consists of small transparent cells through which light can pass.

3. The **stratum granulosum** (granular layer) consists of cells which look like distinct granules. These cells are al-

*Some histologists refer to the subcutaneous tissue as a continuation of the dermis, while others consider it as a separate layer.

most dead and undergo a change into a horny substance.

4. The **stratum mucosum** (Malpighian layer) is composed of several layers of cells. Its deepest layer is sometimes called the stratum germinativum. (See footnote *.)

5. The **stratum germinativum** (basal layer) is composed of a single row of columnar cells often called mother cells, responsible for the reproduction or growth of the epidermis. These cells contain a pigment called melanin which is responsible for the coloration of the skin.

The **dermis** is the true skin. It is also called **derma, corium** or **cutis.** In this layer is found an elastic network of cells through which are distributed blood and lymph vessels, nerves, sweat glands and oil glands. It contains the following layers:

1. The **papillary layer,** which lies directly beneath the epidermis, contains the papillae, or little cone-like projections, made of fine strands of elastic tissue which extend upward into the epidermis. Some of these papillae contain looped capillaries, others contain terminations of nerve fibers called **tactile corpuscles.** This layer also contains some of the melanin skin pigment.

2. The **reticular layer,** in whose network is contained the fat cells, the blood and lymph vessels, the sweat and oil glands, and the hair follicles.

The **subcutaneous tissue** (subcutis) is regarded by some histologists as a continuation of the dermis. It varies in thickness according to the age, sex and general health of the individual. This fatty (adipose) tissue gives smoothness and contour to the body, besides providing a reservoir for fuel and energy and also acting as a protective cushion for the outer skin layers. This fatty layer contains a network of arteries, and a superficial and deep network of lymphatics.

Blood and Lymph Supply to the Skin

From 1/2 to 2/3 of the total blood supply of the body is found distributed to the skin. The blood and lymph, as

*Some histologists classify the stratum germinativum and the stratum mucosum as one layer.

they circulate through the skin, contribute essential materials needed for its growth and nourishment. In the subcutaneous tissue are found networks of arteries and lymphatics which send their smaller branches to the papillae, the hair follicles

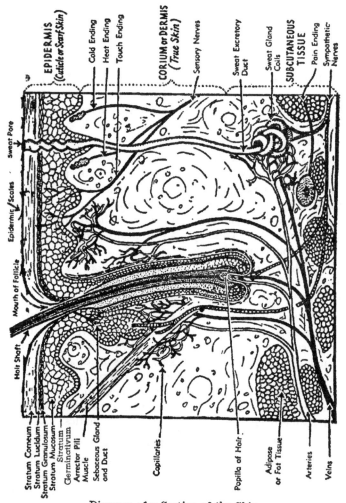

Diagram of a Section of the Skin

and the skin glands. The capillaries are quite numerous in the skin.

Nerves of the skin. The skin contains the surface endings of many nerve fibers classified as follows:

1. Motor nerve fibers which are distributed to the blood vessels and the arrectores pilorum muscle of the hair follicles.

2. Sensory nerve fibers which react to heat, cold, touch, pressure and pain.

3. Secretory nerve fibers which are distributed to the sweat and oil glands of the skin.

Pliability of the skin. It depends upon the elasticity of the fibers of the dermis. For example, after expansion, the skin regains its former shape almost immediately.

The **color of the skin** depends partly upon the blood supply, but more upon the melanin pigment or coloring matter which is deposited in the stratum germinativum and the papillary layer of the dermis. The pigment varies in different people and races.

Sweat and Oil Glands

Glands of the skin. The skin contains two types of glands which extract materials from the blood to form new substances.

1. **The sudoriferous (sweat) glands** excrete sweat.

2. **The sebaceous (oil) glands** secrete sebum, an oily substance.

The **sweat glands** (tubular type) consist of a coiled base or **fundus** and a tube-like **duct** which terminates at the skin surface to form the **sweat pore.** Practically all parts of the body are supplied with sweat glands, being more numerous on the palms, soles, forehead and under the armpits. The sweat glands function like a miniature kidney and help to eliminate waste products from the body. Their activity is greatly increased by heat, exercise, mental excitement and certain drugs. The excretion of sweat is under the control of the nervous system.

The oil glands (sacular type) consist of little sacs whose duct opens into the neck of the hair follicle. They secrete sebum which lubricates the skin and preserves the softness of the hair. With the exception of the palms and soles, these glands are found in all parts of the body, particularly the face.

Functions of the Skin

The principal functions of the skin are:

1. Protection.   4. Sensation.
2. Heat Regulation.   5. Absorption.
3. Secretion and Excretion.

1. **Protection.** The skin protects the body from injury and bacterial invasion.

2. **Heat Regulation.** The healthy body maintains a constant internal temperature of about 98.6 degrees Fahrenheit. As changes occur in the outside temperature, the blood and sweat glands of the skin make necessary adjustments in their functions.

3. **Secretion and Excretion.** By means of its sweat and oil glands, the skin acts both as a secretory and excretory organ.

4. **Sensation.** The skin has a rich nerve supply which responds to the influences of heat, cold, touch, pain and pressure, thereby permitting the body to adapt itself to varying conditions of the environment.

5. **Absorption.** The skin has limited powers of absorption through its pores. Small amounts of lanolin creams or fatty substances can be absorbed by the skin, whereas water and alcohol are not absorbed at all.

Respiration. Some textbooks still list **respiration** among the functions of the skin. Recent studies have disproved this theory. However, in animals, there is a definite amount of oxygen gas taken in and carbon dioxide gas discharged directly through the skin, but in man this is negligible.

The appendages of the skin are: hair, nails, sweat and oil glands.

THE SKIN

1. Briefly describe the skin.	The skin is a soft, strong, flexible covering of the body.
2. What are five important functions of the skin?	Protection, heat regulation, secretion and excretion, sensation, and absorption.
3. Name the two main divisions of the skin.	The epidermis and dermis.
4. Briefly describe the structure of the epidermis.	The epidermis consists of five layers and does not contain any blood vessels or nerve endings.
5. Name the layers of the epidermis.	1. Stratum corneum (horny layer). 2. Stratum lucidum (clear layer) 3. Stratum granulosum (granular layer). 4. Stratum mucosum (Malpighian layer). 5. Stratum germinativum (basal layer).
6. Which epidermal layer is continually being shed and replaced?	Stratum corneum.
7. Which epidermal layer consists of small, transparent cells?	Stratum lucidum.
8. Which epidermal layer starts to undergo a change into a horny substance?	Stratum granulosum.
9. Where is the coloring matter of the skin found?	In the stratum germinativum (basal layer) of the epidermis and the papillary layer of the dermis.
10. What is the function of the stratum germinativum?	Starts the reproduction of the epidermis.
11. Describe the structure of the dermis.	Consists of an elastic network of cells containing blood and lymph vessels, nerve endings, sweat glands, oil glands and hair follicles.
12. Name the two layers of the dermis.	The papillary layer and the reticular layer.
13. Which structures are found in the papillary layer?	Papillae or cone-like projections containing either capillaries or nerve endings
14. Which structures are found in the reticular layer?	Fat cells, blood and lymph vessels, sweat and oil glands and hair follicles.
15. Which structures render the skin flexible?	The fibers in the dermis.
16. What is the function of the subcutaneous tissue?	Acts as a protective cushion for outer skin layers, gives smoothness and contour to the body and also contains a reserve supply of fats.

Sweat and Oil Glands

1. What is a gland?	An organ which removes certain materials from the blood and forms new substances.
2. Name two types of glands found in the skin.	Sudoriferous or sweat glands; sebaceous or oil glands.
3. Describe the structure of the sweat glands.	Consist of a coiled base and a tube-like duct which forms a pore at the surface of the skin.
4. Where are sweat glands found?	Over the entire area of the skin, more numerous on the palms, soles, forehead and armpits.
5. What is the function of the sweat glands?	Eliminates waste products in the form of sweat.
6. Name four agents capable of increasing the activity of the sweat glands.	Heat, exercise, mental excitement and certain drugs.
7. Describe the structure of the oil glands.	Consist of small sacs whose ducts open into the neck of the hair follicle.
8. Which substance is secreted by the oil glands?	Sebum, an oily substance.
9. What is the chief function of sebum?	Lubricates the skin and hair, keeping them soft and pliable.
10. Where are the oil glands found?	Oil glands are found in all parts of the body with the exception of the palms and soles.

THE HAIR

The study of the hair is of importance to the barber. The chief purpose of the hair is to protect the body, promote beauty and conserve heat. To keep the hair healthy, proper attention must be given to its care and treatment. The barber who has the knowledge of hair structure, its characteristics and qualities is in a better position to give professional hair treatments.

Hair is a slender thread-like outgrowth of the skin and scalp of the human body.

Composition of hair. Hair, an appendage of the skin, is composed of a horny substance, mainly **keratin.** There is no sense of feeling in the hair of the head or body, owing to the absence of nerves in the hair.

The composition of the hair varies with different races and individuals. Keratin, the chief constituent of the hair, is made up of about 45% carbon and 30% oxygen, with lesser amounts of such chemical elements as hydrogen, nitrogen and sulphur.

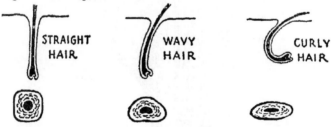

Shapes and Cross-Sections of Different Forms of Hair

Shapes of the hair. The hair takes its shape, size and direction from the shape, size and direction of the follicles. The various shapes of hair are as follows:

1. Straight hair is usually round.
2. Wavy hair is usually oval.
3. Curly or kinky hair is usually flat.

Full grown hair as found on the human body is divided into two principal parts:

1. **The hair root** is that portion of the hair structure found beneath the skin surface.

2. **The hair shaft** is that portion of the hair structure extending above the skin surface.

Structures closely associated with the hair root are the hair follicle, hair bulb and hair papilla.

The hair follicle is a tube-like depression or pocket in the skin, enveloping the hair root. For every hair, there is a follicle. Hair follicles vary in depth from one thirty-second to one-eighth of an inch, depending upon the thickness and location of the skin.

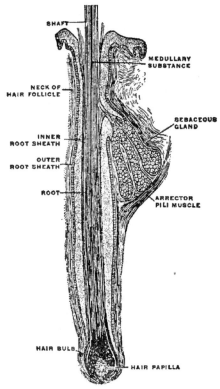

The Hair and Follicle

The hair bulb is a thickened, club-shaped structure forming the lower part of the hair root. The lower part of the hair bulb is hollowed out to fit over the hair papilla.

The hair papilla is a small cone-shaped elevation found at the bottom of the hair follicle that fits into the hair bulb. Within the hair papilla is a rich blood and nerve supply which contributes to the growth and regeneration of the hair.

Hair is found all over the body, with the exception of the palms, soles, and lips. Due to human habits and environmental needs, hair grows long only on the head, and there principally to form a cushion for the skull, which contains the most important organ of the body.

There are three types of hair on the body: **downy** or **lanugo** hair, found on the forehead and body; **short** or bristly hair, such as eyelashes and eyebrows; and **soft, long** hair, growing on the scalp, face, and armpits. Hair kept closely cut as by shaving or trimming, does not coarsen it nor stimulate its growth.

Technical terms given to hair on various part of body:

Hirsuties or **hypertrichosis** means the growth of an unusual amount of hair, or of hair in unusual locations, as on the face of women or the back of men; hairy; superfluous hair.

Capilli—the head.   Barba—the beard.
Cilia—the eyelashes.   Vibrissae—the nostrils.
Supercilia—the eyebrows.   Tragi—the ears.

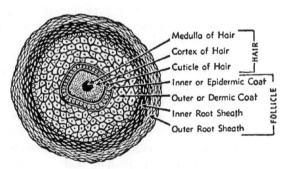

Cross-Section of Hair and Follicle

Hair is composed of three layers: the **medulla,** the center, pith or marrow of the hair shaft; the **cortex,** the middle layer, containing pigment or coloring matter; and the **cuticle,** the outside layer, composed of scale-like cells overlapping like fish scales to give strength and elasticity.

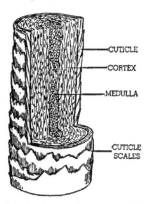

Cuticle Scales and Layers of Hair

Color of hair. The cortex constitutes the chief part of the shaft. It is made up of long, spindle-shaped cells, in which is found coloring matter, minute grains of pigment. The source of pigment has not been definitely settled. It is probably derived from the color-forming substances in the blood, as is all pigment of the human body.

The color of the hair, light or dark, depends upon the color of the grains of pigment. If the granules are dense the color will be deep or dark. If the granules are scarce, the color will be that of the granules, but lighter in tone. The presence of air in the hair will make it a lighter shade. When most of the pigment is gone and air spaces are still more numerous, the hair will be white or gray. Gray hair is really mottled hair-spots of white or whitish yellow scattered about the shafts.

Albino is a person born with white hair, the result of an absence of coloring matter in the hair shaft; accompanied by no marked pigment coloring in the skin or iris of the eyes.

The **arrector pili muscle,** connected to the hair follicle, contracts with fear and cold, thus causing the sensation described by "hair standing on end," and gives the skin appearance of "goose flesh."

Sebaceous (oil) glands are tiny glands emptying sebum at the mouth of the follicle, thereby supplying natural oils to hair and skin, keeping them soft and pliable.

Regeneration of hair. From the papilla comes material for the growth of the hair. As long as the papilla is not destroyed, the hair will grow. If the hair is pulled out from the roots, it will nevertheless grow again, but if the papilla is destroyed, it will never grow again.

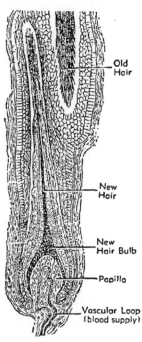

New Hair
Replacing Old Hair

In human beings there is a constant death and replacement of hair. In a hair about to be shed, the bulb becomes cornified and splits up into a number of fibers. The hair then becomes detached from the papilla and the root sheath, and is cast off. The empty root sheath collapses and forms a cord of cells between the papilla and lower end of the shedding hair. If the dead hair is to replaced by a new one, there will soon occur a multiplication of cells in the region of the old papilla. From this "hair germ" the new hair is formed growing upward, under or to one side of the dead hair, which it finally replaces.

If the blood supply to the papilla is weak, due to poor circulation, the new hair produced will be thin, dry and weak in appearance.

Life and density of hair. The average life of a hair on the head is from two to four years, after which time it is replaced by a new one. Eyelashes and eyebrows are replaced every four or five months. The number of hairs on the head varies with the color of the hair, there being about 140,000 for light blonde, 110,000 for brown, and 100,000 for black and titian, the latter two are generally the coarsest.

Hair can be both beautiful and healthy regardless of color or texture if there is a loose scalp, and elasticity in the hair. Normal hair will stretch about one-fifth of its natural length, and will spring back when released.

THE HAIR

1. What is hair?	Hair is a slender thread-like outgrowth of the skin and scalp of the human body.
2. What is the chief constituent of the hair?	Keratin.
3. Name three functions of hair.	Protects the body, promotes beauty and conserves heat.
4. Name three types of hair found on the body.	Long hair; short, stiff hair; soft, lanugo hair.
5. Where is long hair found?	Scalp and face of man.
6. Where is short, stiff hair found?	Eyebrows and eyelashes.
7. Where is soft, lanugo hair found?	On the forehead and other parts of the body.
8. Which parts of the body do not contain any hair?	Palms of the hands, soles of the feet and lips.
9. Name the two parts into which the length of the hair is divided.	The hair root and hair shaft.
10. What is the hair shaft?	That portion of the hair which extends beyond the skin.
11. What is the hair root?	That portion of the hair beneath the surface of the skin.
12. What is the hair follicle?	A tube-like depression or pocket in the skin.
13. Which muscle and gland are attached to the hair follicle?	The arrector pili muscle and oil gland in the skin.
14. What is the hair bulb?	The club-shaped structure forming the lower part of the hair root.
15. What is the hair papilla?	A small cone-shaped elevation at the bottom of the hair follicle that fits into the hair bulb.
16. How does the hair receive its nourishment?	From the tiny blood vessels in the papilla.
17. Which three factors determine the shape of the hair?	The size, shape and direction of the hair follicle.
18. Name three shapes of hair.	Straight hair, wavy hair, and curly or kinky hair.
19. Name three layers found in hair.	Medulla, cortex and cuticle.
20. Which hair layer makes hair elastic?	The cuticle of the hair.
21. Which hair layer contains coloring matter?	The cortex of the hair.
22. Explain the process of hair growth and replacement.	Active hair growth starts at the papilla. When the hair has reached its fullest growth, it begins to shed. If the hair papilla is alive and properly nourished by the blood, a new hair will grow again.

THE NAIL

While the barber is not required to know the procedure for manicuring, the study of the structure and function of the nail will be beneficial.

The condition of the nail, like that of the skin, reflects the general health of the body. The normal, healthy nail is firm and flexible and exhibits a slightly pink color. Its surface should be smooth, curved and unspotted without any hollows or wavy ridges.

The nail, an appendage of the skin, is a horny plate which acts as a protective covering for the tips of the fingers and toes.

Composition. The nails contain a complex substance, called keratin, which imparts a whitish appearance and allows the pink color of the **nail bed** to be seen.

Growth. The average rate of growth in the normal adult is about one-eighth of an inch per month, being faster in the summer than in the winter. The nails of children grow more

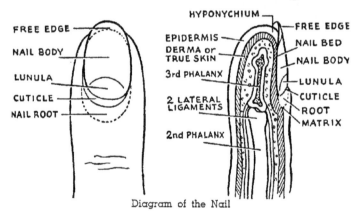

Diagram of the Nail

rapidly; whereas those of elderly persons grow more slowly. The nail grows fastest on the middle finger and slowest on the thumb. Although toe nails grow more slowly than finger nails, they are thicker and harder.

Definitions

Parts of the nail. The nail consists of three parts: the body or plate, the root and the free edge.

The **nail body or plate** is the visible portion of the nail extending from the nail root to the free edge.

The **nail root** is at the base of the nail and is imbedded underneath the skin. The nail root originates from an actively growing layer known as the matrix.

The **free edge** is the terminal portion of the nail body and reaches over the fingers tips.

The **lunula** is the visible half-moon area at the base of the nail body. The pale color of the lunula is due to the numerous cells of the matrix which are less vascular.

The **nail grooves** are furrowed edges on either side of the nail body.

The **skin adjoining the finger nail** includes the nail bed, the matrix, the cuticle, the mantle and the nail walls.

The **nail bed** is the portion of the skin on which the nail body rests. It is composed of vascular tissue corresponding to dermis and stratum mucosum of the skin.

The **matrix** is that part of the nail bed extending beneath the nail root. The matrix produces the nail, the cells of the matrix constantly undergoing a reproducing and hardening process.

The **cuticle** is the overlapping part of the skin of the finger around the nail.

The **eponychium** is the extension of excess cuticle at the base of the nail.

The **hyponychium** is that portion of the epidermis, under the free edge where the nail leaves the nail bed.

The **mantle** is the deep fold of the skin in which the nail root is lodged.

The **nail walls** are the small folds of skin overlapping the nail body.

ELECTRICITY

The beneficial effects of electricity have long been recognized to be of value in barbering. Electricity is a valuable servant, provided it is used intelligently and safely. Not only does it supply light and heat, but it can operate various kinds of electrical machines and appliances to the advantage of the barber and the customer. Thus, time and energy are saved and the effectiveness of barber services is improved.

Although the exact nature of electricity is not yet completely understood, its generating sources and effects are known. It is generally believed that electricity is a form of energy, which when in motion, produces magnetic, chemical or heat effects.

Electricity cay be **produced** chemically or mechanically. **Battery cells,** either dry or wet, change chemical energy into electrical energy. **Dynamos and magnetos** are mechanical generators which convert the energy released by waterfalls or burning coal into electricity.

A **current of electricity** is a stream of electrons (negatively charged particles) moving along a conductor.

A **conductor** is a substance which readily transmits an electric current. Metals (copper, gold, silver, aluminum, zinc), carbon and watery solutions of acids and salts are good conductors of electricity.

A **non-conductor or insulator** is a substance, such as rubber, silk, dry wood, glass, cement or asbestos, which resists the passage of an electric current.

An **electric wire** is composed of metal (conductor) which is surrounded by rubber or silk (insulator or non-conductor).

Electrodes, composed of good conductors, serve as points of contact when applying electricity to the body.

Two forms of electricity are employed for commercial purposes, the direct and alternating currents.

1. **Direct current (D.C.)** is a constant and even-flowing current, traveling in one direction.

2. **Alternating current (A.C.)** is a rapid and interrupted current, flowing first in one direction and then in the opposite direction.

If necessary, one type of current can be changed to the other type by means of a converter or rectifier.

A **converter** is an apparatus used to convert a direct current into an alternating current. A **rectifier** is used to change an alternating current to a direct current, which is required to generate galvanism.

A **complete circuit of electricity** is the entire path traveled by the current from its generating source through various conductors (wire, electrode, body) and back to its original source.

A **closed circuit** is one in which the current flows after proper connections have been made.

A **ground circuit** is one in which one pole is used to deliver current and the other pole is connected to a ground (a water pipe or radiator).

An **open circuit** is one in which the flow of electricity has been interrupted or disconnected.

A **short (broken) circuit** occurs when the current is diverted from its regular path by faulty connections or by frayed wires.

A **fuse** is a safety device which prevents the overheating of electric wires. It will blow out because of overloading (too many connections on one wire) or through a short circuit. To re-establish the circuit, disconnect apparaus before inserting a new fuse.

SAFETY PRACTICES

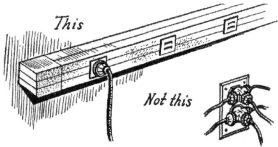

This

Not this

Use only one plug to each outlet. Overloading may cause fuse to blow out.

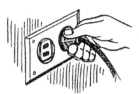

To disconnect current, remove plug without pulling cord. Never pull on cord as the wires may become loosened, and may cause a short circuit.

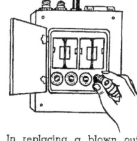

In replacing a blown out fuse, make sure to:
1. Use new fuse with proper rating.
2. Stand on a dry surface.
3. Keep hands dry.

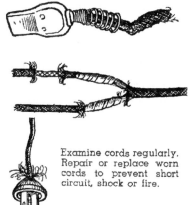

Examine cords regularly. Repair or replace worn cords to prevent short circuit, shock or fire.

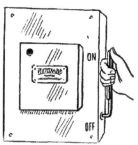

In an emergency, turn off main switch, as illustrated, to shut off electricity for entire shop or building.

ELECTRICAL MEASUREMENTS

Electrical measurements are expressed in terms of the following units:

The **volt** is a unit of electrical **pressure.**

The **ampere** is a unit of electrical **strength.**

The **ohm** is a unit of electrical **resistance.**

An electrical current flows through a conductor when the pressure is sufficiently great to overcome the resistance offered by the wire or body to the passage of the current. According to **Ohm's law,** it takes one volt of pressure to drive one ampere of strength through one ohm of resistance in one second's time.

Instead of the ampere which is too strong, the **milli-ampere,** 1/1000th part of an ampere, is used for facial and scalp treatments. The **milliamperemeter** is an instrument for measuring the rate of flow of an electric current.

The **voltmeter** is an instrument for measuring the exact voltage of an electric current.

The **transformer** is a device for changing (either increasing or decreasing) the voltage of an electric current It can be used only on alternating current.

The **frequency** of a current is the number of complete cycles or waves occurring in one second. The ordinary alternating current operates at a rate of 60 cycles and at a voltage of 110.

A **high-frequency current** refers to a current with 10,000 or more cycles per second.

A **watt** is a unit of electrical power which flows at the rate of one ampere under a pressure of one volt. It takes approximately 746 watts to make one **horsepower.**

A **kilowatt** is a unit of quantity, representing 1000 watts. It is used to figure the cost of power consumed in the barber shop.

HIGH-FREQUENCY CURRENT

There are three types of high-frequency current: d'Arsonval, Oudin and Tesla currents, named after their respective discoverers. These currents are characterized by a high rate of vibration, ranging from 10,000 or more cycles per second. Of chief interest to the barber is the **Tesla current,** commonly called the **violet ray.** The other two types are used in the practice of medicine.

The Tesla current is of medium voltage and amperage and can be connected to either the direct or alternating currents. The primary action of this current is thermal, or heat producing. Because of its rapid vibrations, there are no muscular contractions. The physiological effects are either stimulating or soothing, depending on the method of application.

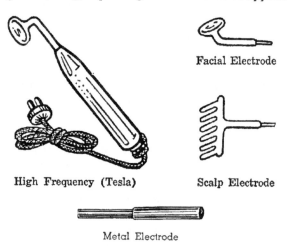

Facial Electrode

High Frequency (Tesla)

Scalp Electrode

Metal Electrode

The electrodes for high-frequency are made of glass or metal. Their shapes vary, the facial electrode being flat and the scalp electrode being rake-shaped. As the current passes through the glass electrode, tiny violet sparks are emitted when the electrode is held about half an inch from the skin. All treatments given with high-frequency should be started with a mild current, and gradually increased to the required strength. The length of the treatment depends upon the condition to be treated. For a general facial or scalp treatment about five minutes should be allowed.

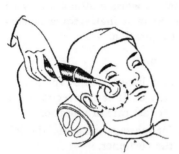 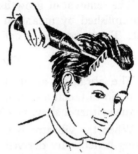

Applying High-Frequency to Face   Applying High-Frequency to Scalp
Using Facial Electrode.   Using Rake Electrode.

There are three methods of using the Tesla current:

1. **Direct surface application.** The barber holds the electrode and applies it over the customer's skin. For effective facial treatments, the electrode should be applied directly over the cosmetic cream.

2. **Indirect application.** The customer holds the electrode, while the barber uses his fingers to massage the surface being treated. At no time is the electrode attached to the barber. To prevent shock, the current is turned on after the customer has the electrode firmly in his hand; the current is turned off before removing the electrode from the customer's hand.

3. **General electrification.** By holding a metal electrode in his hand, the customer's body is charged with electricity without being touched by the barber.

To obtain sedative, calming or soothing effects with high-frequency current, the general electrification treatment is used, or the electrode is kept in close contact with the parts treated by the use of direct surface application.

To obtain a stimulating effect, the electrode is lifted slightly from the parts to be treated by using it through the clothing or a towel.

In using high-frequency with hair tonics, never use a tonic with a high alcoholic content. If it is desirable to use this type of tonic, use the electricity **first,** and the tonic **after** the electricity has been applied.

The removal of growths such as warts and moles may be accomplished by means of sparks of a high-frequency current. This treatment is called **fulguration.**

The Vibrator

The vibrator is an electrical appliance used by the barber as an aid in facial and scalp massage. It can be regulated to produce either a slow, medium or fast rate of vibration.

When the vibrator is used for massage purposes, the following benefits are derived by the customer.

1. Stimulates the functions of the skin.
2. Stimulates muscular tissues.
3. Increases the blood supply to the parts being massaged.
4. Increases glandular activities.
5. Soothes the nerves.

The vibrator may be used in two ways:

1. **Indirectly with an applicator attached to the barber's wrist or hand.** When in use, the vibrations are transmitted through the barber's fingers to the parts being treated.
2. **Directly with a rubber applicator.** The rubber applicator transmits the vibrations directly to the parts being treated. For sanitary reasons, a new rubber applicator should be used on each customer. Used rubber .applicators cannot be effectively sterilized; therefore must be replaced with a new one for each customer.

Although the vibrator produces beneficial results when properly used, it should never be used if the customer has a weak heart, fever, inflammation or an abscess.

WALL PLATE

A wall plate is a device used to adapt the different types of current supplied by the power plant or battery cells to suit the requirements of electrical appliances used in the barber shop. By adjusting certain switches, it is possible to obtain the type of current desired.

GALVANIC CURRENT

The galvanic current is a constant and direct current generated by a direct current (D.C.) or by battery cells. It possesses polarity as manifested by the chemical changes produced when this current is passed through certain solutions containing acids or salts. Chemical effects are also produced when a galvanic current is passed through the tissues and fluids of the body.

The negative pole of the galvanic current has a special use in electrolysis, and is employed for the permanent removal of unsightly hair from the body.

SHORT-WAVE DIATHERMY

The short-wave diathermy is another form of high-frequency current, and is also used for the rapid and permanent removal of undesirable hair from the body.

FARADIC CURRENT

The faradic current is an alternating and interrupted current capable of producing a mechanical reaction without a chemical effect. It is used principally to cause muscular contractions.

SINUSOIDAL CURRENT

The sinusoidal current resembles the faradic current in many respects. It is an alternating current which produces a mechanical effect on the body. The manner of application is the same as for the faradic current.

ELECTRICITY

1. What is the nature of electricity?	A form of energy capable of producing magnetic, chemical or heat effects.
2. What is a conductor? What substance is usually used as a conductor in an electric wire?	A substance which readily carries an electric current. Copper is usually used as a conductor.
3. What is a non-conductor or insulator? Give three examples.	A substance which resists the passage of an electric current, such as rubber, silk and glass.
4. What are electrodes?	Applicators used in applying electricity to a customer.
5. What is a direct current (D.C.)?	A constant and even-flowing current, traveling in one direction.
6. What is an alternating current (A.C.)?	A rapid, interrupted current, flowing first in one direction and then in the opposite direction.
7. Which apparatus changes a direct current into an alternating current?	Converter.
8. Which apparatus changes an alternating current to a direct current?	Rectifier.
9. Define a closed circuit.	A closed circuit is one in which the current flows after proper connections have been made.
10. Which type of circuit will not operate an electrical appliance?	An open circuit or a short circuit.
11. Which safety device is needed to correct a short circuit?	Fuse.
12. Which three defects may cause a fuse to blow out?	Overloading an electrical outlet, faulty connections, and frayed wires.
13. What is a volt?	A unit of electrical pressure.
14. What is an ampere?	A unit of electrical strength.
15. What is an ohm?	A unit of electrical resistance.
16. What is a high-frequency current?	A current having a high rate of vibration, ranging from 10,000 or more cycles per second.
17. Which type of high-frequency current is commonly used in the barber shop?	Tesla current.
18. What effects does the Tesla current produce on the body?	Either stimulating or soothing effects, depending on the method of application.

19. Name three kinds of electrodes.	The facial electrode, the scalp electrode and the metal electrode.
20. Name three methods of applying the Tesla current.	Direct surface application; indirect application; general electrification.
21. Briefly describe how to use direct surface application.	The barber holds the electrode and applies it directly to customer's skin.
22. Briefly describe how to use indirect application.	While the customer is holding the electrode, the barber massages the surface being treated.
23. Briefly describe how to use general electrification.	The customer holds the metal electrode in his hand, thereby charging the body with electricity.
24. Which method of application produces soothing results?	Either direct surface application or general electrification.
25. How are stimulating effects produced?	By lifting the electrode slightly from the part being treated or by using it through a towel or clothing.
26. How long should a general facial or scalp treatment last?	About five minutes.
27. What safety precaution should be observed in using hair tonics having a high alcoholic content?	Use the high-frequency current first, followed by the application of hair tonic.
28. What is a vibrator?	An electrical appliance used as an aid in massage.
29. Name five benefits produced by vibratory massage.	1. Stimulates the functions of the skin. 2. Stimulates muscular tissues. 3. Increases the blood supply to the part being massaged. 4. Increases glandular activities. 5. Soothes the nerves.
30. Under what conditions should a vibrator never be used?	If the customer has a weak heart, fever, inflammation or abscess.
31. Describe the methods of using the vibrator.	The vibrator may be used directly or indirectly. It can be used directly with the rubber applicator to the parts to be treated. Or it may be used indirectly, by placing the vibrator on the back of the barber's hand, or wrist—the vibrations are thus transmitted through the fingers to the parts to be treated.

LIGHT THERAPY

Light therapy refers to the application of light rays for treatment of disease. Light or electrical waves travel at a tremendous speed—186,000 miles per second. The Angstrom Unit (A.U.) has been adopted to simplify the measurement of these waves.

There are many kinds of light rays, but in barber shop work we are concerned with only three—those producing heat, known as infra-red rays; those producing chemical and germicidal reaction, known as ultra-violet rays; and visible lights, all of which are contained within the spectrum of the sun.

If a ray of sunshine is passed through a glass prism, it will appear in seven different colors, known as the **rainbow,** arrayed in the following manner: red, orange, yellow, green, blue, indigo and violet. These colors which are visible to the eye, constitute the **visible spectrum,** comprising about 12% of sunshine.

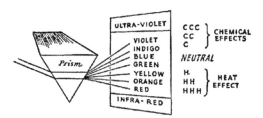

Dispersion of Light Rays by a Prism

Scientists have discovered that at either end of the visible spectrum are rays of the sun which are **invisible** to us. The rays beyond the violet are the **ultra-violet rays,** also known as **actinic** rays. These rays are the shortest and least penetrating rays of the spectrum, comprising about 8% of sunshine. The action of these rays is both chemical and germicidal.

Below the red rays of the spectrum are the **infra-red rays.** These are pure heat rays, comprising about 80% of sunshine.

Ultra Violet Rays			Solar Spectrum	Infra Red Rays
1847 AU to 3900 AU			3900 AU to 7700 AU	7700 AU to 14,000 AU
Far 1847-2200	Middle 2200-2900	Near 2900-3900	Violet Indigo Blue Green Yellow Orange Red	Penetrating
Germicidal	Therapeutic	Tonic		Analgesic
Cold Invisible Rays			Visible Rays	Invisible Heat Rays

Natural sunshine is composed of:
8% ultra-violet rays; 12% visible light rays; 80% infra-red rays.

Properties of ultra-violet rays:
1. Short wave length.
2. High frequency.
3. Weak penetrating power.

Properties of infra-red rays:
1. Long wave length.
2. Low frequency.
3. Deep penetrating power.

How Light Rays Are Reproduced

A therapeutic lamp is an electrical apparatus capable of producing certain rays of the spectrum. There are separate lamps for infra-red and for ultra-violet.

Types of Ultra-Violet Lamps

There are three general types of ultra-violet lamps.

1. The glass bulb.
2. The hot quartz.
3. The cold quartz.

ULTRA-VIOLET GENERATORS

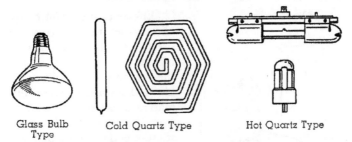

Glass Bulb Type   Cold Quartz Type   Hot Quartz Type

The **glass bulb lamp** produces mostly longer ultra-violet rays. It is used mainly for cosmetic or tanning purposes.

The **hot quartz lamp** produces both short and long ultra-violet rays. It is a general all purpose lamp suitable for tanning, tonic, cosmetic or germicidal purposes.

The **cold quartz lamp** produces mostly short ultra-violet rays. It has a limited use in the barber shop.

Infra-red rays are best reproduced by metal generators, giving no light whatsoever, only a rosy glow when active. Special glass bulbs are also used to produce infra-red rays.

The **visible rays**, sometimes referred to as dermal lights, are reproduced by carbon filament or tungsten bulbs in clear glass which gives the white light, or in colored bulbs giving the various colors.

Protecting the eyes. The customer's eyes should always be protected with cotton pads saturated in a boric acid or witch hazel solution, placed on the eyelids during such treatments. The barber and customer should always wear goggles when using ultra-violet rays.

ULTRA-VIOLET RAYS

Ultra-violet rays are invisible rays beyond the violet of the spectrum. Their action is both chemical and germicidal. Plant and animal life need ultra-violet rays for healthy growth. In the human body, these rays produce changes in the chemistry of the blood and also stimulate the activity of body cells.

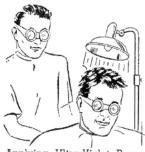

Applying Ultra-Violet Rays

Effects of ultra-violet rays. Ultra-violet rays increase resistance to disease by increasing the iron in the blood and the red and white cells in the blood. They also increase elimination of waste products; restore nutrition to the parts, stimulate the circulation and improve the flow of blood and lymph.

Skin tanning is the result of one or more exposures to ultra-violet rays which stimulate the production of pigment or coloring matter in the skin.

Sunburn may be produced by ultra-violet rays, in various degrees; however, for cosmetic purposes, first degree only is given. This is manifested by a slight reddening, appearing several hours after application, without any signs of itching, burning or peeling.

Treating diseases. Ultra-violet rays are used effectively in the treatment of acne, tinea and seborrhea. They may also be used to combat dandruff. They are beneficial in the process of healing, as well as to the growth of hair, because they increase the number of active tissue cells.

How applied. Ultra-violet rays are the shortest light rays of the spectrum, and the farther they are from the visible light region, the shorter they become. In practically all skin and scalp disorders there is manifested a deficiency of calcium. The long ultra-violet rays tend to increase the fixation of calcium in the blood. If the lamp is placed from 30 to 36 inches away, practically none of the shorter rays will reach the skin, so that the action is then limited to the effect of the longer rays.

The shorter rays are obtained when the lamp is within twelve inches from the skin. These rays are not only destructive to bacteria, but to tissue as well, if allowed to remain in use for too long a period of time.

Average exposure may produce redness of the skin, and overdoses may cause blistering. It is well to start with a short exposure of two or three minutes, and gradually increase the time to seven or eight minutes. **The barber and customer must wear eye goggles to protect their eyes.**

The slightest obstruction, of any nature whatever, will hinder ultra-violet rays from reaching the skin Consequently the skin must be entirely cleansed of creams, oils, powders, etc., before being subjected to ultra-violet rays.

INFRA-RED RAYS

Generally speaking, infra-red rays, which are the longest rays of the spectrum, produce a soothing and beneficial type of heat which extends for some distance into the tissues of the body.

Use and effect of infra-red rays:

1. Increase metabolism in general.
2. Relieve pain.
3. Increase oxidation in tissues.
4. Increase perspiration and secretion of sebum on skin.
5. Dilate blood vessels, and therefore increase blood flow.
6. Relax dermal tissues.
7. Heat tissues in area of exposure to high temperature without increasing body temperature.

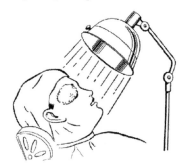

Applying Infra-Red Rays

How applied. The lamp is operated at an average distance of thirty inches. It is placed closer at the start, and then moved back gradually as the surface heat becomes more pronounced. Always protect the eyes of the customer during exposure.

VISIBLE LIGHTS

The **lamp** used to reproduce visible lights is usually a dome-shaped reflector, mounted on a pedestal with a flexible neck. The dome is finished with highly polished metal lining capable of reflecting heat rays. The bulbs used with this lamp come in various colors for different purposes. As with all other lamps, the customer's eyes must be protected from the glare and heat of the light. For proper eye protection, the customer's eyes are covered with pads.

Use and effect of the white light:

1. Relieves pain, especially in the congested areas; more particularly around the nerve centers, such as the back of the neck and around and within the ear.

Use and effect of the blue light:

1. Has a tonic and irritating effect on the bare skin.

2. Is deficient in heat rays.

3. Has a soothing effect on the nerves.

4. To obtain the desired result, it is only used over the **bare skin.** Creams, oils, powders, etc., must not be present on the skin.

Use and effect of the red light:

1. Has strong heat rays.

2 Has a stimulating and tonic effect when used over the bare skin.

3. Penetrates more deeply than the blue light.

4. Heat rays aid the absorption of cosmetic creams by the skin.

5. Is recommended for dry, scaly, and shriveled skin.

LIGHT THERAPY

1. What is light therapy?	The application of light rays for the treatment of disease.
2. At what speed does light travel?	About 185,000 miles per second.
3. Which unit measures the wave length of light?	Angstrom Unit (A.U.)
4. What is the average composition of natural sunshine?	80% infra-red rays; 12% visible rays; 8% ultra-violet rays.
5. Name the colors composing the visible light rays.	Red, orange, yellow, green, blue, indigo, and violet.
6. Which rays of the sun are invisible?	Ultra-violet rays and infra-red rays.
7. What is a therapeutic lamp?	An electrical apparatus used in producing various rays of the sun.
8. Name three characteristics of ultra-violet rays.	Short wave length, high frequency and weak penetrating power.
9. Name three types of therapeutic lamps which produce ultra-violet rays.	Glass bulb lamp, hot quartz lamp and cold quartz lamp.
10. Which ultra-violet lamps are desirable for the barber shop?	Glass bulb lamp and hot quartz lamp.
11. What benefit does the blood receive from ultra-violet rays?	The blood becomes enriched by an increase in the number of red and white cells.
12. What effects do ultra-violet rays have on the body?	Increases the blood and lymph flow, restores nutrition and increases the elimination of waste products.
13. Which skin and scalp disorders are helped by ultra-violet rays?	Acne, tinea, seborrhea and dandruff.
14. What benefit does the hair receive from ultra-violet rays?	Stimulates the growth of hair.
15. How far should the ultra-violet lamp be kept from the skin?	About twelve inches.
16. Why should the eyes be covered with goggles during exposure to ultra-violet rays?	To prevent irritation and injury to the eyes.
17. How long should the skin be exposed for the first time?	About two or three minutes.
18. For how many minutes can exposure be gradually increased?	Seven or eight minutes
19. Why should prolonged exposure be avoided?	May cause severe sunburn and blisters.

20. Which degree sunburn is safe for customers?	First degree sunburn.
21. What are the signs of first degree sunburn?	Slight reddening of the skin, appearing several hours after application, without any signs of itching, peeling or burning.
22. What causes the skin to tan?	The ultra-violet rays stimulate the production of pigment or coloring matter in the skin.
23. Why should the skin be clean before exposure to ultra-violet rays?	The slightest covering on the skin prevents these rays from reaching the skin.
24. Name three characteristics of infra-red rays.	Long wave length, low frequency and deep penetrating power.
25. Which types of therapeutic lamps produce infra-red rays?	Metal generators or special glass bulbs.
26. How should the eyes be protected during exposure?	Cover the eyes with pads dipped into boric acid or witch hazel solution.
27. How far should the infra-red lamp be kept from the skin?	About thirty inches from the skin.
28. What are the effects of infra-red rays on the body?	1. Heats and relaxes dermal tissues. 2. Increases blood flow. 3. Increases formation of sweat and sebum. 4. Increases oxidation and metabolism. 5. Relieves pain.
29. Which types of therapeutic lamps produce visible lights?	Dermal lights, having a tungsten or carbon filament in clear or colored bulbs.
30. Why should the eyes be protected during exposure?	To protect the eyes from the heat and glare of the light.
31. What are the benefits of using a white light?	The heat relieves pain in congested areas.
32. Which visible light lacks heat rays?	Blue light.
33. What are the benefits of using a blue light?	Tones the bare skin and soothes the nerves.
34. What are the benefits of using a red light?	The heat penetrates the skin, and has a stimulating or tonic effect on the bare skin.

CHEMISTRY

It is necessary for the barber to be familiar with the fundamentals of chemistry, a subject that has a direct bearing upon the composition and use of various cosmetics in the barber shop.

Chemistry is the science which deals with the composition, characteristics, and changes of matter.

Organic chemistry is that branch of chemistry which treats of carbon and its compounds, which may be derived from the animal and vegetable kingdoms.

Inorganic chemistry is that branch of chemistry that treats of substances found in or on the earth and are generally of mineral origin.

Matter is any substance which occupies space and has weight. It may exist in any or all of three forms:

1. **Solid**—having definite shape.
2. **Liquid**—having volume but no definite shape.
3. **Gaseous**—having neither volume nor definite shape.

Changes in matter may be either physical or chemical.

A physical change is one in which the identity of the substance remains the same both before and after the change. There is merely a change in the physical combination of the substance. Example: Mixtures such as powders, solutions, etc., represent different combinations of matter. It is possible to separate the ingredients from each other by physical means.

A chemical change is one in which the chemical nature and characteristics of the substance are permanently lost and an entirely new substance is produced. Example: Soap is formed from the chemical reaction between an alkaline substance (potassium hydroxide) and an oil or fat. The soap does not resemble the alkaline substance or the oil from which is it formed.

Matter may be separated into two or more simple substances which cannot be decomposed by any known agents. These substances are called **elements.** There are about ninety-two elements recognized at the present time, of which the most common are hydrogen and oxygen. Each element is identified by a letter or combination of letters, known as its **symbol**. Thus, the symbol for oxygen is O; for hydrogen, H.

A substance formed by the chemical union of two or more elements is known as a **compound**. For example, water is formed by the union of hydrogen and oxygen through the agency of electricity. Compounds may possess characteristics differing from any of the elements composing them. Hydrogen and oxygen are gases, but the water resulting from their chemical union is a liquid.

A chemical reaction involves a change in the identity and characteristics of the substance participating in the reaction.

Analysis is a chemical reaction in which a substance or compound is separated into its component parts or elements.

Synthesis is a chemical reaction in which two or more substances or compounds combine to form an entirely new product.

A combination of elements which retain their identities as separate substances, however thoroughly mingled, is called a **mixture**, such as salt water.

Chemical compounds are known by the symbols of the elements composing them. One **atom**, or smallest unit, of the element sodium (Na) combined with one atom of chlorine (Cl) makes one **molecule** (smallest particle of the compound) of the resulting product, sodium chloride (NaCl) or common salt. Two atoms of hydrogen (H) combined with one atom of oxygen (O) form one molecule of water, for which the formula is H_2O.

Acids, Bases and Salts

The barber should observe certain elementary chemical reactions of acids, bases and salts. For purposes of study, absorbent litmus paper, dyed with a violet blue coloring matter obtained from lichens, is used for testing.

Acids are sour substances containing hydrogen and some other non-metallic element such as nitrogen, sulphur, etc.

An acid solution will turn blue litmus paper red. Well known acids include: Hydrochloric (HCl), Sulphuric (H_2SO_4), Nitric (HNO_3), Acetic ($HC_2H_3O_2$), and Oxalic ($C_2H_2O_4$).

Bases are bitter tasting substances containing hydrogen, oxygen and some metal, such as sodium or potassium. They are soapy to the touch and in solution will turn red litmus paper blue. Bases are also known as **alkalies.** Sodium hydroxide (NaOH), potassium hydroxide (KOH) are common bases, both being used in the manufacture of soaps.

When there is any doubt regarding the nature of any solution, litmus paper can be used to determine its acid or alkaline content.

Salts are formed by the addition of acids to bases. Water is also formed in this manner, because of the natural alteration of hydrogen and oxygen. **Acids** are said to be neutralized by their contact with bases which is proved by the fact that litmus paper is not affected by salt solution. Salts contain metal and non-metal, and in some cases oxygen Remembering the formulas of the acids and bases previously given, the barber will readily see how water is a natural by-product in the forming of salts. Hydrochloric acid + sodium hydroxide :: water + sodium chloride (HCl + NaOH :: H_2O + NaCl).

Some common salts and their formulas are as follows: **sodium chloride** (NaCl) contains sodium and chlorine; **magnesium sulphate** ($MgSO_4$) contains magnesium, sulphur and oxygen; and **potassium nitrate** (KNO_3) contains potassium, nitrogen and oxygen.

Chemistry of Water

Water is the most abundant substance known. It covers about 75% of the earth's surface and comprises about 65% of the human body. Many foods are largely composed of water. It is the universal solvent. It can absorb more heat than any other substance and it is a good conductor of electricity.

Water serves many useful purposes in the barber shop. Only water of known purity is fit for drinking puposes. Suspended or dissolved impurities render water unsatisfactory for cleansing objects and for use in barber treatments.

Impurities can be removed from water by the following methods:

Filtration: passing through a porous substance, such as charcoal.

Boiling: heating to a temperature of 212° Fahrenheit to destroy microbic life and drive off gases.

Distillation: heating in a closed vessel arranged so that the resulting vapor passes off through a tube and is cooled and condensed to a liquid. This process is usually employed to purify water used in the manufacture of cosmetics.

Soft water, such as rain water or distilled water, contains little or no minerals. It is very important that soft water be used for shampooing, bleaching or dyeing the hair. **Hard water** contains mineral substances that curdle soap instead of permitting a lather to form. Hard water may be softened by **boiling, distillation,** or by the use of **borax** or **washing soda.**

For the latter method of softening water, a large vessel, with a faucet near the bottom, is filled with water and placed on a low platform. One pound of borax or washing soda is dissolved in two quarts of water; and for each unit of twenty gallons of water in the tank, one ounce of borax solution is added. The water in the vessel is stirred vigorously with a clean wooden paddle. Any cloudiness appearing should be allowed to settle and then a small amount of the water drawn off for testing.

A good **test for soft water** employs a standard soap solution made by dissolving three-quarters of an ounce of pure powdered castile soap in a pint of distilled water. A pint bottle should be half filled with fresh water, and one drop of soap solution added. The bottle is then shaken vigorously. If a lather forms at once and lasts for a few minutes, the water is very soft. If a lather does not appear at once, another drop of soap solution is added and the shaking repeated. If more than a few drops of the soap solution are needed to produce a good lather, the water must be softened.

Softened water is tested as described, and another ounce of the borax solution to each twenty gallons of water must be added if a lather lasting two minutes cannot be produced. A record of the findings in this test is helpful in softening the next large quantity of water.

United States Pharmacopeia (U.S.P.)

The barber needs to become familiar with certain drugs used in cosmetics. The United States Pharmacopeia is a book defining and standardizing drugs and is therefore in the possession of every druggist. The initials U.S.P. following the name of any drug is an indication that it is listed in the above mentioned volume.

Alcohol (grain or ethyl) is a colorless liquid obtained by the fermentation of certain sugars. It is a powerful antiseptic and disinfectant, a 70% solution being usable for sterilization of instruments, and 60% solution for the skin.

Alum is an aluminum derivative, supplied in the form of crystals or powder, which has a strong astringent taste and action. It is used as a styptic in cases of small cuts by dusting the powder over the injury.

Ammonia water, as commercially used, is a colorless liquid with a pungent, penetrating odor. It is a by-product of the manufacture of coal gas. As it readily dissolves grease, it is valued as a cleansing agent, and is also used with hydrogen peroxide in bleaching hair. A 28% solution of ammonia gas dissolved in water is commonly employed in the barber shop.

Sodium carbonate (washing soda) is prepared by heating **sodium bicarbonate.** In the barber shop, it is used for water softening and to prevent the rusting of metallic instruments in sterilization.

Bichloride of mercury is usually sold in tablet form, about $7\frac{1}{2}$ grains, shaped peculiarly for ready identification. As it is a very strong poison, it should be employed very sparingly in barber shops. It may be used for the sterilization of the hands in the proportion of 1/2500.

Boric acid, also called boracic acid, is a powder obtained from sodium borate. It is a mild, healing and antiseptic agent. It is sometimes used as a dusting powder, and in solution, as a cleansing lotion or eyewash.

Formaldehyde is a gas, but in a water solution containing from 37% to 40% of the gas by weight, it is known as **formalin.** The gas is rendered inactive by the addition of ammonia. Formaldehyde has a very disagreeable strong odor, and is very irritating to the eyes and the mucous linings of the nose and mouth. In barber shops formalin is used both in wet and dry sterilizers for sterilization of instruments.

Glycerine is a clear, colorless, odorless, syrupy liquid with a sweet taste. It is a type of alcohol formed by the decomposition of oils, fats or molasses. It is an excellent skin softener, and is an ingredient of face creams and lotions, brilliantine, etc. In sterilization, glycerine is added to the chemical solution to keep metal instruments from corroding.

Iodine is obtained from seaweed which is burned and the ashes washed, yielding iodides of potassium and bromine. Iodine is only slightly soluble in water, when it appears gray, but is readily soluble in alcohol, when it appears dark brown, and is called tincture of iodine. The 2% tincture of iodine can be safely used on the skin to treat minor cuts and bruises. Iodine stains are readily removed with alcohol.

Hydrogen peroxide (H_2O_2) is a colorless oily fluid, heavy, with slight odor and sharp taste. It is very unstable, and since it decomposes readily in the presence of heat and light, it is kept in dark glass bottles, in a cool place. The 17 or 20 volume hydrogen peroxide solution is used as a bleaching agent for the hair. A 3% or 10 volume solution of hydrogen peroxide possesses antiseptic qualities.

CHEMISTRY AS APPLIED TO COSMETICS

Chemistry as applied to cosmetics is both a science and an art. The science of chemistry consists in knowing what to do in the correct manner, art involves the proper methods of preparing and applying the cosmetic to the body.

A barber will be better equipped to serve the public

if he has an understanding of the chemical composition, preparation and uses of cosmetics which are intended to cleanse, beautify and improve the hygiene of the external portions of the body.

Cosmetics used in the barber shop may be classified according to their physical and chemical nature and the characteristics by means of which they are recognized.

Physical and Chemical Classification of Cosmetics

1. Powders
2. Solutions
3. Emulsions
4. Ointments
5. Soaps

Powders

Powders are a uniform mixture of insoluble substances which have been properly blended, perfumed and/or tinted to produce a cosmetic which is free from coarse or gritty particles.

Solutions

A **solution** is a preparation made by dissolving a solid, liquid or gaseous substance in another substance, usually liquid.

A **solute** is a substance dissolved in the fluid.

A **solvent** is a liquid used to dissolve a substance.

Solutions are clear and permanent mixtures of solute and solvent which do not separate on standing. Since a good solution is clear, filtration is often necessary, particularly if the solution is cloudy.

Water is called a universal solvent because it is capable of dissolving more substances than any other solvent. Grain alcohol and glycerine are frequently used as solvents. Water, glycerine and alcohol readily mix with each other.

Emulsions

Emulsions (creams) are permanent mixtures of oil and water which are united with the aid of a binder (gum) or an emulsifier (soap). Emulsions are usually milky white in appearance.

Creams differ from ointments in the large amount of water contained therein.

Ointments

Ointments such as sulphur ointment are semi-solid mixtures of organic substances (lard, petrolatum, wax) and a medicinal agent. No water is present. For the ointment to soften, its melting point should be below that of the body temperature (98.6° Fahrenheit).

Soaps

Soaps are compounds formed in a chemical reaction between alkaline substances (potassium or sodium hydroxide) and the fatty acids in the oil or fat. Besides the soap, glycerine is also formed. Potassium hydroxide produces a **soft soap**, whereas sodium hydroxide forms a **hard soap**. A mixture of the two alkalies will yield a soap of intermediate consistency.

A **good soap** does not contain an excess of free alkali and is made from pure oils and fats.

Shaving Soaps

Shaving soaps can be purchased in various forms and shapes. Hard shaving soaps include those sold in cake, stick or powdered form, and are similar in composition to toilet soaps. Available as **soft soap** is shaving cream in tube or jar. Liquid soap can also be used by the barber.

Whatever form of shaving soap is used, it usually contains animal and vegetable oils, alkaline substances and water. The presence of **cocoanut oil improves the lathering qualities** of the shaving soap.

Cosmetics for the Skin, Scalp and Hair

NAME	COMPOSITION	USE
Soap	Contains oils and fats combined chemically with alkalies such as potassium hydroxide.	Cleanses the skin.
Shaving soap	Contains soap combined with water and glycerine.	Softens the hair and lubricates the skin prior to shaving.
Cold cream	Contains oil, borax, wax, water and perfume.	All-purpose cream used to cleanse, protect and lubricate the skin.
Cleansing cream	Contains a cold cream base with a high content of mineral oil.	Melts quickly and cleanses the skin.
Tissue cream	Contains oil, water, lanolin, wax and perfume.	Softens the skin and replaces any natural deficiency of oil.
Massage cream	Contains a cold cream base with starch or casein.	Cleanses the skin and aids in facial massage.
Muscle oil	Contains vegetable or mineral oil, lecithin or cholesterol.	Softens and lubricates the skin and aids in facial massage.
Astringent (after-shave) lotion	Contains alcohol, astringent and perfumed water.	Closes the pores, and corrects an oily skin.
Witch hazel	Contains alcohol, water and extract of witch hazel bark.	Cools and refreshes the skin after shaving.
Bay rum	Contains alcohol, oil of bay or other fragrant oils.	Cools and refreshes the skin after shaving.
Talcum powder	Contains insoluble magnesium compounds and perfume.	Soothes and dries the skin after shaving or used on back of the neck before and after haircutting.
Shampoo	Contains soap in liquid form.	Cleanses the scalp and hair.
Hair rinse	Contains water, a mild acid or coloring agent.	Removes insoluble soap residue from the hair, or tints the hair a definite shade.
Hair tonic or scalp lotion	Contains alcohol, water, oil, perfume and medicinal agent (either antiseptic or irritant).	Stimulates circulation, reduces dandruff, keeps scalp clean and healthy, and dresses the hair.
Scalp ointment or dandruff ointment	Contains lanolin, petrolatum and medicinal agents.	Used to correct dandruff and stimulate circulation of blood to the scalp.
Brilliantine or pomade	Available in liquid and solid form and contains vegetable or mineral oil, wax and perfume.	Used as a hair dressing to keep the hair in place.

COSMETICS

1. What are cosmetics?	Cosmetics are preparations used to cleanse and improve conditions of the skin, scalp, and hair.
2. Why should the barber have a knowledge of cosmetics used in the barber shop?	In order to select the right kind of cosmetic to meet the customer's requirements.
3. What is the composition of water?	Water contains the elements of 2 parts hydrogen and 1 part oxygen, known by the formula H_2O.
4. What is soft water?	Water containing little or no minerals, such as rain water or distilled water.
5. What is hard water?	Water containing small amounts of mineral salts.
6. Which type of water does not lather freely with soap?	Hard water.
7. Name three methods for softening hard water.	Boiling, distillation or the use of borax or washing soda.
8. Which ingredients are used in making soaps?	Alkalies such as sodium hydroxide or potassium hydroxide are added to fats or oils to form a soap.
9. What are the qualities of a good soap?	A good soap does not contain an excess of free alkali and is made from pure fats or oils.
10. Which soap preparations may be used by the barber?	Powdered soap, stick soap, cake soap, liquid soap and shaving cream.
11. What is the composition of creams?	Creams are a uniform mixture of oils, fats, waxes, soap, water and other special ingredients.
12. Name four kinds of creams used by the barber.	Cold cream, cleansing cream, tissue cream and massage cream.
13. What is the composition of ointments? Give an example.	Ointments are semi-solid mixtures of fatty substances, waxes and medicinal agents. Sulphur ointment.
14. What is the composition of face powders?	Face powders consist of a powder base, perfume and with or without a tint.
15. What is the composition of facial lotions?	Facial lotions are solutions of alcohol, water, astringent and perfume.
16. What is the composition of witch hazel?	Witch hazel is a solution of alcohol, water and an extract from witch hazel bark.
17. What is the composition of bay rum?	Bay rum is a solution of alcohol combined with oil of bay or other fragrant oils.
18. What is the composition of hair tonics?	Hair tonics are solutions of alcohol, oil, water and an antiseptic or irritant.
19. What is the composition of hair dressings?	Hair dressings are a mixture of vegetable or mineral oil, wax and perfume.

20. Which cosmetics are generally used after shaving?	Cold cream, facial lotion, witch hazel, bay rum and talcum powder.
21. Which cosmetics are generally used after haircutting?	Hair tonic or hair dressing.
22. Which agents are generally used to cleanse the hair?	Shampoo and water .
23. Which agents are generally used to cleanse the skin?	Soap and water, and cleansing cream.
24. Name two types of shaving creams.	The brush shaving cream and the brushless shaving cream.

DISEASES OF THE SKIN, SCALP
AND HAIR

The barber should be able to recognize readily the common disorders of the skin and scalp so that preventive measures may be used to avoid more serious affections. Unusual or unfamiliar symptoms of disorder should be immediately referred to a physician for treatment.

Dermatology is the science of the skin, its nature, structure, functions, diseases and treatment.

Dermatologist is a skin specialist.

Trichology is the science of the hair and its diseases.

Etiology is the science of the causes of disease.

Diagnosis is the recognition of a disease from its symptoms.

Prognosis is the foretelling of the probable course of a disease.

Pathology is the science which treats of modifications of function and changes in structure caused by disease.

LESIONS OF THE SKIN

A lesion is a structural change in the tissues caused by injury or disease. There are three types: primary, secondary and tertiary. The barber is concerned with primary and secondary lesions only

Symptom is a sign of disease. The symptoms in diseases of the skin are divided into two groups.

1. **Subjective**—symptoms that can be felt, as in itching, burning, pains, etc.

2. **Objective**—symptoms that can be seen, as in pimples, pustules, etc.

Primary Lesions

1. **Macule**—a small discolored spot or patch on the surface of the skin, neither raised nor sunken, usually found in rashes, such as measles.

2. **Papule**—a small elevation of the skin containing no fluid, but which may so develop that it will later contain pus.

3. **Wheal**—a raised ridge on the skin, usually caused by the blow of a whip, bite of an insect, or as the characteristic eruption of urticaria.

4. **Tubercle**—a solid elevation of the skin, varying in size from that of a flaxseed to about the size of a hickory nut.

5. **Tumor** (phyma)—an external swelling, varying in size, shape and color.

6. **Vesicle**—a small circumscribed elevation of the skin containing a serum-like fluid, such as a blister.

7. **Bulla** (bleb)—a blister containing a serum-like fluid, similar to a vesicle, but larger.

8. **Pustule**—an elevation of the skin having an inflamed base, containing pus.

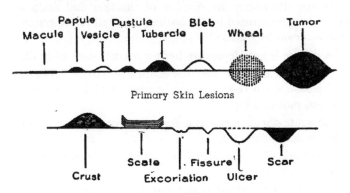

Primary Skin Lesions

Secondary Skin Lesions

Secondary Lesions

1. **Scale** (squama)—a dry or greasy separated portion of the epidermis.

2. **Crusts** (scabs)—three varieties:
   a) Blood crusts (red-black in color).
   b) Pus crusts (yellow-green).
   c) Serum crusts (honey-colored).

3. **Excoriation** (abrasion)—a raw surface due to the loss of the superficial skin after an injury.

4. **Fissure** (rhagade)—a crack in the skin penetrating into the derma, as in the case of chapped hands or lips.

5. **Ulcer**—an open lesion with formation of pus upon the surface of the skin.

6. **Scar** (cicatrix)—the tissue formed after the healing of a wound or an ulcer.

7. **Stain**—an abnormal discoloration remaining after the disappearance of moles, freckles or liver spots, sometimes apparent after certain diseases.

DEFINITIONS OF COMMON TERMS APPLIED TO DISEASE

Before describing the diseases of the skin and scalp so they will be recognized by the barber, it is well to understand what is meant by disease.

A **disease** is any departure from a normal state of health.

A **skin disease** is an infection of the skin characterized by an objective lesion (one that can be seen), which may consist of scales, pustules, etc.

An **acute disease** is one manifested by symptoms of a more or less violent character.

A **chronic disease** is one of long duration, usually marked by no violent character.

An **infectious disease** is one due to a pathogenic microorganism taken into the body as a result of contact with a lesion or contaminated object.

A **contagious disease** is one that is communicable by contact

A **congenital disease** is one that is present in the infant at birth

A **seasonal disease** is one that is influenced by the weather, as prickly heat in the summer, and forms of eczema more prevalent in cold weather.

An **occupational disease** is one that is due to certain kinds of employment, such as dermatitis, caused by coming in contact with chemicals or dyes.

A **deficiency disease** is one that is due to lack of some element in the diet; such as scurvy or rickets.

A **parasitic disease** is one that is caused by vegetable or animal parasites, such as lice, scabies or ringworm.

A **pathogenic disease** is one produced by a disease producing bacteria, such as staphylococcus and streptococcus, pus-forming bacteria.

A **systemic disease** is one that is due to lack or over functioning of the internal glands. One of the main causes may be due to faulty diet.

A **constitutional disease** is one that is associated with or marked by a disturbance of metabolism; a blood disease.

A **venereal disease** is a contagious disease commonly acquired by contact with an infected person during sexual intercourse.

An **epidemic** is the manifestation of a disease that attacks simultaneously a large number of persons living in a particular locality; such as infantile paralysis, Spanish influenza or small-pox.

Allergy is a sensitivity which certain persons develop to normally harmless substances. Skin allergies are quite common. Contact with certain types of cosmetics, medicines and dyes may bring about an itching eruption, accompanied by redness, swelling, blisters, oozing and scaling.

DISEASES OF THE SEBACEOUS (OIL) GLANDS

There are several common diseases of the sebaceous (oil) glands which the barber should be able to identify and understand.

Comedones, or blackheads, are a worm-like mass of hardened sebum, appearing most frequently on the face, forehead and nose.

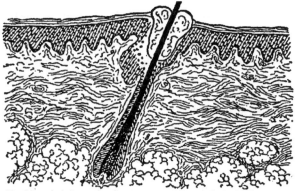

Blackhead (plug of sebaceous matter and dirt) Forming
Around Mouth of Hair Follicle

Blackheads accompanied by pimples frequently occur in youths between the ages of 13 and 20. During the adolescent period, the activity of the sebaceous glands is stimulated, thereby contributing to the formation of blackheads and pimples. Should this condition become severe, medical attention is necessary.

Milia or whiteheads—

A disorder of the sebaceous (oil) glands caused by the accumulation of sebaceous matter beneath the skin. Occurs on any part of the face and may be associated with blackheads.

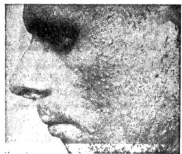

Milia (Whiteheads)

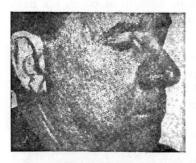

Acne Rosacea

Acne rosacea is a chronic, inflammatory congestion of the cheeks and nose. It is characterized by redness, dilation of the blood-vessels, and the formation of papules and pustules. It is usually caused by poor digestion and over-indulgence in alcoholic liquors. It may also be caused by over-exposure, constipation, faulty elimination and hyperacidity. It is usually aggravated by eating and drinking hot, highly spiced, or highly seasoned foods or drinks. It generally has three stages.

The **first stage** starts with a slight pinkness all over the face, varying with the temperature, and temperament of the individual.

The **second stage** affects the capillaries. Often they become so dilated that they are apparent to the naked eye. At this stage the sebaceous glands are always affected. Large pores, oiliness and comedones invariably result.

The **third stage** is very disfiguring. The entire face becomes congested, and the condition may remain chronic although dormant, for years, even after treatment.

Steatoma (wen) or sebaceous cyst, is a subcutaneous tumor of the sebaceous glands, the contents consisting of sebum, smooth pea to orange size; usually occurring on the scalp, neck and back.

Asteatosis is a condition of dry skin, characterized by absolute or relative deficiency of sebum, due to senile changes (old age) or some constitutional disorder or disease. In local conditions it may be caused by alkalies, such as are found in soaps and washing powders.

Seborrhea is a skin condition due to over-activity and excessive secretion of the sebaceous or oil glands. The appearance of the skin affected is oily and shiny. On the scalp it is readily detected by the unusual amount of oil on the hair. Seborrhea exists in two forms:

1. **Seborrhea oleosa,** an oily condition.

2. **Seborrhea sicca,** a dry condition.

Acne is a chronic inflammatory disease of the skin, occurring in or around a sebaceous gland, characterized by pustules, papules or tubercles, affecting chiefly the face. The cause of acne is generally held to be microbic, but predisposing factors are age and disturbances of the digestive tract.

The different forms of acne are as follows:

Acne vulgaris or simplex. The common pimple. An inflammatory skin disorder involving the sebaceous (oil) glands. Appears chiefly on the face and is often associated with blackheads and an oily skin. Acne (pimples) occur among adolescent youth.

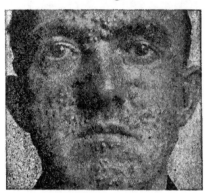

Acne Vulgaris
(The Common Pimple)

Acne papulosa—vulgaris in which the papular lesions predominate.

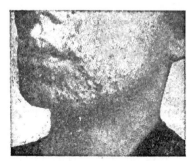

Acne pustulosa — vulgaris in which the pustular lesions predominate.

Acne Pustulosa

Acne punctata—red papules in which blackheads are usually found.

Acne albida—the presence of milia (whiteheads) in acne.

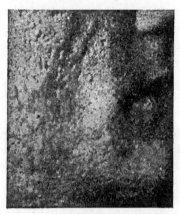

Acne hypertrophica

(acne scars)—Scar formation in acne varies with the severity of the lesions. Surface lesions give rise to little scar formation. Pitted scars result from deep-seated lesions affecting the sebaceous glands.

Acne Scars

Acne artificialis—caused by the application of external irritants, or drugs taken internally.

Acne indurata—deep seated with hard tubercular lesions occurring chiefly on the face, neck and back.

Acne cachecticorum—occurring in the subject of anemia, or of some weakening constitutional diseases.

Acne keratosa—an eruption of papules consisting of horny plugs projecting from the hair follicles, accompanied by inflammation.

Acne urticaria—a skin disease in which the lesions often lead to marked scar formation.

DISEASES OF THE SUDORIFEROUS (SWEAT) GLANDS

Anidrosis (lack of perspiration) is often a result of fever or certain skin diseases.

Bromidrosis or **osmidrosis** refers to foul smelling perspiration, usually noticeable in the armpits or on the feet.

Hyperidrosis (excessive perspiration) is caused by excessive heat or general body weakness. The most commonly affected parts are the armpits and joints.

Chromidrosis (discolored perspiration), which is very rarely seen, is usually caused by nervous disorders. The excretion is brown, yellow or bluish in color. It should be referred to a physician for treatment.

Hemidrosis (bloody sweat) is an affection similar to chromidrosis except that the excretion is of a bloody fluid. It is very rare; usually follows hysteria or extreme nervous excitement. It should be referred to a physician for treatment.

Hydrocystoma (cysts of the coil-ducts) is a chronic, non-inflammable disorder, characterized by the presence on the face of scattered, isolated, deep-seated, persistent, clear vesicles.

Uridrosis is an affection of the sweat glands having the characteristic odor of urine. It may occur with chromidrosis. It should be referred to a physician for treatment.

Sudamen is a non-inflammatory affection of the sweat glands, consisting of tiny pimples that do not contain pus, but are filled with perspiration. It is accompanied by intense itching.

Miliaria rubra (prickly heat), which is noticeable in burning and itching skin, is usually caused by exposure to excessive heat.

Miliary fever (sweating sickness) is an infectious disease characterized by fever, profuse sweating and the production of sudamina.

DANDRUFF

Dandruff is the presence of small, white scales usually appearing on the scalp and hair. Dandruff is also known by such medical terms as pityriasis and seborrhea sicca.

Just as the skin is continually being shed and replaced, in a similar manner, the uppermost layer of the scalp is being cast off all the time. Ordinarily, these horny scales are loose and fall off freely. The natural shedding of the horny scales, too infrequently removed, is often mistaken for dandruff.

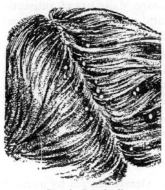 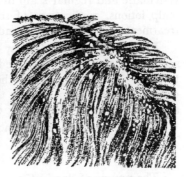

Simple Dandruff   Excessive Dandruff

Long neglected dandruff frequently leads to baldness.

The causes of dandruff are as follows:

1. A direct cause of dandruff is the excessive shedding of the epithelial cells. Instead of growing to the surface and falling off, the horny scales accumulate on the scalp.

2. Indirect or associated causes of dandruff are a sluggish condition of the scalp occasioned by poor circulation, lack of nerve stimulation, improper diet and uncleanliness. Contributing causes are the use of strong soaps and insufficient rinsing of the hair after a shampoo.

The two principal types of dandruff are:

1. **Pityriasis capitis simplex,** dry type.
2. **Pityriasis steatoides,** a greasy or waxy type.

Pityriasis capitis simplex (dry dandruff) is characterized by the presence of an itchy scalp and small, white scales usually attached in masses to the scalp or scattered loose in the hair, occasionally they are so profuse that they fall to the shoulders.

Treatment—Frequent oil treatments and oil shampoos, systematic and regular scalp massage, daily use of antiseptic scalp lotions, applications of scalp ointments and electrical treatments will correct this condition.

Pityriasis steatoides (greasy or waxy type of dandruff) is scaliness of the epidermis mixed with sebum which causes it to stick to the scalp in patches. The associated itchiness causes the person to scratch the scalp, and if the greasy scales are torn off, bleeding or oozing of sebum may follow.

Medical treatment is advisable.

Precaution

The nature of dandruff is not clearly defined by medical authorities. It is generally believed to be of infectious origin Some authorities hold that it is due to a specific microbe. However, from the barber's point of view, both forms of dandruff are to be considered contagious and may spread by the use of common brushes, combs or hair pins. Therefore, the barber must take the necessary precautions by sterilizing everything that comes in contact with the customer.

INFLAMMATIONS

Dermatitis

The term **dermatitis** is used to denote an inflammatory condition of the skin. The lesions come in various forms, such as vesicles, papules, etc.

Dermatitis venenata is an eruptive skin affection caused by external applications of medicaments, such as lotions, powders, iodine, hair dyes, etc.

Dermatitis medicamentosa is an eruption of blebs, papules, etc., caused by internal introduction of bromides, antitoxins, etc.

Dermatitis combustionis is a variety of dermatitis produced by extreme heat, or by the sun's rays.

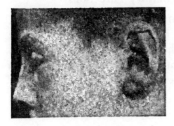

Dermatitis Seborrheica

Dermatitis seborrheica is an inflammation of the skin co-existent with seborrhea. It is sometimes called **eczema seborrheicum**. It may be distinguished from other forms of dermatitis and from simple eczema by its origin on the scalp, its oily secretion and crusts, and the yellowish color and sharp outline of its lesions. It should be referred to a physician for treatment.

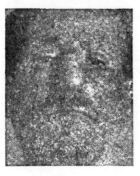

Eczema

Eczema

Eczema is an inflammation of the skin of acute or chronic nature, presenting many forms of dry or moist lesions. It is frequently accompanied by itching, burning, and various other unpleasant sensations. All cases of eczema should be referred to a physician for treatment.

The **difference** between **dermatitis** and **eczema** is that dermatitis usually refers to skin eruptions due to a **known** cause, while eczema refers to dermatitis of **unknown** origin.

The unsatisfactory explanation of this condition by medical authorities makes it almost impossible to describe eczema with any great degree of certainty. A great majority of physicians class eczema under the general head of dermatitis.

In general, eczema is not contagious. However, the stage of eczema where pustules are present (usually found on the scalp and supposed to result from poor nourishment) is sometimes classed as infectious eczema or dermatitis, and is also known as **eczema contagiosa.**

Miscellaneous Inflammatory Affections

Psoriasis is a chronic inflammatory skin disease which, when appearing on the scalp, forms patches of dry, white scales. These scales when scratched leave tiny bleeding points. Its cause is associated with internal disorders and certain foods. It should be referred to a physician for treatment.

Herpes simplex is a virus infection commonly known as "fever blisters". It is characterized by the eruption of a single or group of vesicles on a red swollen base. The eruption may appear on the lips, nostrils, face or any part of the body. An attack rarely extends over a period of a week.

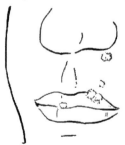

Herpes Simplex or Fever Blisters
involving the lips and nostrils

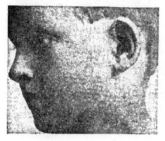

Pityriasis Pilaris

Pityriasis pilaris is a chronic inflammatory disease characterized by an eruption of papules surrounding the hair follicles, each papule being pierced by a hair, and tipped with a horny plug or scale. This condition should be referred to a physician.

Impetigo contagiosa (scrum-pox) is an inflammatory skin disease. Pustules appear in isolated form as in small pox; the eruptions of pustules, which open, rupture or become crusted. They occur chiefly on the face, around the mouth and nostrils. Usually associated with

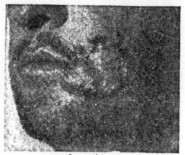

Impetigo

general weakness, faulty nutrition or hygienic neglect.

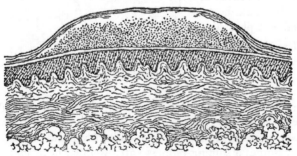

Impetigo Contagiosa, showing formation of Skin Blister Filled with Pus Cells and Bacteria

Variola or smallpox—A contagious skin disease identified by the presence of papules, vesicles and pustules and associated with fever, headache and pains.

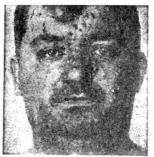

Variola (Smallpox)

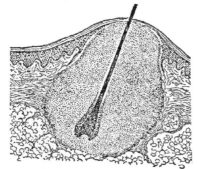

Furuncle or Boil

Furuncle or boil is an acute staphylococci infection of a hair follicle producing constant pain. A furuncle is the result of an active inflammatory process limited to a definite area and subsequently producing a pustule perforated by a hair.

Carbuncle is the result of an acute deep-seated staphylicocci infection larger than a furuncle, or boil. It should be referred to a physician.

Erysipelas, also known as St. Anthony's fire, is an acute, infectious disease

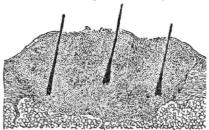

Carbuncle appears as a Deep Skin Infection, involving several Hair Shafts

characterized by intense inflammation of the skin and subcutaneous tissue; it is limited in area, and attended by many constitutional symptoms, such as chills, fever and nausea. The skin assumes a shining redness with swelling, heat, and pain, and in many cases shows a tendency to vesicular or bleb formation. This disease is uncommon today.

Urticaria (hives or nettle-rash) is an affection of the skin, characterized by eruptions of itching and stinging wheals or red elevations. Causes: external contact with herbs or shrubs of the nettle family, by eating shellfish, strawberries, etc., or the use of cosmetics which do not agree with the individual skin.

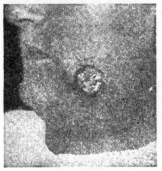

Anthrax

Anthrax—An inflammatory skin disorder caused by the use of an infected shaving brush. Detected by the presence of a small, red papule, followed by the formation of a pustule, vesicle and hard swelling. Accompanied by itching and burning feelings at the point of infection.

Ivy dermatitis — A skin inflammation caused by exposure to the poison ivy, poison oak or poison sumac leaves. Blisters and itching develop soon after contact occurs. The infection spreads from one part of the body to another. It is very contagious and should be referred to a physician for treatment.

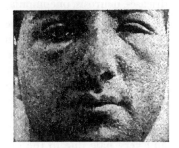

Ivy Dermatitis (Poison Ivy)

Alopecia

Alopecia refers to the abnormal loss of hair arising from any cause, usually affecting the scalp. It is the technical term for any form of baldness.

The natural falling out of the hair should not be confused with alopecia. When hair has grown to its full length, it comes out by itself and is replaced by a new hair. The natural shedding of the hair occurs most frequently in spring and fall. On the other hand, the hair lost in alopecia does not come back, unless special treatments are given to encourage hair growth.

Alopecia adnata is the technical term for congenital baldness. It is the complete absence, or partial absence, of hair, occurring at or soon after birth, due to a more or less completely arrested development of the hair follicle.

Alopecia senilis is the form of baldness occurring in old age. The loss of the hair is permanent.

Alopecia premature. There are two types, as follow:

1. **Alopecia prematura idiopathica** is the form of baldness beginning any time before middle age by a slow thinning process, due to the fact that the first hairs that fall out are replaced by regrowth of weaker ones.

2. **Alopecia prematura symptomatica** is the form of baldness resulting from some local or general disease, either of the scalp or body, such as fevers, shocks from operations, blood diseases, neurosis, pneumonia, etc.

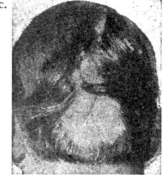

Alopecia areata is the sudden falling out of hair in round patches, or baldness in spots, sometimes caused by anemia, scarlet fever or typhoid fever, grippe, erysipelas or syphilis. Affected areas are slightly depressed, smooth and very pale due to the decreased blood supply. Patches may be round or irregular, and vary in size from ¼ inch to 2 or 3 inches in diameter.

Alopecia Areata, caused by a syphilitic infection attacking the central nervous system.

In most conditions of alopecia areata, the nervous system has been subjected to some injury. And since the flow of blood is influenced by the nervous system the affected area is poorly nourished as well.

Alopecia seborrheica (or seborrhea capitis) is loss of hair caused by a disease of the sebaceous glands.

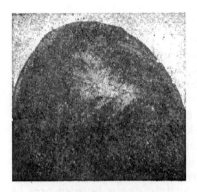

Alopecia Cicatrisata

Alopecia cicatrisata—A scalp disorder identified by the presence of circular, oval or irregular patches of baldness. The main lesions are small, reddish, inflammatory papules or pustules located at the mouth of hair follicles and pierced by hairs. Crusts and scars also form on the scalp and permanent baldness may result.

Alopecia syphilitica is loss of hair resulting from syphilis occurring in the second stage of this disease.

Alopecia dynamica is hair loss due to destruction of the hair follicle by ulceration or some disease process.

Alopecia follicularis is hair loss occasioned when the hair follicle becomes inflamed, resulting in the loss of hair in the affected area.

Alopecia localis is hair loss occurring in patches on the course of a nerve at the site of an injury.

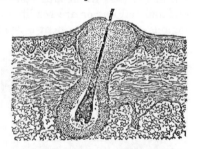

Folliculitis, infection of hair follicle

Alopecia maligna is a term denoting a form of alopecia that is severe and persistent.

Alopecia universalis is a condition manifested by general falling out of the hair of the body.

Alopecia follicularis is hair loss occasioned when the hair follicles become inflamed, resulting in the loss of hair in the affected area.

Alopecia localis is hair loss occurring in patches on the course of a nerve at the site of an injury.

PARASITIC AFFECTIONS

Tinea is the medical term for **ringworm.** The following are the different forms of ringworm:

Tinea tonsurans or **trichophytosis capitis** (ringworm of the scalp) is a contagious, vegetable parasitic disease of the hairy scalp, characterized by red papules or scalp spots at the opening of the hair follicles. The patches spread, the hair becomes brittle and lifeless and breaks off, leaving a stump, or falls from the enlarged open follicles. It is very contagious and should be referred to a physician.

Tinea sycosis or **trichophytosis barbae** (barber's itch) is a fungus infection occurring chiefly over the bearded area of the face. Beginning as small, rounded, slightly scaly, inflamed patches, the areas enlarge, clearing up somewhat centrally with elevation of the borders. As the parasites invade the hairs and follicles, hard lumpy swellings develop. In severe cases, pustules form around the hair follicles and rupture, forming crusts. In the later stage, the hairs become dry, break off, and fall out or are readily extracted. Being highly contagious, medical treatment is required.

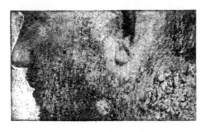 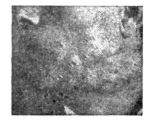

Tinea Sycosis (Barber's Itch)

Sycosis vulgaris (folliculitis barbae) is a chronic staphylococci infection involving the hair follicles of the beard and mustache areas. Caused by the use of unsterilized towels or barber implements, and made worse by irritation such as shaving or a continual nasal discharge. The main lesions are papules and pustules pierced by hairs. The surrounding skin is tender, reddened, swollen at times, and tends to itch. Medical care is required. (This affection must not be confused with tinea sycosis, which is due to ringworm fungus.)

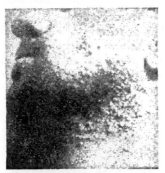

Sycosis Vulgaris

Differential Diagnosis

Tinea Sycosis

Typical case presents large lumpy or nodular tumefactions due to trichophyton fungus infection.

Beard area affected but the mustache is rarely affected.

Hairs broken and easily extracted. Roots usually dry.

Course rapid. Marked changes from week to week.

Not so chronic.

Very contagious—medical attention required.

Sycosis Vulgaris

Typical case presents small discrete papules or pustules pierced by hairs due to staphylococci infection.

Beard area affected and mustache is frequently affected.

Hairs firmly attached until loosened by suppuration.

Course slow. Little change from week to week.

Very chronic.

Very contagious—medical attention required.

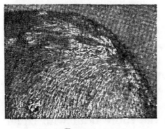

Favus

Favus (tinea favosa or honeycomb ringworm) is an infectious fungus growth due to a vegetable parasitic disease that is characterized by dry sulphur-yellow, cup-like crusts, called scutula, on the scalp, having a peculiar mousy odor. Scars from favus are bald patches; pink or white and shiny. It is very contagious, and should be referred to a physician.

Scabies (the itch) is a highly contagious animal parasitic skin disease, due to the itch mite. From the irritation of the parasite and still more from the scratching of the affected areas, vesicles and pustules may form.

Ringworm (tinea) of the hands. A highly contagious disease caused by a fungus (vegetable parasite). The principal symptoms are papular, red lesions occurring as patches or rings over the hands. Itching may be slight or severe. Ringworm may also affect the nails.

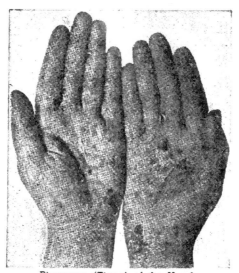

Ringworm (Tinea) of the Hands

Pediculosis capitis is a contagious condition caused by the head louse (animal parasite) infesting the hair of the scalp. As the parasites feed on the scalp, itching symptoms are felt. The head louse is transmitted from one person to another by intimate contact with infested hats, combs, brushes or other personal articles.

To treat head lice, shampoo the entire head with equal parts of larkspur tincture and ether before retiring. The next morning, shampoo again with germicidal soap. Repeat treatment as necessary.

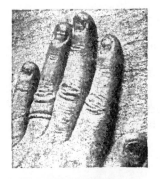

Ringworm (Tinea)
of the Nails

Tinea unguium (ringworm of the nails)—A local infectious disease. As the disease spreads, the nails become thickened, brittle and lose their natural shape. It is very contagious.

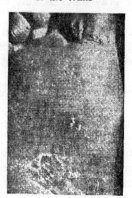 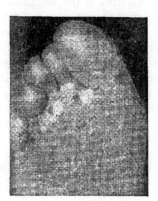

Ringworm (Tinea) of the Foot
(Athlete's Foot)

Ringworm (tinea) of the foot. (Athlete's foot)—A local infectious disease. The inflamed areas on the sole of the foot and between the toes show signs of redness, blisters and cracking of the skin. Itching and excessive sweating are also present. It is very contagious.

Precaution

Ringworm of the feet may spread and infect other parts of the body. Every barber infected must take special precaution to prevent the spread of this disease by sterilizing his hands, feet and socks until cured.

NON-CONTAGIOUS AFFECTIONS OF THE HAIR

There are six non-contagious affections of the hair, as follows:

Canities—grayness of hair.
Trichoptilosis—split hair.
Hypertrichosis (hirsuties)—superfluous hair.
Trichorrhexis nodosa—knotted hair.
Monilethrix—beaded hair.
Fragilitas crinium—brittle hair.

Canities

Canities is the technical term for gray hair. It may be either of three types, as follows:

1. Congenital canities—occurs in albinism and occasionally in persons with perfectly normal skin. The patchy type of congenital canities may develop slowly or rapidly, according to the cause of the condition.

2. Accidental canities—grayness of hair resulting from fright.

3. Acquired canities—may be due to old age; or premature, as in early adult life.

Several causes of acquired canities are worry, anxiety, nervous strain, prolonged illness, various wasting diseases and hereditary tendency. All these play an important part in acquired canities.

Ringed hair—A rare form of canities, due to the alternate formation of medulla and no medulla, in which the hairs appear silvery gray and dark in alternating bands. Usually seen in several members of the family.

Hair losing its color is due to the absence of pigment in the cortex and the presence of air particles. As the pigment lessens in the cortex, the white color increases. No treatment is available, unless dyes are used.

Trichoptilosis is the technical name for split hair. Treatment: The hair should be well oiled to soften and lubricate the excessively dry ends. The ends may also be removed by clipping or singeing.

Hypertrichosis (hirsuties) means superfluous hair; an abnormal development of hair on areas of the body normally bearing only lanugo hair. Treatments:

1. Dark hairs—bleached to render them less conspicuous.
2. Severe cases—by electrolysis, shaving or epilation.

Trichorrhexis nodosa, or knotted hair, is a dry, brittle condition with the formation of nodular swellings along the hair shaft. The hair breaks easily and shows a queer brush-like spreading out of the fibers of the broken off hair while the underlying tissues are normal. Shaving the head or softening the hair with ointments may prove beneficial.

Monilethrix is the technical term for beaded hair. The hair breaks between the beads or nodes. Scalp treatment may be beneficial.

Fragilitas crinium is the technical term for brittle hair. The hairs may split at any part of their length. The hair should be brushed to distribute the natural oil, and scalp treatments may be given.

Pigmentations of the Skin

Tan is caused by excessive exposure to the sun.

Lentigines (singular, lentigo) (freckles) are manifested by small yellowish to brownish colored spots occurring on those parts of the body exposed to sunlight and atmosphere, principally the face, hands and arms.

Chloasma (moth patches or liver spots) is characterized by increased deposits of pigment in the skin that have taken in a more or less localized portion of the body, mainly on the forehead, nose and cheeks.

Naevus (nevus) is commonly known as birthmark. It is a small circumscribed malformation of the skin due to pigmentation or dilated capillaries.

Leucoderma refers to abnormal whiteness in patches, a congenital condition of defective pigmentations of the skin. It is a colorless condition of the skin, classified as follows:

1. **Vitiligo**—an acquired condition of leucoderma. There is no treatment for this condition except to bleach the surrounding parts, thus making them less conspicuous.

2. **Albinism**—a congenital absence of pigment in the body including the skin, hair and eyes. This condition may be partial or entire.

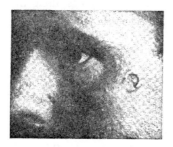

Deep-Seated Epithelioma
(Skin Cancer)

Epithelioma—A destructive skin cancer present on the skin. The new growth may appear on the surface of the skin or be deep-seated. It should always be referred to a physician.

Hypertrophies (New Growths)

Keratoma (callous) are acquired, superficial, circumscribed, thickened patches of epidermis, occurring for the most part in regions of pressure and friction on the hands and feet.

Verruca is the technical term for wart.

Xanthoma is a wart-like growth commonly located on the eyelids.

Keloid, a growth that develops in the subcutaneous tissue, is a dense fibrous growth usually forming at the site of a scar after an operation.

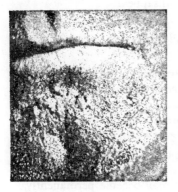

Acne keloid of the chin— An inflammation of the subcutaneous tissue of the skin, starting as pinhead papules which come together to form irregularly shaped scars. Also affects the subcutaneous tissue of the skin along the hair line at the back of the neck.

Acne Keloid of the Chin

Fibroma is a tumor composed mainly of fibrous connective tissue and is non-malignant.

Adenoma sebaceum is a small tumor of translucent appearance, usually occurring on the face in multiples, originating in the sebaceous glands.

NAIL DISORDERS

The barber should be able to recognize and tell the difference between normal and abnormal conditions of the nail.

Nail Irregularities

Corrugations or **wavy ridges** are caused by an uneven growth of the nails, usually resulting from illness. This condition is benefited by soaking the finger tips in warm olive oil for five minutes each day.

Leuconychia or **white spots** are caused by bruises or air bubbles in the nail body. Sometimes the white spots are caused by injuring the nail root. As the nail continues to grow, these white spots eventually disappear.

Onychauxis or **hypertrophy** is an overgrowth of the nail, either in length or thickness, usually caused by a local infection or other bodily disturbance.

Onychatrophia, atrophy or **wasting away** of the nail causes the nail to lose its lustre, become smaller and may shed entirely. Injury or disease may account for this nail irregularity. The nail should be protected from injury or exposure to strong soaps and washing powders.

Onychophagy or **bitten nails** is an acquired nervous habit which prompts the individual to chew the nail or the hardened cuticle. As a result, the nail may become permanently deformed. Oil should be applied to the cuticle regularly.

Onychorrhexis or **brittle nails.** This condition is caused by strongly alkaline soaps or chemicals and by rough manual labor. To correct this condition, discontinue the use of drying agents on the nails. Hot oil treatments are recommended. Cream or oil applied to the nail base, is also recommended.

Hangnails (**agnails**) is a condition in which the cuticle splits around the nail. Failure to correct dryness of the cuticle or cutting the cuticle too short or unevenly may result in hangnails. The cuticle should be softened with warm oil and then trimmed carefully.

Pterygium is a forward growth of the cuticle which adheres to the base of the nail. To remove the adhering growth use a sharp knife or instrument.

A bruised nail may be kept from discoloring, by placing it alternately in bowls of hot and cold water, immediately after the accident. A tablespoonful of epsom salt, added to the hot water, has a healing effect.

Nail Diseases

Any nail disease which shows signs of infection or inflammation (redness, pain, swelling or pus). Medical treatment is required for all nail diseases.

Onychosis (onychonosus) is a technical term applied to any nail disease.

Onychomycosis, tinea unguium or **ringworm of the nails** is an infectious disease caused by a vegetable parasite. The nails tend to become thick, furrowed and brittle in appearance.

Paronychia or **felon** is an infectious and inflammatory condition of the tissues surrounding the nails. This condition is traceable to bacterial infection.

Onychia is an inflammation of the nail matrix accompanied by pus formation. Improper sterilization of nail imstruments and bacterial infection may cause this disease.

Onychocryptosis or **ingrown nails** may affect either the finger or toe. In this condition, the nail grows into the sides of the flesh and may set up an infection. Rounding nail corners and failing to correct hangnails are often responsible for ingrown nails.

Blue nails may be attributed to poor blood circulation or a cardiac disorder.

SYPHILIS

Syphilis probably kills more people than any other contagious disease. It may have serious consequences for the infected person if not properly treated. If neglected, it may cause grave complications such as heart trouble, blindness, paralysis or insanity. Besides causing harm to the individual, syphilis is also a menace to the community. This disease may be carried from one person to another.

Syphilis is a dangerous disease caused by tiny germs known to doctors as the treponema pallida (also called the spirochaeta pallida). The disease germs enter the body through the skin or mucous membranes of the body. The most common way of infection is through sexual intercourse with a person having the disease. Other channels of infection are kissing an infected person and the use of infected materials.

The barber can do his part in preventing the spread of this harmful disease. Through his friendly help, the barber can direct a customer to seek competent advice if there is the slightest suspicion of syphilis. Delay reduces the chances of cure. Only a physician is qualified to diagnose and prescribe treatment for this condition. The infected person must never get into the hands of a quack doctor, or try to cure himself with patent medicines. If in doubt as to who is qualified to treat syphilis consult with your local Health Department.

The symptoms or signs of syphilis appear in three stages.

First stage. Several weeks after the disease germs get into the body, a sore or chancre usually appears at the spot where they entered. Little discomfort is experienced in early syphilis. After a few weeks, the chancre heals and leaves a scar. In the meantime, the disease germs reach the bloodstream and are carried to all parts of the body where they begin to do their damage.

Second stage. This stage of syphilis develops about three to six weeks after the chancre has appeared. As the disease

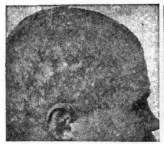 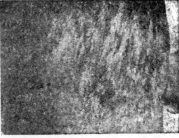

Patchy Syphilitic Alopecia
Occurring during the second stage of syphilis

progresses, the following symptoms may occur in a mild or severe form.

1. Skin rash.   4. Loss of hair.
2. Sores in mouth and throat.   5. Fever and headache.
3. Swollen glands.

Third stage. If syphilis has not been treated and cured at this stage, it may damage the vital organs such as the heart and brain.

Syphilis is most infectious in the primary and secondary stages, especially when the lesions (chancre and mucous patches) are located on an exposed part of the body or in the mouth. The open sores or chancres in syphilis contain the germs of the disease. Syphilis can be readily spread from the infected to the healthy person by direct, or immediate body to body contact; and by indirect means through contact with infected objects. The barber has a responsibility to himself and his customers and should refuse to serve any person known or suspected of having syphilis in its early stages. If in doubt whether a person has syphilis, take every precaution to sterilize all objects coming in contact with the customer.

GONORRHEA

Gonorrhea is a contagious disease which generally attacks the mucous membranes covering the mouth, eyes, sex organs and other internal structures of the body. It is caused by a tiny germ called the diplococcus (gonococcus) of Neisser. Gonorrhea, like syphilis, is usually spread by sexual relations with an infected person or contact with infected objects harboring the disease germs.

The first symptoms of gonorrhea usually appear in from two to five days after exposure. At first, itching and burning feelings are experienced in the affected parts. Shortly afterward, a discharge of pus begins to come from the inflamed organ. The pus discharge from an infected person contains an abundance of disease germs. At this stage, gonorrhea is highly contagious and the barber should take every precaution to prevent the spread of the disease to others.

As with syphilis, the barber should refuse to serve any person known or suspected of having gonorrhea. The best assistance the barber can give is to recommend medical treatment as soon as possible.

Failure to treat gonorrhea in its early stages may cause the disease to spread to adjacent or remote tissues, thereby causing further complications. Occasionally, in the later stages, gonorrhea attacks the lining of the heart, the joints and the lining around the liver.

THE CONTROL OF VENEREAL DISEASE

The success of any program to eliminate syphilis and gonorrhea depends upon the wholehearted cooperation of every barber and member of the community.

An effective program of venereal disease control is based upon prevention, diagnosis and treatment.

The aim of every health program for control of venereal disease is to find infected persons and start treatment soon after the infection. The person who receives prompt treatment is more likely to be cured, besides preventing the spread of the infection to other people. If every infected person would refrain from exposing others to the disease, begin early treatment and continue treatments until cured or rendered non-infectious, venereal disease would soon be conquered.

Medical science has introduced the use of penicillin and sulfa drugs for the treatment of venereal diseases. Patients may now be treated in hospitals and rendered non-infectious within a short period of time. Health Departments are now offering free treatments to those who cannot afford the services of a private doctor.

Syphilis and gonorrhea can be cured if treated by a skilled physician as soon as the first sign of infection is detected. If treatment is either neglected or delayed, the cure may take a long time and permanent damage may be the final result. Only a reliable physician can safely decide which treatment is best for the patient.

The barber can make his contribution to public health by:

1. Eliminating the sources of infection in the barber shop.

2. Encouraging early medical treatment for those who need it.

3. Urging the infected person to follow the doctor's instructions.

4. Cooperating with health officials on any campaign to control venereal diseases.

DISORDERS OF THE SKIN

1. a) Define dermatology. b) What is a dermatologist?	a) Dermatology is the science of the skin, its nature, structure, functions, diseases and treatment. b) A dermatologist is a skin specialist.
2. a) What is the most common disease of the oil glands? b) What causes it?	a) Comedones or blackheads. b) A worm-like mass of hardened sebum obstructing the duct of the oil gland.
3. Name the primary lesions of the skin.	Macule, papule, wheal, tubercle, tumor, vesicle, bulla, pustule.
4. Differentiate between objective lesion and subjective lesion.	An objective lesion is one that can be seen, such as pimples, while a subjective lesion is one that can be felt, as in itching, pains, etc.
5. Define acne rosacea; is it contagious?	Acne rosacea is a chronic congestion of the skin, usually confined to the nose and cheeks. It is not contagious.
6. What are freckles, and what causes them?	Freckles are yellowish to brownish colored spots occurring on those parts of the body exposed to sunlight and atmosphere, and are caused by excess pigmentation.
7. Name the secondary lesions of the skin.	Scale, crust, excoriation, fissure, ulcer, scar and skin stain.
8. What is acne? Give three suggestions for its prevention.	Acne is a chronic inflammation of the oil glands. Prevention—extreme cleanliness, proper diet, and regular and thorough evacuation.
9. Define hyperidrosis; what parts of the body are most commonly affected?	Hyperidrosis is excessive perspiration. The most commonly affected parts are the armpits and joints.
10. Name a disease of the skin caused by a vegetable parasite.	Ringworm.
11. Matching test: freckles cicatrix warts furuncles scar lentigines blackheads verrucae boils comedones	Freckles—lentigines. Warts—verrucae. Scar—cicatrix. Blackheads—comedones. Boils—furuncles.
12. Name six different forms of acne.	Acne vulgaris or simplex, acne punctata, acne papulosa, acne pustulosa, acne indurata, and acne rosacea.
13. Matching test: milia tumor phyma fever blister squama whiteheads dermatitis inflammation herpes scale simplex impetigo scrum-pox	Milia—whiteheads. Phyma—tumor. Squama—scale. Dermatitis—inflammation. Herpes simplex—fever blister. Impetigo—scrum-pox.

14. What is a carbuncle, and what causes it?	Carbuncle is a boil, caused by bacterial infection.
15. Define the following: a) eczema. b) albinism.	a) Eczema is an inflammation of the skin accompanied by itching, burning, and other unpleasant sensations. b) Albinism is a congenital condition, a deficiency of the pigment in the skin, hair and eyes.
16. Place the medical term after the common name in the list below: a) birthmark. b) liver spots. c) hives. d) callous.	 a) naevus. b) chloasma. c) urticaria. d) keratoma.
17. Name six diseases of the sebaceous (oil) glands.	Seborrhea, asteatosis, comedones, acne, milia and steatoma.
18. What causes urticaria? Describe its appearance.	Urticaria is caused by eating shellfish, strawberries, etc., or by contact with herbs or shrubs of the nettle family. It is characterized by eruptions of itching wheals or red elevations.
19. Name the common diseases of the sweat glands, and briefly describe each.	Hyperidrosis—excessive sweating. Bromidrosis—foul-smelling sweat. Miliaria rubra—prickly heat. Anidrosis—lack of perspiration. Sudamen—non-inflammatory eruption containing perspiration.

DISORDERS OF THE SCALP AND HAIR

1. Define trichology.	Trichology is the science of the hair and its diseases.
2. Is the ordinary falling out of hair considered a disease? Explain.	No; a certain amount of hair, that has grown to its full length, falls out when it is replaced by new hair.
3. At what time of the year is falling out of the hair most noticeable?	In the spring and fall.
4. Define the following: a) trichoptilosis. b) trichophytosis. c) trichorrhexis nodosa.	a) trichoptilosis—split hair. b) trichophytosis—ringworm of the scalp. c) trichorrhexis nodosa—knotted hair.
5. What is meant by: a) canities? b) name three types.	a) Canities is the technical term for gray hair. b) Congenital canities, accidental canities and acquired canities.
6. What is meant by ringed hair?	Ringed hair is a form of canities in which the hair shows alternate pigmented and white segments.
7. Give several causes for acquired canities.	Worry, anxiety, nervous strain, prolonged illness, various wasting diseases, and hereditary tendency.

8. How is dandruff recognized?	Dandruff is recognized by the presence of white scales in the hair, and on the scalp.
9. What is a direct cause of dandruff?	A direct cause of dandruff is the excessive shedding of the epithelial cells. Instead of growing to the surface and falling off, the horny scales accumulate on the scalp.
10. Give the medical term for: a) dandruff. b) dry type of dandruff. c) greasy or waxy type of dandruff.	a) Pityriasis. b) Pityriasis capitis simplex. c) Pityriasis steatoides.
11. What is meant by alopecia? Can it be cured?	Alopecia is the technical term for baldness. It is curable only in the early stages of the disease.
12. What is alopecia senilis?	Alopecia senilis is baldness occurring in old age.
13. What is the common name for each of the following medical terms? a) pediculosis capitis. b) tinea sycosis. c) tinea favosa. d) tinea tonsurans. e) scabies.	a) Head louse. b) Ringworm of the bearded area. c) Honeycomb ringworm of the scalp. d) Ringworm of the scalp. e) The itch.
14. How is pediculosis capitis treated?	The entire head is shampooed with equal parts of larkspur tincture and ether before retiring, and shampooed with germicidal soap the next morning. If necessary, the treatment should be repeated.
15. What is alopecia areata?	Alopecia areata is baldness in spots.
16. What is hypertrichosis?	Hypertrichosis is superfluous hair.
17. What does oily condition of the hair indicate?	A disturbance of the sebaceous glands, due to an excessive discharge of sebum.
18. What is favus? What treatment would you suggest?	Favus is an infectious parasitic fungus growth characterized by round crusts on the scalp, having a peculiar mousy odor. The customer should be referred to a physician.
19. Name three contagious nail diseases.	Onychomycosis, paronychia, and onychia.
20. Name two contagious venereal diseases.	Syphilis and gonorrhea.

PART IV

WOMEN'S HAIRCUTTING

The art of haircutting or bobbing requires thorough instruction in the proper way to shorten, thin and shape the hair by means of shears, razor or clipper. Skill can be developed only after patient practice on living models. A good haircut is important because it serves as a foundation for beautiful coiffures. The barber's education is not complete until he has acquired artistic skill and judgment in haircutting.

Modern haircuts are styled to bring out the customer's individuality and to accentuate her good points while con-

VARIOUS SHAPES OF HEADS

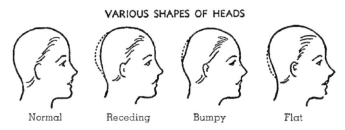

Normal   Receding   Bumpy   Flat

cealing her poor features. The barber must be guided by the customer's wishes as well as what is best for her personality. In selecting the proper hair style, the barber should take into consideration the customer's head shape, her facial contour, her neck line and hair texture.

Preparation of Customer

A hydraulic chair is used for hair cutting, and a tissue neck band is adjusted closely around the customer's neck. A hair cloth is then adjusted, allowing the tissue band to protrude for about half its width.

The hair is then carefully combed straight down on the sides and in the back, and the contour of the head studied carefully.

Cutting Virgin Hair

In cutting a virgin head of hair, it is customary to cut off the long hair with a few clips of the haircutting shears at a point about half an inch below the desired length. This will create a long straight bob. If this type of cut is desired, the shears are used to trim off any projecting ends. In case the hair is very thick, this straight bob must be thinned out, as described later.

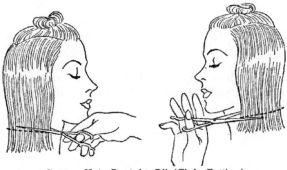

Cutting Hair Straight Off (Club Cutting)

Slithering

To bring out the graceful curves of the head, the hair must be thinned and tapered by slithering. This is accomplished by either of the following methods.

Method 1—Using regular haircutting shears, hold a small strand of hair between the thumb and index finger, and insert the hair in the shears so that only the underneath section of the hair will be shortened. Slide the shears up and down the strand, closing them slightly each time the shears is moved towards the scalp. Slither enough to allow the hair to lie close to the scalp wherever needed.

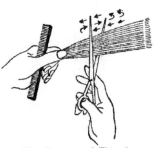

The Process of Thinning the Hair (Slithering)

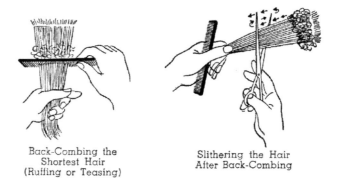

Back-Combing the
Shortest Hair
(Ruffing or Teasing)

Slithering the Hair
After Back-Combing

The short hair may be ruffed or back-combed as shown
in illustration, and then slithered as explained above.

STRANDS OF HAIR

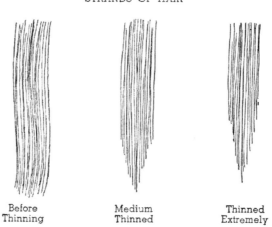

Before
Thinning

Medium
Thinned

Thinned
Extremely

Method 2—Holding the hair between the index and middle fingers. In this method more hair is slithered, thereby hastening the process.

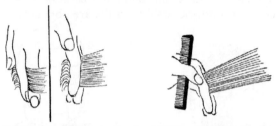

Holding the Hair between the Middle and Index Fingers

In order to avoid the slipping out of the hair, the middle finger should overlap the index finger a trifle.

Method 3—Using thinning shears, take a strand of hair between the **index** and **middle fingers**. Spread it well, and

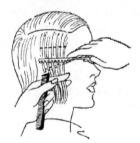

Thinning the Hair, using the
Thinning (Serrated) Shears

cut by means of simply closing the thinning shears held at right angles. The cuts are made starting about one inch from the scalp and repeated toward the ends of the hair, at regular intervals; then the hair strands are combed out to remove the cut hair ends.

Method 4—Using the razor for thinning and tapering. For detailed instructions, see Razor Cutting on page 371.

Layer Haircutting with Scissors
and Thinning Shears

Layer haircutting is the thinning operation repeated all over the head until the desired results are obtained.

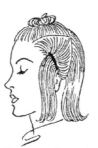

The Hair Correctly
Sectioned

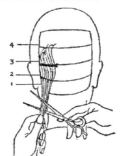

Thinning the Lowest Layer
Using Shears
Top Layer Held Out of Way
with Comb

Before the hair can be properly cut, it is combed and brushed free from tangles.

Part the hair across the crown from back of ear to back of ear, and then from each temple to crown. Pin the remaining hair on top of the head. The hair on each side of the head is held out of the way with combs.

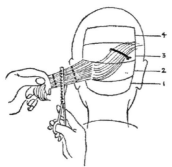

Thinning the Lowest Layer Using
Serrated Shears
Top Layer Held Out of Way
with Comb

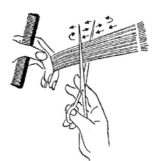

Thinning the Hair by Holding it
between Index and Middle
Fingers

Starting at the lowest layer, the thinning is done by dividing the hair into small sections and parting and lifting each resulting lock separately. The length of the stroke in slithering depends upon the thickness or thinness of the hair. For instance, if the strand is thick the stroke is short, and if the strand is thin the stroke is long.

After the lowest layer is completed, repeat the thinning process on the second layer, and continue with each layer until you have reached the crown.

To thin the sides, part the hair previously pinned to the top of the head and slither the hair on the sides in layers, as directed for the back of the head.

Suggestions for Deformed Heads

For a long neck—Do not expose the neck by giving a bob or shingle cut; leave the hair longer.

For a narrow head—Thin the hair at the back of the head and leave it tapered and fluffy at the sides.

For a broad head—Thin the hair at the sides and leave it full or fluffy at the back.

For a short, round head—Taper the neck line into a V shape; do not give a bob with a round neck line.

Razor Haircutting

Haircutting with a razor differs from other methods of haircutting in that a sharp razor is used when cutting hair that has been dampened by water. This method of haircutting is preferred by many hairstylist. Much care and skill are required to know where and how to cut the hair properly.

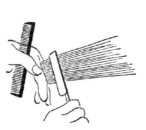

Proper way to Hold the Hair
for Razor Haircutting

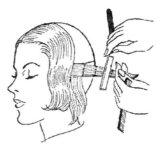

Layer Haircutting the Back
Part of the Head

After the hair has been dampened, combed, blocked and sectioned, it is ready to be cut with a razor. As the hair strand is drawn towards the operator, the razor is placed flat, not erect, about one inch from the scalp. Using short, steady, downward strokes towards the ends, the hair is tapered to the necessary thickness and length. Many hairstylists prefer to taper both on top and bottom of the strand.

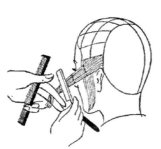

Layer Haircutting the
Sides of the Head

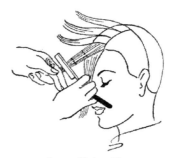

Layer Haircutting
the Bangs

THE BOYISH BOB
Also Known as The Shingle Bob

The Boyish Bob may be parted on the side or in the middle. It is cut in the following manner:

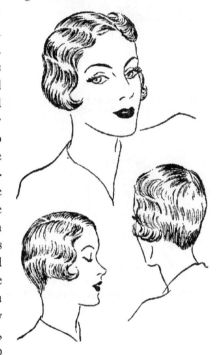

First part the hair as desired and smooth down with comb and brush. If the hair is too long, cut evenly all around, about one and one-half inches below the ear lobe. Start to cut at the back of the head about three-quarters up from the nape of the neck. Continue this operation with graduating shortness as you go down toward the neck, increasing the length gradually as you go toward the side. How long the hair should be, or how close to the scalp it should be cut, must be decided in each case, depending upon the desire of the customer and the shape of the head.

If thinning or tapering is desired, follow directions as previously explained.

After establishing a hair line, taper upward, being careful to leave the ears well covered. Taper the side below the ear lobe slightly upward, and taper the hair below and in back of the ears to create a smooth contour.

Helpful Hints On Shingling
For The Boyish Bob

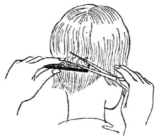

Shingling the back of the head
in a graduating effect

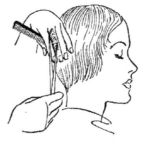

Trimming the hair ends over
forefinger and middle finger to
even up any irregularities or
protruding ends

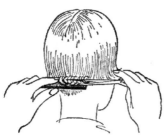

Trimming the neckline upward
in a graduating effect

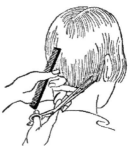

Shaping the neckline with the
points of the scissors

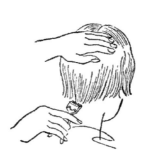

Cleaning the Neck
with Clippers

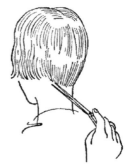

Cleaning the Neck with the
Points of the Shears

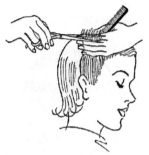

Tapering the Hair Ends by
Cutting the Hair held in an
Upward Position

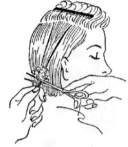

Trimming and Tapering the
Hair Ends by Using the
Slithering Method

Shaping Neck Line

The neck lines of short bobs can be shaped into natural, "V," oval or round shape first, then followed by shingling the hair to conform with the neck line, taking care not to allow too much of the neck exposed. The neck lines of conservative bobs are shaped after the thinning is done.

Completing the Haircut

The customer is then given the opportunity of viewing her head in the mirror with the aid of a large hand mirror. The hair cloth is loosened, the tissue removed and discarded, and the hair cloth carefully removed so that no cut hair falls onto the customer's clothes. If any short hairs remain on the neck after the tissue band is removed, they can be removed with tissues sprinkled with talcum powder.

Hair requiring waving. Should the hair require waving, leave the hair one inch longer to allow for the waves.

Concerning the Clippers

There is a mistaken idea amongst women that the use of the clippers to clean the neck line has a tendency to make the hair grow in thicker at the neck. This is not true, however, as the amount of human hair can only be as great as the number of follicles on the neck, and these do not increase by the use of the clippers or any other instrument.

POPULAR HAIR STYLES FOR YOUNG GIRLS

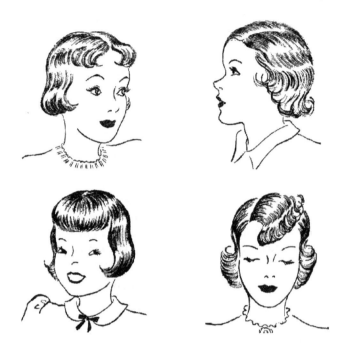

Special consideration should be given to children. Knowing how to handle the children is where their mothers go and have their own hair done.

SPECIAL PROBLEMS
Correcting Split Hair Ends

Trichoptilosis is the technical term for **split hair ends**. When the hair becomes dry and brittle, due to several causes, the hair ends frequently split. Temporary relief for this condition may be obtained either by singeing or clipping the hair ends.

Singeing is the process of burning off split ends of the hair, and should be given just before a shampoo.

The hair is combed thoroughly and divided into small, equal sections. Each section or strand is twisted tightly from the scalp to the ends, and left for an instant while the wax taper is lighted.

The twisted strand is then held in the left hand while the extended fingers of the right hand ruff the strand upward to the scalp. During this process the lighted taper stands erect and out of the way. This ruffing motion frees the split end, which will now protrude from the tightly twisted strand of hair.

Next the taper is passed under the strand so that the frayed hair ends are ignited. The strands are all treated in the same way, the taper is extinguished, and the hair thoroughly brushed to remove burnt particles. The hair is then shampooed in the usual way.

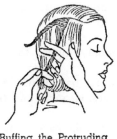

Ruffing the Protruding
Hair Ends

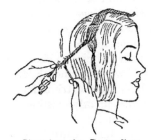

Singeing the Protruding
Hair Ends

Clipping

Split ends may be clipped in case the customer prefers this process to singeing.

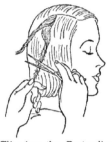

Clipping the Protruding
Hair Ends

The hair is combed, divided, twisted and ruffed as before, but the split hair ends are removed with clipping shears. Beginning near the scalp, cut alongside of the strand all protruding hair ends, gradually moving downward to the end of the strand, where the remaining ends are cut. The hair is then brushed briskly to remove the short hair clippings.

Terms Used in Connection with Haircutting

Hairdressing is the art of arranging the hair into various becoming shapes or styles. The contour of the face, shape of the head, and the current season's styles, must all be considered in this phase of the work.

Hair stylist—A hairdresser who has the artistic ability to suggest and create a becoming new hair fashion.

Haircutting—The shortening, thinning and tapering of the hair, using comb and shears, to mold the hair into a becoming shape.

Hair bobbing—The term commonly applied to the cutting of women's and children's hair.

Hair trim or trimming—Cutting the hair lightly in going over the already existing formed lines, cleaning and tidying the neckline.

Shingling—Cutting the hair close to the nape of the neck, leaving the hair gradually longer as you go higher toward the crown of the head, without showing a definite line.

Thinning—Decreasing the thickness of the hair where it is too heavy.

Tapering—Shortening and thinning the hair at the same time.

Feathering—Another term for thinning and tapering.

Slithering—The process used in tapering and thinning the hair.

Shredding—Another term for slithering.

Effileing—A French term for slithering.

Clipping—The operation of removing the hair by the use of hair clippers. Removing split hair ends or cutting the extreme ends of the hair with the shears is also known as clipping.

Singeing—Burning the hair ends by the quick passing of a lighted wax taper over the split ends of the hair.

Club cutting—Cutting the hair straight off, without thinning or tapering.

Layer cutting—Tapering and thinning the hair by dividing it into many thin layers.

Razor cutting—The use of the razor in thinning or cutting the hair.

Natural hair line—Where no artificial hair line is created; the hair at the nape of the neck is left in its natural hair line.

Artificial hair line—A neck line which has been changed by cutting into a V, oval, or round shape.

Featheredge—When the hair line at the nape of the neck is carried smoothly upward into a graceful, straight effect, and the neck is cleaned at the base with clippers, a little higher than the natural hair line.

Back-combing—Combing the short hairs towards the scalp. Other terms used for back-combing are: teasing, ruffing.

FINGER WAVING AND PIN CURLING

Finger Waving

Finger waving is popular in the designing of artistic hair styles. No expensive equipment nor complicated procedures are required for finger waving. With the aid of water, comb and his own fingers, the barber can employ finger waving anywhere and anytime. A barber who is competent as a finger waver can always command a good paying position.

Finger waving is the art of shaping the hair, wetted with waving lotion, into becoming waves with the aid of the fingers and comb. Better results in producing soft, natural waves are obtained with hair that has a natural wave or has been permanently waved, rather than with straight hair.

The use of the right kind of **waving lotion** is an aid to better finger waving. Besides making the hair more pliable, the application of a waving lotion holds the hair in place while the hair is drying. A good waving lotion is harmless to the hair and should not flake upon drying.

A pleasing finger wave should harmonize with the shape of the customer's head, as well as her features.

Practice on Dressing Block

It is very much easier for beginners to learn finger waving by practice on hair pieces before attempting to wave living hair, and for that reason preliminary instructions are given for work on hair pieces.

Preparation of hair. An ordinary switch or weft may be used, the support is fastened firmly to a dressing block. The hair piece is thoroughly moistened with water, using the fine teeth of a dressing comb to comb the water through the hair until the hair piece lies flat on the block.

Movements For A Right-Going Wave

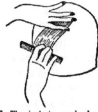
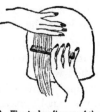
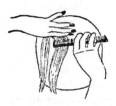

1. The hair is combed at a slightly slanted angle to the left.

2. The index finger of the left hand is placed directly above the position for the first ridge and the hair under the index finger is combed downward.

3. With teeth pointing slightly upward, the comb is inserted directly under the index finger. In one motion, draw the comb ¼" away from the index finger and direct the hair ¾" to the right.

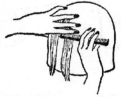
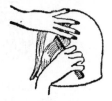

4: With the teeth still inserted in the ridge, the comb is flattened against the dressing block in order to hold the ridge in place. (The left hand is not shown in the illustration so that you may see the ridge and position of comb.)

5. Remove the left hand from the dressing block and place the middle finger above the ridge and the index finger on the teeth of the comb. Emphasize the ridge by closing the two fingers and applying pressure to the dressing block. **DO NOT SQUEEZE THE RIDGE UPWARD.**

6. Without removing the comb, the teeth are turned downward and the hair combed in a right semi-circular effect to form a dip in the groove of the right-going wave.

Left-going wave. The fingers of the left hand are now moved carefully. The index finger is placed directly above the position for the second ridge (to give the average size wave the index finger is placed about 1½ inches from the ridge just formed) the comb and fingers are now used to build another ridge by repeating the movements, **except that the hair is directed to the left.** The movements are repeated for the entire length of the hair strand.

The index finger and the middle finger have the double duty of holding down the waves already made and forming the ridges between them.

Matching Waves

When the student has learned to finger wave a straight hair piece, he is ready to learn the matching of waves.

Part the hair into 2½-inch sections for convenience in waving. Special care must be taken to match the waves exactly so that the finished work will show no line of demarcation between the sections. This will require considerable practice before the waves can be matched perfectly without disturbing the complete section.

The ends of the hair may be coiled into pin curls.

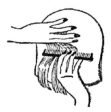 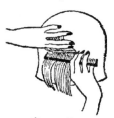

Matching
Right-going Waves

Connecting
Right-going Waves

Place forefinger ¼" to the left and above the ridge already made. With teeth upward, place comb under the forefinger and repeat the finger waving movements described previously, allowing the comb to work over part of the adjoining ridge and wave.

 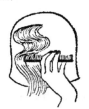

Left Wave
Begin on Left

Connecting the
Second Wave

For a left-going wave, begin work on the left side of the hair piece or weft.

The time spent in matching waves on the dressing block will be profitably expended as the student will learn to make even-sized, regular waves, and will become accustomed to the way in which hair lies on the human head.

FINGER WAVING ON A LIVE MODEL

The barber washes his hands and has available sterile implements and clean supplies. The customer is seated comfortably and a neck strip and shampoo cape are properly adjusted. The proper amount of waving lotion to use should be based on the following factors:

Naturally or **permanently waved hair** requires either light, medium or heavy waving lotion, governed by the texture and condition of the customer's hair.

Shaping the Finger Wave

1. Comb hair on heavy side away from the face.
2. Place index finger of left hand on the front part of the head, from two to three inches from the part.

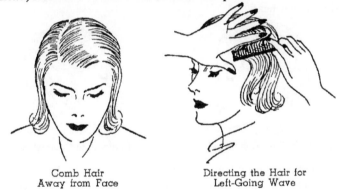

Comb Hair
Away from Face

Directing the Hair for
Left-Going Wave

3. With comb in right hand, insert the teeth under index finger and direct hair for a left-going wave towards the face as previously explained on pages 380-381.

4. To emphasize the ridge, press the fingers against the head. (Do not pinch the ridge as the hair would be pushed upward and out of position.)

5. Roll the index finger upward and re-insert the fine teeth of the comb, and comb hair smooth.

6. Follow the line of this ridge to crown where it is lost. (See illustration on next page.)

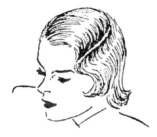

The First Ridge
Completed

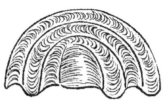

Diagram for Side Part
Wide Wave Hair Style

7. Now move to the opposite side of the customer.

8. Comb hair on thin side away from face.

9. Proceed for a right-going wave and continue this ridge around the head. This will complete the first wave on heavy side of the head.

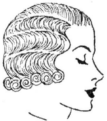

Light Side Completed

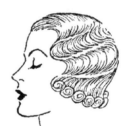

Heavy Side Completed

10. Begin second wave at the hair line on the heavy side, directing the hair towards the face. Continue this ridge around the head to the thin side. Work from one side to the other until the entire head of hair is waved.

11. Finish the ends of the hair with pin curls.

Completing the Finger Wave

1. Attach net to hair and safeguard customer's forehead and ears with rubber discs and paper protectors.

2. Adjust the dryer to medium and allow hair to dry thoroughly.

3. Remove dryer, hair net and pins from hair.

4. Comb out curls and reset waves into a soft coiffure.

Popular Finger Waved Hair Styles

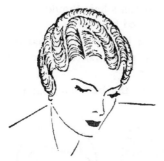

Side Part Medium Wave
Hair Style

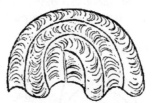

Diagram for Side Part
Medium Wave Hair Style

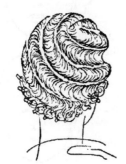

Semi-Swirl Finger Wave
Hair Style

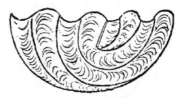

Diagram for
Semi-Swirl Hair Style

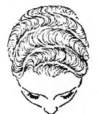

Pompadour
Hair Style

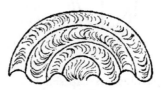

Diagram for
Pompadour Hair Style

PARTING THE HAIR

The manner of parting the customer's hair should be adjusted to her facial type and the desired hair style.

The hair stylist should be guided by the natural parting of the customer's hair. To locate this part, first comb the hair back tightly and then push it forward.

The following illustrations reveal the best hair partings for various facial types.

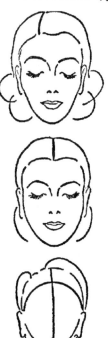

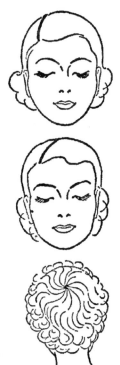

Side part. A high side parting is suitable for the oval facial type, whereas the low side parting is advisable for the triangle, round or square facial type.

Center part. Usually suggested for the oval facial type.

Diagonal part. Recommended for the round or square facial type.

Ear to ear . crown parting. Suggested for hair styles with high and low effects and forward movement of bangs.

Center back parting. Creates length to the head. Suggested for warm weather.

Cap shape crown. Some heads dress better without back partings. A cap shape wave that combs from the crown is suggested. This style requires a well-shaped head, and the face needs a halo effect of curls to frame it.

PIN CURLS

Pin curls, also called sculpture curls, are suitable for naturally curly or permanently waved hair. There are many methods of making pin curls. The ones described here are the most commonly used. The hair must be in a moist condition with water or with waving lotion.

Hair Ends Inside of Curls

Winding from Hair Ends to Scalp

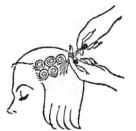

1—Separate the hair into small strands and comb smoothly.

2—Place index finger about two inches on the strand from hair ends.

3—Wind the hair ends around index finger, remove the wound hair off finger, pull slightly to insure a tight curl.

4—Roll the curl towards the scalp.

5—Pin the curl securely (left or right) in the direction in which it is to be combed.

Winding from Scalp to Hair Ends

1—Separate the hair into small strands, and comb smoothly.
2—Place back of index finger of left hand against scalp.
3—Wind hair with right hand around tip of finger, in the direction in which the resultant curl is to be set.
4—Force curl off fingers with hair ends inside of curl and pin it securely.

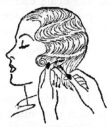

Illustration shows clockwise (c) winding. To obtain counterclock (cc) curl reverse the winding.

Hair Ends Outside of Curls

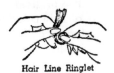

1—Separate the hair into small strands, and comb smoothly.
2—Place tip of left index finger in center of square and at right angles to the scalp.
3—Wind the hair flat with right hand around the index finger, in the direction in which the resultant curl is to be set.
4—Remove finger from curl and pin it securely.

Overlapping Curl

Hair Line Ringlets

A small strand of hair is rolled between the thumb and index fingers of both hands, and adjusted in a circular form with the hair ends on the inside of the circle. Pin securely until dry.

Hair Line Ringlet

MEN'S HAIR BLEACHING

Hair bleaching is a profitable source of income to the barber who possesses the necessary knowledge, experience and skill of this specialty. Men are prompted to have their hair bleached mostly because of necessity, and to improve their appearance. The man who is satisfied with the initial treatment, is bound to come back for a retouch at periodic intervals.

Hair bleaching removes color, upon application, and there is partial or total removal of the natural pigment.

Hair bleaching involves the application of chemical agents for the purpose of:

1. Lightening darker hairs so that gray hairs will not be too obvious.
2. Restoring hair to its original shade (if hair had been previously tinted).
3. Producing an entirely new shade of hair.

Hair bleaching **corrective treatments** are recommended for:

1. Men with prematurely gray hair. (Light complexion.)
2. The business man.
3. Men who must maintain a youthful appearance.
4. Changing an unattractive shade of hair.

To bleach hair successfully, one must have a knowledge of:

1. The general structure of hair and skin.
2. The composition, merits and limitations of all bleaching agents and formulas.
3. The chemical reactions following their application.
4. The correct method of application.

It is of great advantage to the barber to be capable in the art of hair coloring. His services become unlimited, and his customers do not have to look elsewhere for this service. The barber has a big advantage over the beautician when it comes to coloring hair. The application of bleach on women's hair is much more involved than the application to men's hair. Although the fee for the coloring service may be the same for both men and women, the cost of material for women's hair bleach is at least twice as much as that of men; plus the fact that there is less than half the time involved for the application of bleaching men's hair.

Hair Bleaching

Hair bleaching is the process of partially removing the natural pigment from the hair. Hair that is not in the best possible condition, may be damaged by bleaching treatments. Hence, the barber should carefully examine the texture and condition of the hair. A bleach should never be given to a customer whose scalp is not free from eruptions or abrasions.

The customer who has had his hair bleached for the first time, will appreciate good service by coming back for a retouch to the same shop and the same barber. If a written record is kept of the bleaching treatments, the work of the barber, in giving the retouch, will be simplified.

Prepared Bleaches

Many of the prepared bleaching agents in use today contain coloring matter. As a hair coloring technician, you should use these products as directed by the manufacturer in order to achieve the most satisfactory results.

Essentials For Hair Bleaching

To produce the best results in hair bleaching, the technician barber must be equipped with:

1. Various sizes of glass or porcelain dishes or flat cups.
2. Swab sticks and brushes.
3. Measuring cup.
4. Dropper.
5. Fresh peroxide—17 to 20 volume.
   (Some barbers prefer to use 25 volume hydrogen peroxide for quicker bleaching results.)
6. Ammonia water—28%.
7. White henna.
8. Oil bleaches.
9. Absorbent cotton.
10. Soap flakes.
11. Cream rinse.

There are many formulas for bleaching hair in use today, but professionally, the following agents are used:

1. Peroxide—17 to 20 volume. 25 volume for a quicker bleaching process.
2. Peroxide and ammonia.
3. Peroxide, ammonia and white henna.
4. Prepared bleaching powder and peroxide.
5. Colored oil bleaches.
6. Peroxide, ammonia and soap flakes.

Hydrogen Peroxide

The chemical composition of hydrogen peroxide is H_2O_2, which is two parts of hydrogen and two parts of oxygen. Hydrogen peroxide is a safe and dependable bleaching, softening and oxidizing agent, provided it is a fresh product, having 17 to 20 volume strength. It is available in two forms, liquid and tablet.

1. When **tablets** are used, it is important that they be completely crushed and dissolved, otherwise the full strength of the 20 volume hydrogen peroxide will not be released.
2. **Liquid** hydrogen peroxide deteriorates, and should be purchased in pint sizes, kept closed when not in use, and stored in a cool, dark, dry place.

Uses of Hydrogen Peroxide

As a **bleaching agent,** hydrogen peroxide solution, whose **function** is to soften the cuticle of the hair shaft, oxidizes to a lighter shade the grains of pigment or coloring matter in its inner cortical layer. If a solution of less than 17 volume is used, it will act too slowly. Some barbers prefer to use 25 volume hydrogen peroxide for quicker bleaching results.

Bleaching makes the hair porous, as well as lighter in color. The shades that may be obtained range from light brown and golden brown to straw color and platinum, depending upon the basic color of the hair and the formula of the bleach. Continued use of bleaches will make some hair over-dry and brittle. The addition of 28% **ammonia water hastens** the bleaching action of hydrogen peroxide.

An excess of ammonia is undesirable, since it imparts a reddish tint to the hair.

As a softening agent, hydrogen peroxide solution softens the outer cuticle of the hair and makes it more receptive to the penetrating action of an aniline derivative dye. Care must be taken to control the softening process so that the hair is not bleached.

As an oxidizing agent, hydrogen peroxide solution is used in all penetrating hair dyes. It acts as a developer to liberate oxygen gas which changes para-phenylene-diamine into a dark-colored compound capable of dyeing the hair.

Testing For Volume Content

There are two methods for testing the volume content of peroxide.

1. The hydrometer method.
2. The J tube method.

The most popular and quicker of the two is the hydrometer method because it requires the least amount of equipment.

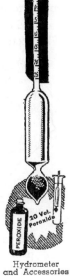

The hydrometer method. Pour a little of the liquid peroxide into a test tube. Immerse hydrometer into peroxide so that it floats in the peroxide. The reading on the hydrometer reveals the strength of the peroxide.

The J tube method. With the second method, peroxide may be tested by the use of a small instrument, consisting of a J tube, marked off in graduations, each representing one unit volume of gas. A solution of copper sulphate (blue vitriol), containing free ammonia, is added to the tube. The pipette (a slender, transparent glass tube) is filled with peroxide to be tested. One cubic centimeter of the peroxide is then released very slowly into the solution in the J tube, where oxida-

Hydrometer
and Accessories

tion immediately begins. Oxygen bubbles immediately form
and come to the surface at the top of the long arm of the
J tube.

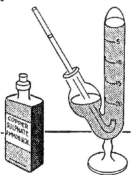

When the last bubble has
formed, note the number of the
graduations to which the oxygen
has forced the blue liquid. This
number shows precisely the number of cubic centimeters of oxygen
gas, or unit volumes, contained in
the original cubic centimeter of
peroxide. If the number noted is
less than "15 volume," it is not
satisfactory for hair dyeing or
hair bleaching purposes.

J Tube and Accessories

Procedure for Bleaching Virgin Head

A virgin head of hair is one which has not been previously
bleached or tinted.

It is desirable to bleach the hair before giving a haircut
in order to have more hair to work with.

1. Examine scalp and hair; shampoo and dry hair.
2. Section hair into quarters.

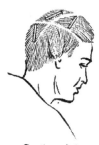
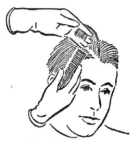
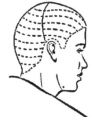

Sectioned in quarters

Subdividing hair into quarter inch strands

Approximate number of quarter inch strands

3. Prepare bleaching formula and use immediately to
   prevent deterioration. Note: The order of applying the
   bleach around the head is immaterial. If the hair

seems resistant or especially dark around the crown, then it is advisable to start at the back of the head to allow for extra time of contact at this region.

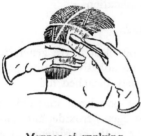

Manner of applying bleach

4. Apply bleach with swab or brush in quarter inch strands, proceeding from scalp to within one inch of the hair ends.

5. Continue to apply the bleach until the entire head is completed.

6. At the sides of the head where the hair is extremely short, the bleach is applied directly to hair without any attempt at sectioning.

7. Comb the bleach through to the hair ends.

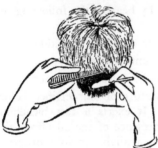

Applying bleach to neck hair with swab

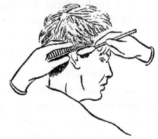

Applying bleach to sideburns with swab

8. Watch carefully for the development of proper shade.
9. Rinse hair with water and shampoo lightly.
10. Apply cream rinse. After 3 minutes rinse with warm water.
11. Dry hair and comb or dress hair as desired.

Causes of Unsatisfactory Hair Bleaching

1. Weakened peroxide.
2. Too much ammonia water in the bleach.
3. Bleaching formula left on the hair too long.

4. Bleaching formula removed too soon.
5. Poor application (overlapping).
6. Too slow in applying bleaching formula.
7. Using too large a swab for application.

Bleach Retouch

White henna, bleach cream or oil bleach, are generally used for a bleach retouch because its adhesive quality prevents the overlapping of the previously bleached hair.

White henna is made by mixing powdered magnesium carbonate with 17 to 20 volume hydrogen peroxide, and correct amount of 28% ammonia water to the consistency of a paste. To each ounce of peroxide add 3 to 5 drops of ammonia water, depending on the texture and color of the hair.

For quicker bleaching results, 25 volume peroxide is used, provided the patron can tolerate the stronger peroxide.

A bleach cream is prepared by beating the following ingredients into a creamy foam:

Half ounce of 17 to 20 volume hydrogen peroxide.

One to three drops of 28% ammonia water.

Add enough soap flakes to make a creamy mixture.

A colored oil bleach is a mixture of oil, certified color, ammonia water and peroxide. It exerts a fast bleaching action and does not run. The presence of the oil offsets the harsh action of the bleach. It is available in four different shades (neutral, gold, red, drab). Use only as directed by the manufacturer.

Procedure for a Bleach Retouch

The procedure for a bleach retouch is the same as that for bleaching a virgin head, except that the mixture is applied only to the new growth of hair and not to the rest of the bleached hair. A swab is employed to apply the bleach mixture from the scalp to a point where the new growth ends, being careful to prevent overlapping. Using a swab, the bleach may be applied freely at the sides of the head and at the neckline where the hair is extremely short.

In keeping records of retouch bleaching, include such information as date, bleaching mixture, what section of the

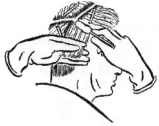

head application was started and length of time bleach remained on the hair.

Bleaching Shampoos

Bleaching shampoos are used to lighten the hair, but not to the extent where a retouch would be necessary. The effects of a bleaching shampoo fade out within a four week period,

Manner of applying
a bleach retouch

at which time, another application may be given. The fact that a retouch would not be necessary, indicates that a large range of shades cannot be produced with this process. Bleaching shampoos highlight and brighten the hair while the range of natural color remains the same.

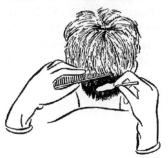

Apply the bleach on the neck
with a swab

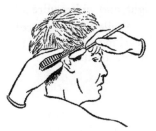

Apply the bleach to sideburns
with a swab

Bleaching shampoo is prepared with the following ingredients:

Three parts of 20 volume peroxide.

One part of concentrated shampoo.

Five drops of 28% ammonia water.

The mixture is applied as a regular shampoo treatment.

Bleaching shampoos should be recommended to all customers who feel that their hair is lacking in color, but do not wish a drastic change in hair color. The only disadvantage of bleaching shampoos is that frequent application will leave a line of demarcation.

Bleaching Rinses

The bleaching rinse is similar to the bleaching shampoo, with the exception of application. The bleaching rinse is applied on dry hair and is allowed to remain on the hair from two to four minutes before it is shampooed. The more porous the hair, the less time it remains on the hair. Although the mixture is the same as the bleaching shampoo, the action on the hair is twice as fast because it is applied on dry hair and is allowed to remain there from two to four minutes. Bleaching rinses are only recommended for the customer who wishes a noticeable change with one treatment.

Caution must be taken not to repeat bleaching rinses too frequently. The effects of the rinse last approximately four to six weeks. If a second application is given before the effects of the first rinse wears off, the change in color will be too light, and will require a touch-up as in regular hair bleaching.

While the actual color of the hair remains the same, the bleaching rinse will highlight and lighten the hair noticeably in one treatment.

Special Problems in Hair Bleaching

Reconditioning bleached hair. No matter how well hair has been treated during a bleaching process, it becomes very much affected by exposure to sun or salt water. Therefore, it is necessary to give reconditioning treatments at regular intervals. Commercial products are available for this treatment. Regular oil or cream treatments, although much slow-in responding, can be used for reconditioning. Hair that has been rendered very dry, brittle or porous, by excessive bleaching, requires reconditioning treatments to restore it to its normal condition. Remember that in giving reconditioning treatments, you are treating the hair itself, rather than the scalp. Take the hair between the palms of the hands and with a rotary movement, rub the oil well into the hair. After the application of oil or cream, the hair may be steamed or the therapeutic lamp or heating cap may be used. This treatment should be continued over a period of time until the hair is reconditioned.

Over-bleaching. The hair becomes over-bleached because it has been abused by the use of a strong bleaching formula, overlapping, or by retaining the bleach too long on the hair. If the hair is coarse, spongy and mats easily when wetted, it is over-bleached. Such hair should be given oil treatments, cream treatments or egg shampoos until such time as this condition has been corrected.

Testing for copper. Hair that is suspected of having been dyed with copper salts should be tested to reveal the presence or absence of copper before giving a bleaching treatment. Prepare a mixture of one-half ounce of hydrogen peroxide and 5 drops of 28% ammonia water. Holding a small strand (preferably in the front of the head underneath the part) between two fingers, apply the mixture and observe if the hair becomes warm to the touch. If it does, it indicates that copper salts have been used on the hair and should, therefore, be removed before bleaching is attempted; otherwise, breakage is likely to occur.

Bleaching Streaked Hair

Streaks of discoloration often appear on the hair, caused in part by unsuccessful and unskillful bleach applications.

To correct streaked hair:

1. Prepare bleach solution as for virgin head.
2. Apply mixture only to the darker streaks.
3. Work one strand at a time.
4. Allow to remain until all streaks are removed.
5. Shampoo hair.

Removing Yellow Streaks

Yellow streaks often appear in gray hair caused principally by strong soaps and exposure to sun.

To remove streaks caused by soap or sun:

1. Prepare bleach solution of one ounce 17 to 20 volume hydrogen peroxide with equal parts of alcohol, and one-quarter ounce of table salt.
2. Apply with brush only to yellow streaks.
3. Allow to remain, rewetting if necessary, until all traces of yellow disappear.
4. Witch hazel rinse may be used to remove the salt after the hair has had one soaping. Avoid the use of colored rinses until the hair has had time to recover from treatments.

Bleaching Partly Gray Hair

Partly gray hair, particularly if the natural shade was light, may be bleached to a more even shade. While the bleach mixture will not affect the color of the gray hair, it will lighten the still natural color hair. Commercial products are available under the name of Drab Bleach for this treatment. Follow directions of manufacturer when using these products.

Mustache and Eyebrow Bleaching

The formula for mustache and eyebrow bleaching consists of:

1. 1 ounce 20 volume peroxide.
2. 3 drops of ammonia water.
3. Enough white henna to make a paste.

It is applied to the hair only. Avoid getting the paste on the skin; allowing it to remain on the skin will result in a peroxide burn. It is dangerous to use any other bleaching formula for this purpose.

Reminders and Hints for Hair Bleaching

1. Always wash your hands, and use sterile swabs, brushes, combs and linens.

2. Be careful in applying bleach so that it does not run over clothing, nor come in contact with skin of the hands, face and neck.

3. To prepare an effective bleaching formula, use fresh materials having the proper strength, measure accurately, and use immediately after mixing.

4. The strength of hydrogen peroxide and ammonia water solutions becomes weakened when such bottles are exposed to the air for a long time, or stored in a warm place.

5. The strength of the bleaching formula and the length of time it is to be left on the hair, vary with the condition and texture of the hair and the shade of hair desired. Oily hair requires more time for bleaching than does dry hair.

6. A preliminary shampoo is advisable if the hair is excessively oily or dirty. Avoid irritation to the scalp during the shampoo.

7. Never use an acid rinse before a bleach.

8. Work as rapidly as possible in applying the bleach to produce a uniform shade without streaks.

9. Overlapping in a retouch can be prevented by using just enough moisture on the swab for the hair to absorb.

10. The final shampoo is given when desired shade has been obtained and all the paste mixture has been removed.

11. Bleached hair is fragile and, therefore, requires special care. A mild cleanser for bleached hair is an egg shampoo, followed by a hand dry.

12. Keep a complete and confidential record of all bleaching treatments.

HAIR BLEACHING

1. What actually takes place when hair is bleached?	The bleaching agent removes or oxidizes some of the original color in the hair.
2. Give three uses for hydrogen peroxide.	Hydrogen peroxide may be used as a bleaching agent, as a softening agent prior to hair tinting, and as an oxidizing agent when mixed with a dye.
3. How is the strength of the peroxide preserved?	Keep bottle closed and store it in a cool, dark and dry place. Use bleaching formula soon after it is prepared.
4. What shades can be obtained with a peroxide bleach?	Light brown, golden brown, straw color and platinum.
5. How long should a peroxide and ammonia bleach be left on the hair?	Until the color of the hair reaches the desired shade.
6. What are the most frequent causes of overbleaching?	Too much ammonia water in the bleach, overlapping, and too long an application of the bleach will cause over-bleaching.
7. What is the best treatment for overbleached hair?	Hot oil treatments, cream treatments or egg shampoos.
8. How can the action of the peroxide be hastened?	The addition of ammonia water to the bleaching formula will hasten the action of peroxide.
9. How can the action of peroxide be slowed down?	Diluting the bleaching mixture with water or antiseptic oil.
10. What will stop the action of the bleach?	Drying of the hair or a shampoo.
11. What is white henna and when is it used?	White henna is a creamy substance of powdered magnesium carbonate with hydrogen peroxide and ammonia water. It is used for a bleach retouch.
12. To what part of the hair is a bleach retouch applied?	A bleach retouch is applied only to the new growth of hair.
13. Name two preparations that can be used instead of white henna for bleach retouch.	Bleach cream and colored oil bleach.
14. a) Give two methods for testing the volume content of hydrogen peroxide. b) Which is the quickest method?	a) The hydrometer method and the J tube method. b) The hydrometer method.

MEN'S HAIR TINTING

Hair tinting is another profitable source of income to the barber who possesses the necessary knowledge, experience and skill. Hair tinting involves the addition of an artificial color to the natural pigment in the hair. The resultant color may duplicate a natural shade or produce an entirely new shade of hair.

Hair Tinting

Hair tinting falls into two main groups, depending upon the action of the colorings, whether they are **temporary or permanent.**

All hair dyes on the market are proprietary products, with the exception of vegetable colorings, the dyes should be used according to the manufacturer's directions.

The routines given here, with minor exceptions, will be found satisfactory with practically every dye manufactured.

Hair tinting involves the application of chemical agents for the purpose of:

1. Covering gray hair.
2. Restoring hair to its original shade.
3. Producing an entirely new shade of hair.

Hair tinting treatments are recommended for:

1. Men with prematurely gray hair.
2. The business man.
3. Men who must maintain a youthful appearance.
4. Restoring bleached hair to its natural shade.
5. Changing an unattractive shade of hair.

Aniline derivative dyes are the most popular with men's hair tinting because they can duplicate a natural shade of hair. A very small percentage of the men tinting their hair use metallic or compound dyestuffs.

The successful barber who has a hair tinting practice, must have the knowledge of:

1. The general structure of the hair and skin.
2. The composition, merits and limitations of softeners, developers, hair dyes and bleaches.

3. The chemical reactions following their application.

4. The correct method of application.

There are unlimited advantages for the barber who maintains a practice in hair tinting. Although his customer may stop off and get his hair cut in another establishment, the chances are that the same customer will never allow any one else to color his hair. This extra service not only insures a better income, but puts the barber on a higher level with his customers.

Men's hair tinting is easier and more profitable than women's. The application of dye on women's hair is much more involved than the application on men's hair. Although the fee for coloring may be the same for both men and women, the cost of material for women's hair tinting is at least twice as much as that for men; plus the fact that there is less than half the time involved for the application on men's hair.

The combination of smaller costs for material and less time for application, means greater profits in men's hair tinting.

Examining Scalp and Hair

The scalp and hair are carefully examined to determine if it is safe to use an aniline derivative dye and whether any special hair dyeing problems exist.

An aniline derivative dye **should not be used** if the following conditions are recognized.

1. Signs of a positive skin test, such as redness, swelling, itching and blisters.
2. Scalp sores or eruptions.
3. Contagious scalp or hair disease.

If the scalp and hair are in a healthy condition, carefully observe and record data relative to:

1. **Type of hair.** Degree of porosity either very receptive, moderately receptive, very resistant or moderately resistant.

2. **Texture of hair.** Coarse, medium, fine or wiry hair.

3. **Color of hair.** Natural or artificial and the percentage of gray hair present.

4. **Forms of hair.** Straight, curly, wavy or permanently waved.

5. **Condition of hair and scalp.** Dry, normal or oily.

The results of such an examination may indicate the need for any of the following:

1. Giving reconditioning treatments.
2. Using the proper strength of softener for the particular type and texture of hair.
3. Using hair dye remover to dissolve accumulated coloring matter on the hair.
4. Selecting an appropriate shade of hair dye.
5. Testing the hair for color or breakage.

Essentials For Hair Tinting

To produce the best results in hair tinting, the barber must be equipped with:

1. Various sizes of glass or porcelain dishes or flat cups.
2. Swab sticks and dye brushes.
3. Measuring cup.
4. Dropper.
5. Fresh peroxide—20 volume.
6. Absorbent cotton.

Temporary Hair Colorings

1. **Colored rinses** are prepared rinses used to clean the hair and bring out its luster, or add color to the hair which will remain on the hair until the next shampoo. They are applied in the manner prescribed under the subject of rinses.

2. **Progressive shampoo tints** are preparations similar to colored rinses compounded with soap. Several applications may be necessary in order to obtain the desired shade. However, these tints must be applied according to the manufacturer's directions.

3. **Crayons** are sticks of coloring, compounded with soaps or synthetic waxes, used to color gray or white hairs between hair dye retouches.

4. **Color blenders** are special hair tinting preparations which serve to blend in gray hair, while giving added color

to the hair. Various colors are available for all shades of hair. Applied as a 15 minute shampoo, the results last for about six weeks. These products have the added advantage of not leaving any line of demarcation. No retouch is necessary.

Permanent Hair Colorings

Permanent hair colorings are grouped according to their chemical composition and their effects on the hair shaft. There are four different classes of permanent hair colorings, as follows·

1. **Aniline derivative dyes** or **synthetic organic dyes** are those dyes having a base derived from aniline, a coal tar product. These preparations penetrate the horny layer of the hair shaft. The action of these dyes is instantaneous and their effect is permanent. **Shampoo tints** come under this classification.

2. **Pure vegetable dyes,** comprised of Egyptian henna, indigo, camomile and sage. They deposit a thin film or coating on the hair shaft.

3. **Metallic or mineral dyes** are of the progressive type and form a metallic coating over the hair shaft. Applications are made successively until the proper shade has developed.

4. **Compound dyestuffs,** such as compound henna, are combinations of vegetable dyes with certain metallic salts and other dyestuffs. The metallic salts are used as a mordant to fix the color. Compound dyes coat the hair shaft and are progressive in action.

Aniline Derivative Dyes

Aniline derivative dyes are also known as organic dyes, synthetic dyes, coal tar dyes, peroxide dyes, or liquid dyes.

The most effective type of hair dye contains, as its essential ingredient, **para-phenylene-diamine,** or a related chemical compound. With this type of preparation, it is possible to duplicate the most unusual shade of human hair without impairing its luster or texture. The color of the hair remains permanent. A small percentage of customers are sensitive to aniline derivative dyes. To identify such individuals, a skin test is required for all customers prior to applying the dye. **This is required by law.** The stock of these dyes should be kept fresh as they deteriorate on standing. When the barber mixes the developer with the dye, a chemical reaction, known as **oxidation,** begins. After the mixture is applied to the hair, the reaction continues as long as the dye remains wet, or until removed when the desired shade has developed. Timing the development of the applied dye requires that the barber have a thorough knowledge of the commercial product, besides consulting the customer's hair dye record.

Hydrogen Peroxide

Its uses, how available, and method of testing for volume content, see page 389.

Skin Test

A skin test is also known as a **patch test** or **predisposition** test. Its purpose is to detect customers who may be sensitive to an aniline derivative dye. It is the duty of every barber to test the skin of every customer. **It is required by law.** The dye used for the skin test must be of the same mixture as the product intended to be used for the hair dyeing.

The following procedure is suggested in giving a skin test:

1. Select test area, either behind ear extending partly into hairline, or on inner fold of elbow.
2. Wash test area, about the size of a quarter, with mild soap and water.
3. Dry test area by patting with absorbent cotton.
4. Prepare test solution by mixing one-half teaspoon of dye and one-half teaspoon of 20 volume peroxide.
5. Apply enough test solution with absorbent cotton-tipped applicator to cover the area previously cleansed.
6. Allow test area to dry. Leave uncovered and undisturbed for 24 hours.
7. Examine test area for either negative or positive reactions.

A **negative skin test** will show no sign of inflammation; hence, an aniline derivative dye may be applied with safety.

A **positive skin test** is recognized by the presence of inflammatory signs, such as redness, burning, itching, blisters or eruptions. A customer, evidencing such symptoms, is allergic to an aniline derivative dye, and **under no circumstances should this particular kind of dye be used.**

Symptoms of hair dye poisoning are as follows:

1. Itchy red spots which may spread to all parts of the body.
2. Tiny blisters from which serum oozes.
3. The customer suffers from headaches and vomiting.

If these warning signs are neglected, and the customer fails to get immediate medical attention, other complications may ensue.

Hair Tinting

For successful hair tinting with an aniline derivative dye, the barber must plan and follow a definite procedure which makes for the greatest efficiency and also suits the customer's needs. A permanent record should be kept of each customer's hair dye treatments. Without a plan, the work takes longer, mistakes are apt to be made, and the customer readily becomes dissatisfied. Customers will have more confidence in the barber's ability if he does his hair dyeing systematically.

It is desirable to tint the hair before giving a haircut in order to have more hair to work with.

The procedure for coloring a virgin head of hair which has not been previously bleached or dyed, is as follows:

1. Preparation.
    a) Examine scalp and hair.
    b) Choose the correct shade of dye.
    c) Give skin test.
    d) Recondition hair, if necessary.
2. Procedure.
    a) Shampoo, dry, and section hair.
    b) Soften or bleach hair, and dry.

   c) Re-section hair.

   d) Prepare and apply hair dye.

3. Completion.

   a) Test for color development.

   b) Give a final shampoo.

   c) Complete with vinegar rinse.

Choosing The Correct Shade of Hair Dye

The customer is always consulted in selecting the best shade to match the existing color of the hair or to impart an entirely new color to the hair. As a general rule, choose the shade which will cause the skin to appear lighter, yet harmonize with the general complexion. For a small percentage of gray hair, select a somewhat lighter shade of hair dye. In every case, follow the directions for selecting the proper shade as outlined by the manufacturer of the hair dye.

Shampooing and Sectioning the Hair

Give a preliminary shampoo with warm water, rinse and dry hair thoroughly.

Water as here mentioned refers to soft water. Do not use hard water unless it is first softened by chemical treatment. Distilled water can be used in place of hard water.

Comb the hair and divide it into four sections, parting the hair from forehead to nape of neck, and from ear to ear. Leave one section free for the application of softener or bleach.

For normal hair. Leave the right front section free.

For partly gray and abnormal hair. Leave the hair section free in which the color of the hair is darkest.

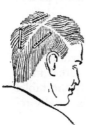

Hair sectioned
in quarters

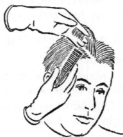

Subdividing hair into
quarter-inch strands

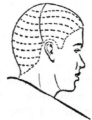

Approximate number
of quarter-inch
strands

Softening or Bleaching the Hair

The hair is **bleached** first only when it is to be dyed to a lighter shade. Otherwise, the hair is **softened** so that it will readily absorb the dye and thereby produce a more lasting shade. Insufficient softening often is the cause of an incomplete development of the dye, and an insufficient coverage of gray hair.

Preparation. Prepare softener or bleach. For coarse hair add 28% ammonia water to the peroxide. Measure the quantities accurately and keep a written record of the formula used.

Procedure for normal hair. Apply softener or bleach on the front right section and continue application all around head. When applying the dye, begin on the same section of hair to which the softener or bleach was last applied.

Procedure for partly gray and abnormal hair. On partly gray hair or hair that has a variable color, the softener or bleach is applied where the color is darkest. Start to apply the dye where the hair is grayest or lightest in color.

Apply softener or bleach with brush to quarter-inch strands. Moisten both sides of strand from the scalp to within one inch of hair ends. When this is completed, comb through the hair to the ends. At sides of head, and at neckline, where the hair is extremely short, apply the softener directly to the hair with a swab but without sectioning the hair. Allow softener to remain for the required length of time (10 to 30 minutes or longer, depending on the type and texture of hair). Finally, dry hair thoroughly.

Preparing and Applying the Hair Dye

Most aniline derivative dyes which are sold without developers, use 20 volume peroxide as a developer. Other manufacturers who use tablets as a developer, supply the tablet with each bottle of dye. One bottle of hair dye is usually required for treating a virgin head of men's hair.

Mix equal parts, dye with 20 volume peroxide, in a glass dish, or cup, and use immediately. If a tablet is used as a developer, crush it to a powder before opening and adding the dye solution.

Applying the dye. The hair is ready to be tinted when it is perfectly dry and re-sectioned in quarters. Wear rubber gloves to avoid staining the hands. Begin application of dye

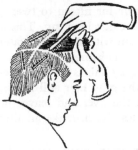

as explained for normal hair or gray and abnormal hair. With a brush, apply an adequate amount of dye to both sides of quarter inch hair strands and stop within one inch of the hair ends. Care must be taken to prevent spilling the dye and having it run over the hairline. Apply the dye freely with a swab at sides and nape of neck without any attempt to sectioning the hair.

Manner of applying dye to quarter-inch strands

When all sections have been treated, comb the dye through to the hair ends. This procedure is modified with extremely porous hair by diluting the remaining portion of

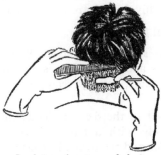

Applying dye to neck hair with swab

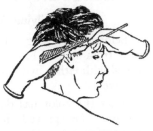

Applying dye to sideburns with swab

the dye with an equal amount of water or shampoo, and then applying this mixture to the hair ends. In this way, the porous hair ends will not develop a darker shade than the rest of the hair.

Judging from the manufacturer's directions and the hair texture, allow the dye to remain on the hair for the required length of time. The action of the hair dye continues so long as the hair and the dye remain in a moist condition.

Test For Color Development

After the dye has been on the hair for fifteen to twenty minutes, it is necessary to test for color development. This is done by wetting a small piece of cotton with soap and water or shampoo, wringing out some of the moisture, and then selecting a section of hair where most gray hair is evident. Remove the dye with wet cotton. If the gray hair still shows, re-moisten this strand of hair with the dye, and leave the dye on for another five to ten minutes. Then make another test for color.

It is impossible to give definite instructions as to the length of time required for color development, as no two heads of hair are alike. The barber will become proficient in determining the necessary time as he progresses with this work, and gains experience in judging hair textures. Again, we must emphasize the necessity for testing the ends of the hair and watching them carefully for color development, as the ends absorb the dye more readily than the rest of the hair.

Giving A Final Shampoo

Before proceeding with the shampoo, remove all dye stains from skin of hairline, ears and neck. This is accomplished with either hydrogen peroxide, hot oil, cream, or left-over dye.

After the color has developed to the desired shade, the hair must be sprayed thoroughly with a strong force of water.* This serves to set the color and removes all excess dye from the hair; the hair is then shampooed lightly with a neutral soap. Pour a vinegar rinse through the hair, to harden the color, and rinse off with warm water immediately. Then dry, or proceed with any other treatment the customer desires.

---

*Some dye manufacturers recommend the use of water that is as hot as the customer can stand it, follow the manufacturer's instructions

Causes of Unsatisfactory Hair Tinting

1. Dye not applied immediately after mixing with developer.
2. Developer (peroxide—20 volume) in weakened strength.
3. Poor application (overlapping).
4. Improper application of softener.
5. Improper mixture of softener.
6. Softener removed too soon from the hair.
7. Hair dye removed too soon from the hair.
8. Hair dye remained on the hair for too long a period.
9. Improper blending of retouch with hair previously dyed.

Retouching Tinted Hair

A "retouch" is the term commonly applied to hair which has been dyed, but where the new growth from the scalp must be dyed to match the rest of the hair. The customer's hair dye record should be consulted to determine the exact shade of dye to use, the strength of softener, and how long to keep it on the hair.

The same procedure is followed as for dyeing virgin hair, except that a swab is used in applying **both** the softener and the dye. Both softener and dye are applied from the scalp to the point where the hair has already been dyed. Great care should be exercised to prevent either the dye or softener from running down on the hair that has already been dyed. Such overlapping would cause a streak which would not only be very ugly, but would make that portion of the hair darker than the rest. Should the dye or softener run, causing overlapping, remove it immediately by lifting the hair with the comb and rubbing a piece

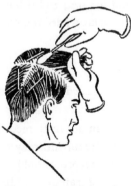

Manner of applying dye retouch with swab to quarter-inch strands

of dry absorbent cotton over it. Keep the wet hair free from the dyed hair as much as possible, otherwise the retouched hair may cause the previous hair coloring to streak. Make a test for color in the usual way, and once the color has sufficiently developed, shampoo and dry the hair. If hair, which had been previously **dyed**, is faded in color, add a little shampoo to the remaining dye mixture and wash through the hair for two minutes before shampooing.

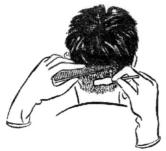
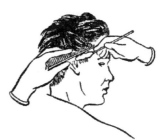

Applying dye to neck hair
with swab

Applying dye to sideburns
with swab

Prevent overlapping. Overlapping will not occur if the barber is careful to use a swab that is not too wet, and if both softener and dye are applied only to the point where the hair has already been dyed.

Hair Dye Records

A permanent record (either a book or a card file) should be kept of all hair dye treatments.

It is of the utmost importance to keep an accurate record so that any difficulties encountered in one treatment, may be avoided in subsequent ones. A complete record should be made with information such as "dries out rapidly," "dye does not develop fast enough," or any other data connected with that particular head.

HAIR DYE RECORD CARD

Name .... Tel. No. ....
Address .... City ....

DESCRIPTION OF HAIR

Form:
☐ straight
☐ wavy
☐ curly
☐ P. W.

Length:
☐ long
☐ medium
☐ short

Texture:
☐ fine ☐ coarse
☐ soft ☐ harsh
☐ silky ☐ wiry

Type:
☐ porous
☐ normal
☐ resistant

Condition: ⎰☐ dry ☐ oily ☐ streaked ☐ faded ☐ % gray
⎱ previously bleached for ....(time)
⎰ previously dyed with .... for ....

(Original sample to be enclosed)

PRELIMINARY TREATMENT

.... Corrective treatments with ....

.... Corrective treatments with ....

(Sample of corrected hair to be enclosed)

Time required for development of color .... minutes

---

HAIR TINTING PROCESS

Whole Head ....   Retouch .... inches   Shampooed ....

Softened with 1 oz. peroxide and ⎰no ⎱ ammonia for ...... minutes
                                 ⎱......dr.⎰

Shade desired: ....

Shade used: .... equal parts of color and developer.
                .... color; .... developer; .... water

Results: ☐ good ☐ poor ☐ too light ☐ too dark ☐ streaked

(Sample of tinted hair to be enclosed)

Date	Operator	Date	Operator
....	....	....	....
....	....	....	....
....	....	....	....
....	....	....	....

Definitions Relating to Hair Tinting

A **virgin head** of hair is a head of normal hair which has had no bleaching or dyeing treatments.

A **touch-up or retouch** is the application of coloring to the new growth of hair, using the same procedure and shade as was employed in the virgin head treatment.

Blending is the application of the same shade of liquid dye to faded hair ends in order to produce a uniform color, or match new dye with the old dye.

Softening is the application of peroxide for a given length of time in order to prepare the hair to absorb the dye.

Dye back is the coloring of the hair to its natural shade, after it has been bleached.

Dye removal is the use of a dye solvent, bleach, or softening treatments to remove an unsatisfactory shade of dye from the hair.

Toning down is the application of a hair dye or shampoo tint on overbleached hair for the purpose of adding more color to the hair.

Color testing is a method of sampling the action of a selected dye on a small strand of hair or the shampooing of a small strand of dyed hair to determine if the color has developed to the desired intensity.

Oxidation is a chemical reaction which takes place when peroxide and dye solution are mixed and applied to softened hair.

A **developer** is an oxidizing agent, such as hydrogen peroxide solution, which supplies the oxygen necessary for oxidation.

Allergy is a condition of increased sensitivity of the body to some chemical substance. Only those people who are susceptible, manifest definite physical reactions or symptoms upon contact with a particular chemical substance.

Susceptible means capable of being allergic.

Idiosyncrasy is an individual peculiarity which makes one susceptible to chemical substances in cosmetics, drugs and foods.

A **skin test** is a procedure for determining whether or not a person is allergic to an aniline derivative dye.

Reminders and Hints for Hair Tinting

1. Always wash your hands and use sterile swabs, brushes, combs and linens.

2. A hair dye should never be used if there is a contagious disease or an eruption present anywhere on the scalp.

3. Keep a complete and confidential record of all hair dyeing treatments. Consult this record whenever necessary.

4. Examine scalp and hair and give skin test before applying dye. If necessary, make a test for color or breakage.

5. Avoid irritating the scalp with sharp fingernails, strong massage movements or hot water during preliminary shampooing.

6 A preliminary shampoo, with a mild soap and soft water, removes dirt and oil which would ordinarily interfere with the action of the dye and the development of the proper shade.

7. Choose a shade of dye which will cause the skin to appear lighter, yet harmonize with the general complexion.

8. If hair is to be dyed to a lighter shade, it is bleached first and then dyed.

9. A glass or porcelain dish is best for mixing the dye with the developer. Use a brush applicator for a virgin head and a swab for retouching. Discard left-over dye.

10. Hair ends are more absorbent, whereas the hair next to the scalp is more resistant to the action of the dye. A full strength is not applied, nor allowed to collect at the hair ends.

11. For brittle and split hair, the action of the dye is slowed down by adding water* or liquid soap, and combing the solution through the hair ends.

12. Before applying dye, drain excess liquid from applicator by pressing it against side of dish. To distribute dye

---

Where hard water is the only kind available, soft water or distilled water must be used instead.

evenly, apply it to hair which is spread out in an upward direction, away from the scalp.

13. Dye stains on the skin are removed with either hydrogen peroxide, hot oil, cream, or left-over dye.

14. The hair must be dry before applying the softener. The softening process takes anywhere from 10 to 30 minutes or longer, depending upon the texture and type of the hair. Resistant hair may require a second application of the softener.

15. Depending upon the quality and condition of the hair, begin the application of the dye to the last strand of hair, wetted by the softener. On partly gray hair, the dye is applied to the grayest part first. At the time the dye is applied, the hair should be thoroughly dry.

16. As long as the hair remains moist, the action of the dye continues.

17. The action of the dye is slowed by the addition of water or shampoo. The color of the dye is lightened by adding hydrogen peroxide.

18. To prevent overlapping in a retouch, use the dye sparingly and apply only to the point where the hair has already been dyed.

19. Tinted hair will be kept in prime condition by the use of oil or cream treatments.

Metallic Hair Tints

Metallic dyes are erroneously referred to as "color restorers" or "hair restorers." They are of the progressive type, and form a metallic coating over the hair shaft. Applications are made successively until the proper shade has developed.

The many disadvantages of metallic dyes limit their usefulness in the barber shop. There is always the danger of absorption and poisoning by the metallic compound. The choice of shades is restricted to colors ranging from dark brown to black. Repeated applications result in unnatural and uncertain shades, besides causing the hair to become brittle.

Metallic dyes are not used professionally by the barbers. They are sold in retail stores for home use. Continued use will leave a strong odor in the hair.

Vegetable Hair Tints

Pure vegetable dyes which deposit a thin film or coating on the hair shaft, are harmless, less effective and less permanent than aniline derivative dyes. They are used as a liquid or paste, and yield a limited range in shades. Repeated applications, at frequent intervals, are required to offset the fading in the color of the hair.

. **Egyptian henna** grows abundantly in Egypt and Asia. On the market it is available as **green** and **brown henna.** The green henna is stronger in staining qualities than the brown henna. Egyptian henna is employed as a tint, pack or rinse, which imparts a red tone to the hair. The exclusive use of henna coarsens the hair.

Indigo is a very dark blue vegetable coloring which is used to modify unsatisfactory henna applications. When added to henna paste, indigo darkens the resulting shade.

Camomile can be used as a rinse or pack to highlight faded blonde hair.

Sage is used mainly as a rinse to darken hair and impart a greenish brown tone.

Application of vegetable hair tints. Follow the manufacturer's instructions.

Henna Pack for Virgin Hair

A henna pack imparts a red tone to hair and is indicated to highlight medium to dark shades of brown hair. The true shade does not develop until two to three days after the henna pack has been applied. For best results in the use of henna, buy a standard and reliable product Henna is not suitable for black hair, nor for hair which has turned gray.

Henna packs are not popular in the barber shop because of their unnatural look, and can only be recommended to one who has had natural red hair, or a complexion that will go with it

The following procedure is recommended for preparing and applying a henna pack.

1. Examine color, condition and texture of the hair.
2. Shampoo hair and partially dry with towel.
3. Comb and section hair into quarters.
4. Consult customer regarding desired shade.
5. Prepare henna pack by mixing 6 ounces of Egyptian henna with 12 ounces of hot water to form a smooth paste. Heat mixture in water bath.
6. Treat each hair strand separately. Start with the right rear section and work clockwise around the head, treating the temple and hairs at the nape of the neck last.
7. Apply hot henna paste with wide paint brush to center of strand of hair, work toward the scalp and then to within one inch of the ends. Comb henna through hair and apply to ends.
8. Cover head with shower cap or waxed paper and place customer under a white therapeutic lamp or heating cap until the desired shade develops. For example: fifteen minutes for a slight tint, and thirty minutes for a brighter shade.
9. Test for shade by sponging a small strand of hair with cotton, wet with shampoo or warm water. More than one test may be necessary before a satisfactory shade develops.
10. Rinse henna from hair and shampoo.
11. Give acid rinse if necessary.

Henna Pack Retouch

The procedure for a henna pack retouch is identical with that of a virgin henna pack, except that the paste is applied only to the new growth of hair. When the desired shade has been obtained, the paste may be rinsed off and a thorough shampoo given, or else dilute the adhering paste with warm water and apply to the remainder of the hair for additional brightening.

Shampoo Tints

Shampoo tints are an innovation which have become increasingly popular with customers who may be reluctant to dye their hair, yet want a simple and quick way to blend gray hairs with the natural shade of their hair. The barber who is prepared and capable of rendering such a service, is not only a great help to his customer, but a valuable asset to his employer. Shampoo tints possess the following advantages over the ordinary hair dyes.

1. Sales are more readily made and repeated.
2. Less time is consumed in completing the treatment.
3. Can be used on all textures, including bleached hair.
4. Can be used over any penetrating dye.
5. Fading of the shade is not very pronounced.

There are various kinds of shampoo tints on the market. Basically, they are a mixture of a soap or soapless shampoo, together with a dye, producing very heavy lather, thoroughly cleansing the hair and scalp, leaving the hair lustrous and beautiful. The soap rinses out easily and no film is left on the hair.

The action of shampoo tints falls into two main groups.

1. **Progressive shampoo tints** which require a series of applications to color the hair to the desired shade. These tints must be applied according to the manufacturer's instructions.

2. **Instantaneous shampoo tints** which color the hair in one application. This type acts exactly like the penetrating (aniline derivative) dyes, allowing for minor differences in manufacturers' directions. They may be used in two ways.

    a) **With softener,** applied to individual strands, as in the standard method. The results are about the same.

    b) **Without softener.** This method requires more time for development of shade and the colors wear off more quickly.

Skin test must be given to determine if the patron can tolerate the aniline derivative type of shampoo tints.

The actual application of shampoo tints is exactly the same as that of hair dyes, whether it be a virgin head or a touch-up.

Color Rinses

Color rinses serve as a temporary tinge of color to the hair, making it appear lustrous and blend in gray hair. There are two types of color rinses. The plain type, which is applied to the hair after a shampoo, and fades out within one week; the other type has a more penetrating effect and remains on the hair until it is shampooed out of the hair.

Color rinses should always be prepared according to the directions given with the product by the manufacturer. Before applying the color rinse, remove excess moisture by towel drying the hair. These color rinses come in about 14 different shades. The barber should recommend them to most all of his customers.

For the man who **does not have gray hair**, the rinse will add color and highlight his natural color of hair. It is applied by pouring the rinse over the head several times, catching what is poured in another pan. Remove excess moisture and comb hair.

For the customer **who has gray hair, or small amounts of gray hair**, we use the penetrating color rinse. Apply by parting the hair in small strands, treating the gray strands first. Continue by working your way from the back of the head to the front hairline, and finally the short hairs at the side of the head.

Allow the rinse to remain on the hair for the length of time specified by the manufacturer, then **rinse off with cool water**. The rinsing action hardens the color and does not come off the hair until the hair is shampooed.

Special Problems In Men's Hair Tinting

Reconditioning hair which has been dyed, is of major importance, no matter how well the hair has been treated during the tinting process. It becomes very much affected by exposure to the sun or salt water. Therefore, it is advisable to give reconditioning treatments at regular intervals. Commercial products are available for this treatment.

Regular oil treatments are also recommended for reconditioning but are much slower in responding.

Hair that has been rendered very dry, brittle or porous, by excessive dyeing, requires reconditioning treatments to restore it to its normal condition. All hair that has been subjected to the use of any metallic substance or discolored from the use of any of the various hair color restorers, etc , must be reconditioned before the hair dye is applied. Remember, that in giving reconditioning treatments, you are treating the **hair itself,** rather than the scalp. Take the hair between the palms of the hands and with a rotary movement, rub the oil well into the hair. After the application of oil, the hair may be steamed or the therapeutic lamp may be used. This treatment should be continued over a period of time until the hair is reconditioned.

Dye Removal

There are three ways in which hair dye can be removed from the hair:

1. Application of dye solvent.
2. White henna preparations.
3. Hydrogen peroxide.

It is a lengthy process and the hair passes through many light red shades before the dye is removed. There are many commercial hair dye removers on the market. When using such a product, follow the directions of the manufacturer.

Correcting Poorly Tinted Hair

With a little study, the barber will soon become familiar with the appearance of the hair when treated by the various hair preparations. Upon first examining the customer's hair, be sure to notice whether any preparations have been used, no matter how vociferously the customer may tell you he has used nothing. Many people do not realize that some of the so-called vegetable rinses and hair color restorers, are really hair dyes in disguise. A prospective customer should be questioned as to the treatment of his hair during the past year. From the customer's description of the preparation used, the barber should be able to tell what treatment should be given. When in doubt, treatments should be given to remove the preparation that was previously used. If there is any question in your mind, it is advisable to make a test for color or breakage.

Take a small strand of hair beneath the part, preferably in front of the head where any unknown preparation has been used most lavishly. Dye the strand as you would if you were dyeing the entire head, going through the same preliminary steps, and taking the same precautions (softening or bleaching, then dyeing). Allow twenty-four hours to elapse. Test the hair for breakage and look for discoloration. If discoloration or breakage occurs, preparations previously used, must be removed from the hair.

Correcting Dark Streaks

Dark streaks in tinted hair may be caused by improper application of softener, overlapping in retouching new growth, and the use of too much dye. To remove streaks, apply hydrogen peroxide, or hydrogen peroxide and ammonia water, and pass a hot iron over the streaked strands only.

Tinting Bleached Hair To Its Natural Shade

An appropriate shade of dye, with which to tint bleached hair, is selected so that it will match the natural shade of hair next to the scalp. A test for color on one or more strands of bleached hair is advisable, since it helps the barber in judging the proper dilution and timing of the dye.

Since the bleached portion of the hair is very porous, the dye is diluted with hydrogen peroxide and water, or with equal parts of shampoo, and applied according to the manufacturer's directions. The new growth of hair, next to the scalp, is neither bleached nor dyed. The development of a very dark color can be prevented by working rapidly and drying each section as it is dyed.

Correcting Over-Bleached Hair

In correcting or toning down over-bleached hair, test first for the color the customer desires. It is advisable always to use two shades lighter than the customer requests, because the hair will appear much darker to the customer who has been accustomed to a light shade. Over-bleached hair should not be softened before the dye is applied, since it is already in a very porous condition, and will accept the dye very quickly.

A drab shade is likely to turn purple on this type of hair due to the fact that the hair accepts the dye too readily, and an off-shade may be the result. It is, therefore, advisable to choose one of the warm shades in preference to a drab shade. Before applying the dye to the entire head, make a test for color as follows:

Apply the dye to a strand of hair from the scalp to the ends. Watch the development carefully until it reaches the desired shade, timing the color development with each test made, and noting the shade and varying dilutions it may be necessary to use. If the action is too fast and the hair immediately turns dark, the action of the dye must be slowed down by adding two to three parts of water to the amount of dye used. If this solution turns a purple or off-shade on the hair, a warm shade should be chosen for testing If this shade in turn is not satisfactory, use one part dye to two parts of hydrogen peroxide, and two parts of water. The addition of water to the dye is not for the purpose of changing the shade, but to slow the action of the dye.

If the original shade decided upon does not develop satisfactorily, another shade must be chosen and experimented with, until the desired result is obtained.

After the correct shade has been determined, enough water should be added to the dye to allow the barber time to do the entire head.

Toning down over-bleached hair correctly is one of the most difficult things to do in hair dyeing. Only through practice and experience will the barber become expert in this particular field.

Tinting Eyebrows and Mustache

An aniline derivative dye should never be used for coloring the eyebrows or the mustache; to do so may cause serious injury. Commercial products are available for this purpose. The choice of color is limited to light brown, dark brown or black. The light brown is used for customers with very light complexions only. Follow the directions given with the product.

Rules For Coloring Eyebrows and Mustache

1. Never shave around the mustache immediately before or after the dye treatment.
2. Use cold instead of warm water to cleanse the skin around the eyebrows and the mustache.
3. To prevent staining the surrounding skin, apply vaseline above and below the hairline of both eyebrows and mustache.
4. The eyebrows and the mustache are colored from the outer end toward the nose.
5. The color development varies with the product used, and is usually from 3 to 5 minutes.
6. To remove grease and free coloring from eyebrows and mustache, use soap and water.
7. Use stain remover solution with small swab if stains do not respond to soap and water.
8. Smooth skin with cream.

REVIEW QUESTIONS ON HAIR TINTING

1. Give three good reasons why a customer might wish to have his hair dyed or shampoo tinted.	To retain a youthful appearance when hair becomes gray, to restore bleached hair to its natural shade, and to change an unattractive shade of hair.
2. Classify hair dyes.	Hair dyes are classified as follows: vegetable products, metallic preparations, compound dyestuffs, and aniline derivatives.
3. What preparations are included under pure vegetable dyes?	Egyptian henna, camomile, indigo and sage.
4. What is the action of metallic dyes?	Metallic dyes form a coating over the hair shafts; applications are made successively until proper shade is obtained.
5. What are compound dyestuffs? Give an example.	Compound dyestuffs are combinations of metallic preparations and vegetable extracts. Example—compound henna, a mixture of henna and metallic salts.
6. What are aniline derivatives? Describe their action.	Aniline derivatives are dyes having a base derived from aniline, a coal tar product. They penetrate the horny layer of the hair shaft, and deposit the coloring in the deeper layers.
7. From what group of dyes should a preliminary 24-hour skin test be given? Why?	The aniline derivative group, in order to determine if the customer is allergic to the ingredients contained in the dye. A skin test is required by law.
8. To be a successful hair dyer, what knowledge is essential?	A knowledge of the general structure of the hair; composition of hair dyes; the chemical reactions following their application, and correct method of applying them.
9. How is a skin test given?	Wash a spot behind the ear or bend of the arm with soap and water, dry, and then paint with a mixture of the dye and peroxide to be used; allow to dry and leave undisturbed for 24 hours. If the spot is free from irritation, it is safe to presume that the individual is not allergic to the dye.
10. Name two ways of using peroxide in dyeing with an aniline dye.	Peroxide is used as a preliminary softener or bleach, and as an oxidizing agent.
11. How long should peroxide be left on the hair as a softener?	From ten to thirty minutes, depending upon how porous or resistant the hair may be.

12. What kinds of hair require reconditioning treatments?	Dry, brittle or porous hair.
13. Why must the hair be moist while the proper shade is developing?	The action of the dye continues only as long as the hair remains moist.
14. Can hair be dyed from a darker to a lighter shade? Explain.	No; it must first be bleached to a light shade, and then dyed to the desired shade.
15. How are dye stains removed from the skin and scalp?	By using hydrogen peroxide, hot oil, cream, or left-over dye.
16. What would you do for hair that has been dyed too dark?	It may be lightened with a dye remover or hot oil treatments.
17. How can the action of the dye be slowed?	Dilute the dye with water or shampoo.
18. What is the difference between hair color restorers and penetrating dyes; which is considered better, and why?	Restorers are usually a metallic form of dye and leave a deposit on the hair shaft which gives the hair its color. Penetrating dyes color the hair by actually penetrating into the hair shaft. The penetrating dyes are most commonly used because they tint the hair in shades which more closely resemble natural hair.
19. State the difference between compound henna and plain Egyptian henna.	Egyptian henna is a vegetable coloring which produces only red shades. Compound henna comes in various shades and usually contains metallic substances to give darker colors.
20. What are dyes called that require a series of applications?	Progressive.
21. What are dyes called that require one application?	Instantaneous.
22. What type of dyes are instantaneous dyes, and by what various names are they commonly known?	Aniline derivative dyes; they are variously known as synthetic dyes, organic dyes, peroxide dyes, and liquid dyes.
23. What type of dyes are progressive dyes?	Metallic dyes.
24. What test should be given to determine whether the customer is allergic to the hair dye?	A skin test.
25. What is the most important factor when considering a hair dye; why?	A preliminary examination of the hair and scalp, to determine whether metallic substances have been used on the hair, and if there are abrasions on the scalp.

26. Which part of the hair absorbs the dye most readily?	The hair ends.
27. To what part of the hair is a retouch applied?	Only to the new growth of hair.
28. What is meant by virgin hair in hair dyeing?	Head of hair that has never been dyed or bleached.
29. Why should a skin test always be given prior to dyeing the hair?	A skin test is given to determine whether the customer is allergic to a hair dye.
30. What does the long continued use of henna do to each hair?	It coats the hair, and makes it coarser.
31. a) What is a henna pack? b) When is it used?	a) A henna pack is powdered Egyptian henna mixed with water to form a paste. b) It is used to highlight medium to dark shades of brown hair.
32. What is a shampoo tint?	A mixture of soap or soapless shampoo together with a dye.
33. What advantages do shampoo tints possess?	They require less time, can be used for all textures of hair, and the fading of the shade is not very pronounced.
34. Why does the instantaneous shampoo tint produce a more permanent color than the progressive shampoo tint?	The instantaneous shampoo tint contains an aniline derivative dye and a developer which penetrate into the hair shaft.
35. What kind of dye should never be used to color eyebrows?	An aniline derivative dye.
36. Why should barbers keep an accurate record card for each customer?	In order to follow the information on the record card when giving a retouch.

BARBER ETHICS

Barber ethics deals with the proper conduct and business dealings of the barber in relation to his employer, customers and co-workers. The essential considerations in barber ethics are honesty, fairness, courtesy and respect for the feelings and rights of others. The ethical barber always gives the best possible service to his customers, keeping in mind their desires, needs and welfare.

Good ethics—To build public confidence and retain a good following, the individual barber should live up to these rules of ethics:

1. Acquire a thorough knowledge and practice of barbering.
2. Believe in barbering sincerely and practice it conscientiously.
3. Keep your word and fulfill all your obligations.
4. Obey all provisions of the Barber State Law.
5. Cherish a good reputation and set an example of good conduct and behavior.
6. Treat all customers fairly; do not show any favoritism.
7. Be loyal to your employer and associates.

Poor ethics—Barber ethics is violated by resorting to questionable practices, extravagant claims and unfulfilled promises which cast an unfavorable light on barbering in general and the individual barber in particular.

BARBER ETHICS

1. What is meant by barber ethics?	Barber ethics deals with the proper conduct and business dealings of the barber in relation to his employer, customers and co-workers.
2. How should the ethical barber treat his customers?	Give the best possible service to his customers; cater to their desires, needs and welfare; treat all customers fairly.
3. How should the ethical barber speak of his fellow barbers?	Speak only good of his fellow barbers.
4. How should the ethical barber behave towards his employer?	Be loyal and conscientious towards your employer; keep your word and fulfill your obligations.
5. Which three practices reflect unfavorably on the barber?	Resorting to questionable barber practices, extravagant claims and unfulfilled promises.

BARBER SHOP MANAGEMENT

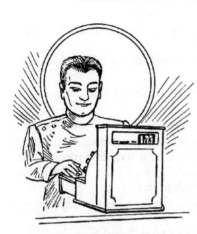

For a barber shop to be successful, it must be carefully planned and efficiently managed. Barber shop management implies the direct control and coordination of all activities that occur while the shop is in operation. Besides being an experienced barber, a prospective owner of a barber shop must have a knowledge of business principles and bookkeeping and must be able to cooperate with his employees in rendering satisfactory service to the public.

Five important functions are performed by every barber shop. They are:

1. Finance or capital investment.
2. Purchasing of equipment and fixtures.
3. Publicity.
4. Salesmanship.
5. Systematic records as an aid in efficient management.

Organizing the Barber Shop

The type of barber shop organization depends largely on the amount of available capital. If the individual has enough money to be the sole proprietor, then the individual form of ownership should be considered. A lack of sufficient capital necessitates either a loan or a partner. When three or more people intend to operate a barber shop, the corporation is the best form of organization.

The **individual** form of organization has certain **merits** over the partnership and corporation.

1. The owner is his own boss and manager.

2. The owner can determine his own policies and decisions.

3. The owner receives all the profits.

The individual form of organization has the following **disadvantages:**

1. The owner's expenditures are limited by the amount of capital investment.

2. The owner is personally liable for all debts in the business

The **partnership,** being a combination of two or three people, has certain advantages over the individual form of ownership. There should always be a written agreement defining the duties and responsibilities of each member. The main **advantages of a partnership** are: .

1. More capital is made available to equip and operate the barber shop.

2. Work, responsibilities and losses are shared.

3. The combined ability and experience of each partner assist in the solution of business problems.

The chief **disadvantages** of a partnership are:

1. Each partner is responsible for the business actions of the other.

2. Disputes and misunderstandings may arise between partners.

A **corporation** has the advantage over a partnership in that its stockholders are not legally responsible in case of loss or bankruptcy. The earning capacity is in proportion to the profits and the number of stocks the individual has in the corporation. Although the corporation has a considerable financial backing, it may only do what is specifically authorized in the charter and approved by the board of directors. The corporation is subject to taxation and regulation by the State.

In **transacting business** for the individual, partnership or corporation, a checking account is a convenient and safe way to make payments and withdrawals. The cancelled checks serve as receipts. If one person is the sole owner, the bank and checking account is in his own name. In a partnership, there is usually a joint account, in which one or both partners may sign checks and withdraw money. A corporation bank account is issued in its own name, with a responsible person authorized to withdraw money and issue checks.

Selecting A Location for the Barber Shop

Just as important as capital investment is the selection of a desirable location for the barber shop. The best kind of store is one that is conveniently located and has the greatest number of people passing its windows. In a residential neighborhood, the main source of customers will be from that vicinity. On the other hand, a transient section supplies patrons both from surrounding and remote places.

Before selecting a store, consult the local bank or real estate agent for assistance. Find out what the earning capacity and the living standards are of the people in a particular neighborhood. This information will help in deciding policies and prices. It is not advisable for a beginner to open a barber shop in a locality where there are many competitors.

In judging the merits of a particular store, consideration must be given to the entrance, the window space, the inside area of the store, the water, lighting and heating facilities, the presence of a sanitary toilet and a sufficient number of windows for adequate ventilation.

A **lease** is protection against any possible increase in rent. There should be a provision in the lease concerning alterations and painting of the barber shop. Before signing a lease, it should be read carefully to avoid any misunderstanding.

Equipping The Barber Shop

After the best site has been chosen by comparing various locations, the store is then ready to be furnished with fixtures and equipment Standard and durable supplies, either new or renovated, are the best. If in the future, equipment has to be replaced or increased, it is easy to duplicate standard supplies. Electrical appliances should be able to work with various types of current and under different conditions. Insurance of the store's contents is a protection against theft and fire.

The main requisites for an attractive barber shop are cleanliness and comfortableness. The equipment should be easily accessible and arranged in an orderly manner. The electric lighting must be neither too dull nor too bright. Dirty towels or linens are not to be used again, but kept in closed containers. Sanitation and sterilization rules must be enforced for the public's protection.

Advertising The Barber Shop

The right kind of publicity is important because it acquaints the public with the various services rendered by the barber shop. The best kind of publicity is that which reaches the greatest number of people at the cheapest cost. The choice of **advertising medium** is either a direct mailing, the distribution of circulars, an advertisement in the local town paper, or over the radio. For advertising to be effective, it must be repeated to make a lasting impression. Once a customer is attracted to the barber shop, **only courteous and efficient service will bring him back and have him recommend others.**

A **pleased customer** is the best form of advertising. A **pleasing personality** is a priceless asset that creates good will and a friendly atmosphere. The barber must be mindful of his **hygienic habits,** being clean and tidy in his clothing and extremely careful to avoid **body odor** and **bad breath.** It is frequently necessary to sense the thoughts and feelings of customers so as not to antagonize them by word or action.

Salesmanship In The Barber Shop

The satisfaction of customers depends on the extent to which their needs are fulfilled. Besides trying to improve the quality of haircut and shave, the barber should practice the selling of additional services such as shampoo, facial and scalp massage, hair tonics, etc. The barber should be acquainted with the types of service offered, the names of the various cosmetic products, their costs and manner of application. By selling extra services the barber will make himself of greater value to the customer, besides helping to increase the profits of the barber shop.

The barber has occasion to use the art of salesmanship in convincing customers as to the merits and benefits of various facial and scalp preparations and treatments. A good salesman knows all about the service or product he is selling. After a basis for confidence has been established, suggestive language, without any high-pressure tactics, may create a desire in the customer to try the new service or product. An attractive feature is to offer combination services at special prices.

Records In The Barber Shop

One of the causes for failure in operating a barber shop is the lack of complete and systematic records. All business transactions must be recorded in order to judge the condition of the business at a particular time. Records are valuable to the proprietor for the following reasons:

1. Efficient operation of the barber shop.
2. Indication of income, expenses, profits and losses.
3. Proves value of barber shop to prospective buyer.
4. Arrange for a loan from the bank.
5. Basis for such reports as income tax, social security, unemployment insurance, minimum hour law and accident compensation.

If a barber shop is to operate profitably, a simple system of bookkeeping must be instituted. An easy plan is to keep a daily account of income and expenses. The cash register indicates the daily income, whereas the receipts and cancelled checks constitute proof of payments. By adding the daily total income and expense, the weekly and monthly totals can be obtained. The difference between the total income and the total expense is the net profit. A profit accrues when the income is greater than the expense. When the expense is greater than the profit, a loss occurs. Continued profits spell success, and continued losses may finally result in bankruptcy.

A budget must be kept so that the income of money will be sufficient to cover the expenses. The following list of expenses are commonly met in the barber shop:

Operating and Administrative Expenses

Salaries	Advertising and printing
Rent	Heat, light and water
Taxes	Sundry supplies such as soaps,
Insurance	tonics, towels, etc.
Repairs	Telephone
Cleaning	Miscellaneous

The payments made on debts, equipment and fixtures are not classified as expenses, but are considered as a reduction in indebtedness which in turn adds to the value of the barber shop.

From time to time, an inventory must be taken of all sundry supplies in the barber shop. This record will show what supplies have been consumed and what new supplies are needed. It is a better policy to have a slight excess of materials rather than a deficiency.

BARBER SHOP MANAGEMENT

1. Name five important functions performed by a barber shop.	Finance or capital investment, purchase of equipment and fixtures, publicity, salesmanship and the keeping of systematic records.
2. Name three forms of ownership.	Individual ownership, partnership and corporation.
3. What is the best location for a barber shop?	A barber shop that is conveniently located and has the greatest number of people passing its windows.
4. Of what protection is a lease for a barber shop?	A lease is a protection against any possible increase in rent and defines the rights and responsibilities of the tenant.
5. What is the best form of advertising?	A pleased customer.
6. Of what value are records in the barber shop?	Indicates the income, expenses, profits and losses. Necessary for income tax, Social Security, unemployment insurance, minimum hour law and accident compensation.
7. When is first aid necessary?	In cases of accidents or emergencies before the arrival of medical assistance.

FIRST AID

Emergencies arise in every line of business, and a knowledge of first aid measures is invaluable to shop managers and employees.

A physician should be called as soon as possible after any accident has occurred, both as a courtesy to the patient and as a protection to the barber shop. There are certain first aid treatments, however, which the layman can give while awaiting medical assistance.

Burns. Burns may be caused by electricity, hot irons, or flames, while scalds are usually due to exposure to hot liquids or live steam. Burns are classified as first degree, characterized by redness; second degree, having watery blisters; and third degree, involving deeper structures of the flesh with possible charring of tissues. First degree burns are treated by an application of cloths saturated with a solution of salt or baking soda. A mild dusting powder, such as boric acid, or a 5% boric acid ointment, may be applied. 10% boric acid, vaseline or 10% ichthyol ointment is used for second degree burns. A 1% solution of picric acid may be used as a wet dressing for second and third degree burns. If a burn is caused by a mineral acid, the flesh should be washed with running water, if possible, followed by a sodium bicarbonate solution. An alkali burn should also be flushed with water, and a dilute solution of vinegar and water applied.

Electric shock. Severe electric shock seldom occurs in a barber shop, but in case such an accident should take place, the barber should be prepared for the emergency. The clothing should be loosened and the patient removed to a cool place. The head should be raised, and the tongue drawn forward to prevent strangulation. Artificial respiration should be administered as outlined below, and massage given over the heart. Alcoholic stimulants should not be given.

Artificial respiration. The Schafer method of artificial respiration, to be employed in severe electric shock, prolonged fainting, drowning, poisoning, gas suffocation, etc., is outlined as follows:

Place the patient on his abdomen with his face turned toward one side. Kneel beside or astride the patient, with the knees at his hips, facing his head.

Place the palms of the hands on the small of his back, with the fingers extended and palms in line with his spine.

First bear forward and bring the weight of your body on your hands, avoiding roughness. Hold this position for two seconds.

Release all pressure and swing back to rest on your heels. Hold this position for two seconds.

Repeat the above movements, alternating the application and release of pressure, at the rate of twelve to fifteen a minute until natural breathing is resumed.

In obstinate cases, artificial respiration should be continued for at least two hours before hope of revival is abandoned.

Epileptic fit. An epileptic fit is a nervous disorder, characterized by unconsciousness, convulsions, contortions of the face, foaming at the mouth, and rolling of the eyes.

Treatment consists of placing the patient in a flat position and fixing a wad of cotton between the teeth to prevent biting the tongue. Mild stimulants may be administered in moderation after recovery. If the patient falls into a deep sleep after the attack, he should not be disturbed until he awakens naturally.

Fainting. Fainting is caused by lack of blood flowing to the brain, bad air, indigestion, nervous condition and unpleasant odors. It is characterized by pallor and loss of muscular control. There is temporary suspension of respiration and circulation. If there is a sign of fainting before it actually occurs, the patient should hold his head between his knees, as this action may check the faintness by causing the blood to flow quickly to the head. Treatment for fainting consists of loosening all tight clothing, changing the air in the room, and placing the patient in a reclining position with the head slightly lower than the body. If the patient is conscious, he should take aromatic spirits of ammonia and stimulants such as hot coffee, tea or milk. If the patient is unconscious, cold applications to the face, chest, and over the heart are given, but cold water should not be dashed in the patient's face.

Heat exhaustion. Heat exhaustion is a general functional depression due to heat. It is characterized by a cool, moist skin, and collapse. Clothing should be loosened and the patient removed to a cool, dark, quiet place. If conscious, the patient should take aromatic spirits of ammonia. He should be kept lying down for several hours, as rest and quiet will hasten recovery.

Nose bleed. Nose bleed is a hemorrhage from the nose, and is treated by loosening the collar and applying ice or pads saturated with cold water to the back of the neck. A solution formed by adding a teaspoonful of salt or vinegar to a cup of cold water may be snuffed up the nose.

THINGS TO CONSIDER
WHEN GOING INTO BUSINESS

CAPITAL
Amount available
Amount required

ORGANIZATION
Individual
Partnership
Corporation

BANKING
Opening a bank account
Deposits
Drawing checks
Monthly statements
Notes and Drafts

SELECTING LOCATION
Population
Transportation facilities
Transients
Trade possibilities
Space required

**DECORATING and
FLOOR PLAN**
Selection of furniture
Floor covering
Installing telephone
Interior decorating
Exterior decorating
    Window displays
    Electric signs

EQUIPMENT and SUPPLIES
Selecting equipment
Comparative values
Installation
Labor saving steps

ADVERTISING
Planning
Direct mail
Newspaper
Radio
Local house organs

BOOKKEEPING SYSTEM
Installation
Record of appointments
Receipts
Disbursements
Petty Cash
Profit and Loss

LEGAL
Lease
Contracts
Claims and law suits

COST OF OPERATION
Rent
Light
Salaries
Supplies
Depreciation
Telephone
Linen service
Sundries
Taxes

MANAGEMENT
Methods of building goodwill
Analysis of materials and labor in relation to service charges.
Greeting customers
Adjusting complaints
Handling employees
Selling merchandise

OFFICE ADMINISTRATION
Office supplies
Stationery
Inventory

INSURANCE
Public liability
Compensation
Disability
Unemployment
Social Security
Fire and burglary

METHODS OF PAYMENT
In advance
C.O.D
Open account
Time payments

**COMPLIANCE WITH
LABOR LAWS**
Minimum wage law
Hours of employment
Minors

ETHICS
Courtesy
Observation of trade practices

BUSINESS LAW FOR THE BARBER SHOP

A barber shop may be owned and operated by an individual, a partnership, or a corporation. Before deciding which type of ownership is most desirable, one should be acquainted with the relative merits of each.

INDIVIDUAL OWNERSHIP

1. The proprietor is boss and manager.
2. The proprietor can determine policies and make decisions.
3. The proprietor receives all profits and bears all losses.

PARTNERSHIP

1. More capital is available for investment.
2. The combined ability and experience of each partner makes it easier to share work and responsibilities and make decisions
3. Profits are equally shared.
4. Each partner assumes unlimited liability for debts and bankruptcy.

CORPORATION

1. A charter has to be obtained from the State.
2. A corporation is subject to taxation and regulation by the State.
3. The management resides in a board of directors who determine policies and make decisions in accordance with the constitution of the charter.
4. The dividing of profits is proportionate to the number of shares of stock possessed by each stockholder.
5. The stockholder is not legally responsible for losses or bankruptcy.

BEFORE BUYING OR SELLING A BARBER SHOP

1. A written purchase and sale agreement should be formulated in order to clarify any misunderstandings or errors between the contracting parties.
2. For safe keeping and enforcement, the written agreement should be placed in the hands of an impartial third person who is to deliver the agreement to the grantee (one to whom the property is transferred) upon the performance of fulfillment of the specified contract.
3. The buyer or seller should take and sign a complete statement of inventory (goods, fixtures, etc.) and the value of each article.
4. If there is a transfer of chattel mortgage, notes, lease, and bill of sale, an investigation should be made to determine any default in the payment of debts.
5. Consult your lawyer for additional guidance.

AN AGREEMENT TO BUY AN ESTABLISHED
BARBER SHOP SHOULD INCLUDE

1. Correct identity of owner.

2 True representations concerning the value and inducements offered to buy the barber shop.

3. Use of shop's name and reputation for a definite period of time.

4. An understanding that the seller will not compete with the prospective owner within a reasonable distance from present location.

PROTECTION IN MAKING A LEASE

1. Secure exemption of fixtures or appliances which may be attached to the store or loft, so that they can be removed without violating the lease.

2. Insert into lease an agreement relative to necessary renovations such as painting, plumbing, fixtures and electrical installation.

3. Secure option from landlord to assign lease to another person; in this way, the obligations for the payment of rental are kept separate from the responsibilities in operating the business.

PROTECTION AGAINST FIRE, THEFT AND LAWSUITS

1. Employ honest and able employees and keep premises securely locked. Follow safety precautions to prevent fire, injury and lawsuits Liability, fire and burglary insurance should be obtained.

2. Do not violate the medical practice law of your state by attempting to diagnose, treat or cure disease.

3. Become thoroughly familiar with the barber law and sanitary code of your city and state.

4. Keep accurate records of number of workers, salaries, length of employment, and Social Security numbers, for various State and Federal laws affecting the social welfare of employees.

Remember — Ignorance of the Law is No Excuse for its Violation

---

CODE—Explanation of numbers and abbreviations on page 439

1—No reciprocity
2—Two years of barber experience
3—Three years of barber experience
4—Four years of barber experience
5—Five years of barber experience
6—Licensed apprentice or barber from another state must have substantially the same requirements as for barbers in this state
7—Attended an approved barber school and completed 2½ years apprenticeship in this state
8—Examination required.
9—Alabama—No law except in Mobile and Jefferson Counties
10—Virginia—No law except in Arlington County
None spec —None specified
Jour —Journeyman

State Boards Educational Requirements
For Barber License

State or Territory	Preliminary Education	Required Training and Education Barber School	Apprenticeship	Reciprocity*
Ala., Mobile Co.-9	8th grade	Pass test in Barber Science & Practice		1
Ala., Jeff. Co.-9				
Alaska	None spec.			1
Arizona	8th grade	1000 hrs.	18 mos.	6, 8
Arkansas	7th grade	1000 hrs. for 6 mos.	18 mos.	8
California	8th grade	1000 hrs. for 6 mos.	18 mos.	6
Colorado	8th grade	1200 hrs. for 6 mos.	24 mos.	1
Connecticut	8th grade	1000 hrs. for 6 mos. AND	30 mos. plus 144 hrs. study	1
Delaware	5th grade		36 mos.	1
Dist. of Col.	None spec.	1000 hrs. AND	24 mos.	1, 8
Florida	8th grade	1000 hrs.		1, 5, 8
Georgia	None spec.	Indefinite		1
Hawaii				
Idaho	8th grade	1000 hrs. for 6 mos. AND	12 mos.	6 or 3, 8
Illinois	8th grade	1248 hrs.	30 mos.	5 or 7, 8
Indiana	None spec.	1000 hrs. AND	18 mos.	6 or 2
Iowa	8th grade	6 mos. AND	18 mos.	1, 5, 8
Kansas	None spec.	1000 hrs.	18 mos.	6, 8
Kentucky	2 yrs. H. S.	1248 hrs. for 6 mos. OR	12 mos.	1, 8
Louisiana	8th grade	1500 hrs. AND	18 mos.	1, 8
Maine	None spec.	1000 hrs. for 6 mos. OR	18 mos.	6
Maryland	None spec.	1200 hrs. for 6 mos. AND	30 or 36 mos.	1, 3, 8
Massachusetts	None spec.	6 mos. AND	24 mos.	1, 2, 8
Michigan	None spec.	1000 hrs. AND	12 mos.	1
Minnesota	8th grade	1200 hrs. for 9 mos. AND	15 mos.	1, 5, 6, 8
Mississippi	8th grade	1500 hrs.	12 mos.	1, 8
Missouri	None spec.	1000 hrs. AND	18 mos.	1, 8
Montana	None spec.	1000 hrs. AND	12 or 18 mos.	1, 8
Nebraska	8th grade	1248 hrs. for 6 mos.	18 mos.	1
Nevada	8th grade	1000 hrs.	18 mos.	Non spec.
New Hampshire	None spec.		12 mos.	1
New Jersey	None spec.	None spec.	18 mos.	6
New Mexico	None spec.	1000 hrs. for 6 mos.		1
New York	8th grade	1000 hrs. for 6 mos. AND	18 or 24 mos.	1
No. Carolina	None spec.	8 mos.		1
No. Dakota	8th grade	1000 hrs. for 6 mos. AND	24 mos.	1
Ohio	8th grade	1000 hrs. AND	18 mos.	6 or 2, 8
Oklahoma	None spec.	1000 hrs. for 6 mos. OR	18 mos.	1
Oregon	8th grade	1000 hrs. for 6 mos. AND	18 mos.	6 or 2, 8
Pennsylvania	8th grade	1250 hrs. for 9 mos. AND	15 mos. (1250 hrs.)	1
Rhode Island	8th grade	1500 hrs. for 12 mos. OR	24 mos.	1, 2, 8
So. Carolina	None spec	6 mos. AND	18 mos.	1
So. Dakota	8th grade	6 mos.	24 mos.	6 or 5, 8
Tennessee	None spec.	1000 hrs. for 6 mos. AND	12 mos.	5, 8
Texas	Read & write	1000 hrs. for 6 mos. AND	18 mos.	1, 8
Utah	None spec.	6 mos.	12 mos.	1, 3, 8
Vermont	None spec.	1800 hrs. OR	12 mos. or comb. of both	1
Virginia-10	No law			
Washington	8th grade	1000 hrs. for 6 mos.		1, 8
W. Virginia	8th grade	1800 hrs.		1, 8
Wisconsin	8th grade		36 mos. Jour. 12 mos.	1, 4, 8
Wyoming	8th grade	1000 hrs.	18 mos.	Non spec.

Explanation of Numbers and Abbreviations, see bottom of Page 438

PART V

REVIEW EXAMINATIONS

HISTORY OF BARBERING

PART I — TRUE OR FALSE TEST

DIRECTIONS. *Carefully read each statement Some are true; others are false. If you believe the statement is true, draw a circle around the letter T, if you believe the statement is false, draw a circle around the letter F.*

1. The word barber comes from the Latin word meaning beard .... T F
2. Barbering was never practiced in ancient Egypt or China .... T F
3. The wearing of beards was a part of many religious customs .... T F
4. Soap was first discovered in ancient Rome .... T F
5. Barbering was a highly developed art in ancient Greece and Rome .... T F
6. During the Middle Ages, barbers were not allowed to perform surgical operations .... T F

ANSWERS

1—T   2—F   3—T   4—T   5—T   6—F

PART II — INSERTION TEST

DIRECTIONS: *Read each statement carefully Select one or more words from the following list and insert in proper space provided in the sentence.*

guilds	Chicago	Swedish
England	Minnesota	France
surgeons	Dutch	

1. During the Middle Ages, barbering was regulated by trade ....

2. Barber-surgeons were brought to America by .... and ....settlers

3. The first state in the United States to pass a barber law was ....

4. After 1745, England separated the barbers from the ....

5. The first barber school in the United States was started about 1893 in ....

ANSWERS

1—guilds   4—surgeons
2—Dutch, Swedish   5—Chicago
3—Minnesota

PERSONAL HYGIENE

PART I — TRUE OR FALSE TEST

1. Personal hygiene helps the barber to preserve his health .... T F
2. The mind has no influence on the health of the body ...... T F
3. Cleanliness is an essential part of personal hygiene ...... T F
4. Air, water and food, of good quality, are required by the body to maintain health .... T F
5. The over-eating of good foods is not harmful to health T F

ANSWERS

1—T ·   2—F   3—T   4—T   5—F

PART II — INSERTION TEST

| deodorants | inward | fatigue |
| forward | sleep | circulation |

1. Faulty standing posture tends to increase ....
2. In good standing posture, the chest is kept up and...............
while the abdomen is kept ....
3. Exercise is beneficial because it stimulates breathing and .. ..
4. Rest and ....helps to combat fatigue.
5. The use of ....offsets offensive body odor.

ANSWERS

1—fatigue   4—sleep
2—forward, inward   5—deodorants
3—circulation

BACTERIOLOGY

PART I — TRUE OR FALSE TEST

1. Bacteriology is the science that treats of infection .... T F
2. Streptococci bacteria grow in chains .... T F
3. Bacilli are rod-shaped organisms .... T F
4. Pathogenic organisms produce disease .... T F
5. All bacteria are harmful .... T F
6. Immunity means lack of resistance to disease .... T F
7. Moisture is essential for the growth of bacteria .... T F
8. Infection refers to the entrance of bacteria into the
   tissues .... T F
9. Bacteria are found everywhere .... ·T F
10. Bacteria grow more favorably in dark, damp places .... T F
11. A bacterial spore can be revived under favorable condi-
    tions .... T F
12. Non-pathogenic germs are not disease-producing .... T F
13. Boiling water will destroy most bacteria but not spore-
    forming bacteria .... T F
14 Bacteria are to be found where dirt and unsanitary con-
   ditions exist .... T F
15. The staphylococci bacteria produce boils and abscesses T F
16. Harmful bacteria produce poisons .... T F
17. Blood poisoning is caused by streptococci .... T F
18. Gonorrhea is caused by a gonococcus .... T F
19. A boil is general infection .. .. T F
20. Improperly sterilized razors may cause an infection .... T F
21. Immunity means the ability to get sick .... T F
22. Infection is the destruction of harmful germs in the body T F
23. Toxin means good health .... .T F

ANSWERS

1—F	2—T	3—T	4—T	5—F
6—F	7—T	8—T	9—T	10—T
11—T	12—T	13—T	14—T	15—T
16—T	17—T	18—T	19—F	20—T
21—F	22—F	23—F		

PART II — MATCHING TEST

DIRECTIONS: *Select the appropriate term from the following list and place in parenthesis alongside of statement.*

Bacilli	Streptococci	Bacteria
Cocci	Staphylococci	Pathogenic
Spirilla	Infectious	Non-Pathogenic

1. Bacteria which are rod-shaped ....(........................)

2. Bacteria which grow in chains ....(................ ......)

3. Bacteria which are round-shaped ....(........................)

4. Bacteria which grow in bunches ....(..........................)
5. Bacteria which are spiral-shaped ....(..........................)
6. Bacteria capable of producing disease ....(..........................)
7. A disease spread from one person to another ......(..........................)
8. Bacteria incapable of producing disease ....(..........................)

ANSWERS

1—Bacilli	4—Staphylococci	7—Infectious
2—Streptococci	5—Spirilla	8—Non-pathogenic
3—Cocci	6—Pathogenic	

PART III — INSERTION TEST

immunity	infect	food
infection	cells	broken
dirt	animals	vegetable
reproduce	microscope	unbroken

1. Bacteria are minute one-celled .... micro-organisms.
2. Many dangerous bacteria are found in ....
3. Bacteria can enter the body through the .... skin.
4. Bacteria are living organisms which grow and ....
5. The ability of the body to resist disease is known as ....
6. Bacteria are so small that it is necessary to have a .... to see them.
7. Bacteria consist of single ....
8. First aid care for cuts and wounds helps to prevent ....
9. A human disease carrier can .... other persons.
10. Without .... some bacteria will die.

ANSWERS

1—vegetable	4—reproduce	7—cells
2—dirt	5—immunity	8—infection
3—broken	6—microscope	9—infect
		10—food

SANITATION AND STERILIZATION

PART I — TRUE OR FALSE TEST

1. An antiseptic prevents the growth of germs ....   T   F
2. Borax and formalin are used in a cabinet sterilizer ....   T   F
3. Sanitation applies to public health only .. ..   T   F
4. Spatulas are used for removing creams from jars ....   T   F
5. The headrest on each chair need not be changed for each customer ....   T   F
6. When a comb is not in use, the barber may keep it in his pocket ....   T   F
7. Lump alum as a styptic may be used on several customers ....   T   F
8. The hands must be washed before and after working on each customer ....   T   F
9. An object that has fallen to the floor should be treated as though it had already been used . ...   T   F
10. Cover coughs and sneezes with a handkerchief ....   T   F
11. Keep clean towels in dust-proof cabinets ....   T   F
12. A communicable disease is one which cannot be avoided   T   F
13. For sterilization, water must be heated to 150 degrees Fahrenheit ....   T   F
14. Hydrogen peroxide is used as an antiseptic ... .   T   F
15. Fumigation produces chemical vapors in a cabinet sterilizer . ...   T   F
16. Any implement that cannot withstand heat may be sterilized by chemicals ....   T   F
17. Boric acid solution is used as a germicide ....   T   F
18. Instruments that cannot be boiled may be sterilized by dipping them into 40% alcohol ....   T   F
19. A disinfectant and a germicide can destroy germs ....   T   F
20. Metal instruments, glass, towels and linens may be sterilized by boiling for two minutes ....   T   F
21. Phenol is also known as carbolic acid ....   T   F
22. Hard rubber combs and hair brushes are best sterilized in boiling water ....   T   F
23. Electrodes may be sterilized with alcohol used on cotton pledget ....   T   F
24. Glycerine added to formalin will prevent the rusting of instruments ....   T   F
25. An object is sterile when it is free from germs ....   T   F
26. Disinfectants may be used on the human body ....   T   F
27. 25% formalin solution is a germicide ....   T   F
28. 60% alcohol may be used on the skin as an antiseptic ....   T   F
29. Combs and brushes are sufficiently sterilized by placing them in a cabinet sterilizer .. ..   T   F
30. Complete sterilization is essential in order to destroy all germs and prevent infection ....   T   F

REVIEW EXAMINATIONS

REVIEW EXAMINATIONS 447

ANSWERS

1—T	2—T	3—F	4—T	5—F
6—F	7—F	8—T	9—T	10—T
11—T	12—F	13—F	14—T	15—T
16—T	17—F	18—F	19—T	20—F
21—T	22—F	23—T	24—T	25—T
26—F	27—T	28—T	29—F	30—T

PART II — MATCHING TEST

Sterilization	Dry heat	Styptic
Chemical	Eye pads	Wet sterilizer
Deodorant	Formalin	Cabinet sterilizer
Hygiene	Combs	Tincture of iodine

1. Implements sterilized with disinfectant solution (...........................)
2. A 40% solution of formaldehyde gas in water ....(...........................)
3. A use for cotton moistened with boric acid solution ....(........................)
4. Method of sterilization for objects that cannot be boiled ....(...........................(
5. The science of preserving health ....(........................)
6. The destruction of all germs ....(...........................)
7. An agent which stops minor bleeding on the skin(...........................)
8. An antiseptic for cuts and bruises ....(...........................)
9. Receptacle for keeping sterilized implements ....(...........................)
10. Receptacle for a disinfectant solution ....(...........................)

ANSWERS

1—Combs	4—Chemical	7—Styptic
2—Formalin	5—Hygiene	8—Tincture of iodine
3—Eye pads	6—Sterilization	9—Cabinet sterilizer
		10—Wet sterilizer

PART III — INSERTION TEST

customer	cabinet	soap
closed	asepsis	unsterilized
water	open	protects
barber	infectious	formaldehyde

1. Responsibility for the prevention of disease in the barber shop rests with the ....
2. Customers having an .... disease should not be treated in the barber shop.
3. The active ingredient of formalin solution is .... gas.
4. Sterilized implements are best stored in a closed .... sterilizer.

5. A sanitary barber shop .... the public's health.
6. The opposite of sepsis is ....
7. Boiling .... is an effective agent for sterilizing barber implements.
8. Clean all implements with .... and warm water before immersing them into a disinfectant.
9. All refuse and hair cuttings should be kept in .... containers.
10. Infection can be caused by the use of .... implements.

ANSWERS

1—barber	4—cabinet	7—water
2—infectious	5—protects	8—soap
3—formaldehyde	6—asepsis	9—closed
		10—unsterilized

PART IV — MATCHING TEST

Prophylaxis	Boiling point of water
Asepsis	Disinfectant
Styptic	Formalin
Sepsis	Antiseptic
Deodorant	Fumigation

1. Stops bleeding .... (........................)
2. Prevention of disease .... (........................)
3. Destroys offensive odors .... (........................)
4. Poisoning due to germs .... (........................)
5. Freedom from germs .... (........................)
6. Checks bacterial growth .... (........................)
7. 37-40% solution of formaldehyde .... (........................)
8. Destroys bacteria .... (........................)
9. Disinfect with chemical vapor .... (........................)
10. 212 degrees Fahrenheit .... (........................)

ANSWERS

1—Styptic	6—Antiseptic
2—Prophylaxis	7—Formalin
3—Deodorant	8—Disinfectant
4—Sepsis	9—Fumigation
5—Asepsis	10—Boiling point of water

CELLS, TISSUES, ORGANS AND SYSTEMS

PART I — TRUE OR FALSE TEST

1. An organ is a group of similar cells performing the the same function .... T F
2. The human body is composed of millions of specialized cells .... T F
3. All cells have the same size and shape .... T F
4. Muscle tissue is capable of contraction .... T F
5. Metabolism represents both constructive and destructive processes .... T F
6. Protoplasm is a jelly-like substance found in living cells T F
7. Epithelial tissue serves as a protective covering of body surfaces .. .. T F
8. The skin is a part of the endocrine system .... T F
9. The heart is an example of an organ .... T F
10. Cells do not have the power to grow and reproduce .. .. T F

ANSWERS

1—F	2—T	3—F	4—T	5—T
6—T	7—T	8—F	9—T	10—F

PART II — INSERTION TEST

respiratory	thyroid	organ
circulatory	mitosis	food
excretory	amitosis	tissue
nucleus	nerve	muscles

1. Metabolism is a complex chemical process controlled by the .... gland.
2. Cells of the human body reproduce by a process called ....
3. The stomach is an example of an ....
4. The blood is an example of a liquid ....
5. An injured .... cell is incapable of self-repair.
6. The .... controls the reproduction of the cell.
7. Adequate .... favors the growth of the cell.
8. The movements of the body are due to the action of ....
9. Waste matter is eliminated from the body through the .... system.
10. The heart is an important organ of the .... system.

ANSWERS

1—thyroid	4—tissue	7—food
2—mitosis	5—nerve	8—muscles
3—organ	6—nucleus	9—excretory
		10—circulatory

PART III — MATCHING TEST

Cell   Nucleus
Anabolism   Catabolism
Cytoplasm

1. Less dense protoplasm. ....(......................)
2. Dense protoplasm ....(......................)
3. Unit of living matter ....(......................)
4. Destructive process ....(......................)
5. Constructive process ....(......................)

ANSWERS

1—Cytoplasm   4—Catabolism
2—Nucleus   5—Anabolism
3—Cell

BONES

PART I — TRUE OR FALSE TEST

1. The cranium consists of ten bones ....   T   F
2. The mandible is located at the lower part of the face ....   T   F
3. Bone is composed of organic and inorganic matter ....   T   F
4. The cranium protects the brain ....   T   F
5. The cranium is the bony case which encases the brain ....   T   F
6. The occipital is located at the crown .. ..   T   F
7. The parietal is located at the forehead .. ..   T   F
8. Periosteum is a disease of the bone ....   T   F
9. There are fourteen bones of the face ....   T   F
10. The maxilla is a small bone of the ear ....   T   F

ANSWERS

1—F	2—T	3—T	4—T	5—T
6—F	7—F	8—F	9—T	10—F

PART II — MATCHING TEST

Hyoid   Malar   Periosteum
Marrow   Anatomy   Ethmoid
Mandible   Frontal   Sphenoid
Occipital   Temporal   Physiology

1. The study of the structure of the body ....(............................)
2. A bone forming the back and lower part of the
   cranium ....(............................)
3. The portion of the bone which supports blood
   vessels and nerves and also nourishes the bone....(.................. ......)

4. A soft, fatty substance filling the cavities of the
bone ....(........................)

5. A U-shaped bone at the base of the tongue ....(........................)

6. The cheek bone .. ..(......... ....)

7. A bone at the side of the head ....(........................)

8. The lower jaw bone ....(........................)

9. A bone forming the forehead ....(........................)

10. A bone which joins together all bones of the
cranium ....(........................)

ANSWERS

1—Anatomy	4—Marrow	7—Temporal
2—Occipital	5—Hyoid	8—Mandible
3—Periosteum	6—Malar	9—Frontal
		10—Sphenoid

PART III — MATCHING TEST

Base of skull	Ear region
Base of cranium	Bridge of nose
Lower jaw	Forehead
Upper jaw	Front of throat
Cheek	Sides and crown of head

1. Frontal ....(...)

2. Temporal ....(...)

3. Sphenoid ....(...)

4. Occipital ....(...)

5. Parietal ....(...)

6. Hyoid ....(...)

7. Mandible ....(...)

8. Maxilla ....(...)

9. Malar ....(...)

10. Nasal ....(...)

ANSWERS

1—Forehead	6—Front of throat
2—Ear region	7—Lower jaw
3—Base of cranium	8—Upper jaw
4—Base of skull	9—Cheek
5—Sides and crown of head	10—Bridge of nose

MUSCLES

PART I — TRUE OR FALSE TEST

1. The function of muscles is to produce all movements of the body .... T F
2. The heart has no muscular structure .... T F
3. The corrugator causes vertical wrinkles above the nose T F
4. The arrector pili is one of the largest muscles of the face T F
5. The epicranius controls the movements of the scalp, and wrinkles the forehead . ... T F
6. Voluntary muscles are controlled by the will .... T F
7. The cardiac muscle is a voluntary muscle .... T F
8. Aponeurosis is a flat expanded tendon .... T F
9. Muscles may be stimulated by massage, heat, and electric current .... T F
10. Striated muscles are involuntary .... T F
11. The orbicularis oris is the muscle that surrounds the eye T F
12. Muscles are always connected directly to bones .... T F
13. The muscular system relies upon the skeletal and nervous systems for its activities .... T F
14. Contractility means able to be stretched or extended ...... T F
15. Muscles clothe and support the framework of the body T F

ANSWERS

1—T	2—F	3—T	4—F	5—T
6—T	7—F	8—T	9—T	10—F
11—F	12—F	13—T	14—F	15—T

PART II — MATCHING TEST

Tendon	Epicranius	Non-striated
Elastic	Caninus	Trapezius
Aponeurosis	Striated	

1. Meaning the same as voluntary muscle ....(.........................)
2. A broad, flat tendon, which serves to connect one muscle to another ....(............. .... ..)
3. Meaning the same as involuntary muscle . ...(.........................)
4. A fibrous tissue which connects muscle with bone(...................... ..)
5. A muscle which draws the head backwards or to one side ....(.........................)
6. The ability to stretch and return to its natural shape ....(.........................)
7. The scalp muscle ....(.........................)

ANSWERS

1—Striated	3—Non-striated	5—Trapezius
2—Aponeurosis	4—Tendon	6—Elastic
		7—Epicranius

PART III — MATCHING TEST

Anterior	Posterior	Levator
Superior	Inferior	Lateral
		Dilator

1. On the side ....(.........................)
2. Situated lower ....(.........................)

3. Situated higher ....(.....................)
4. In front of ....(.....................)
5. In back of ....(.....................)
6. That which enlarges ....(.....................)
7. That which lifts ....(.....................)

ANSWERS

1—Lateral	3—Superior	5—Posterior
2—Inferior	4—Anterior	6—Dilator
		7—Levator

PART IV — CLASSIFICATION TEST

Platysma	Temporalis	Risorius
Masseter	Orbicularis oculi	Epicranius
Depressor septi	Orbicularis oris	Procerus
		Trapezius

1. Scalp Muscle ....(...................................)
2. Eye Muscle ....(...................................)
3. Nose Muscles ....(..... ....)
4. Mouth Muscles ....(.............. ....)
5. Muscles of Mastication ....(...................................)
6. Neck Muscles ....(..... ....)

ANSWERS

1—Epicranius	4—Orbicularis oris, risorius
2—Orbicularis oculi	5—Masseter, temporalis
3—Depressor septi, procerus	6—Platysma, trapezius

PART V — MATCHING TEST

Cheek region	Side of mouth	Neck
Nose	Around mouth	Entire scalp
Side of head	Around eyes	Back part of scalp
		Front part of scalp

1. Orbicularis oris ....(...................................)
2. Orbicularis oculi ....(...................................)
3. Epicranius ....(...................................)
4. Procerus ....(...................................)
5. Platysma ....(...................................)
6. Occipitalis ....(...................................)
7. Frontalis ....(...................................)
8. Buccinator ....(...................................)
9. Temporalis ....(...................................)
10. Risorius ....(...................................)

ANSWERS

1—Around mouth	6—Back part of scalp
2—Around eyes	7—Front part of scalp
3—Entire scalp	8—Cheek region
4—Nose	9—Side of head
5—Neck	10—Side of mouth

NERVES

PART I — TRUE OR FALSE TEST

1. Nerves can be both motor and sensory .... T F
2. Nerves can be stimulated with massage .... T F
3. The trifacial nerve is the smallest of all the cranial nerves .... T F
4. The facial nerve controls the muscles of expression .... T F
5. The cervical nerves supply the muscles and skin at the back of the head and neck .... T F
6. There are twelve pairs of cerebral (cranial) nerves .... T F
7. The trifacial nerve is the same as the facial nerve .... T F
8. Nerves which respond to heat, cold, pressure, touch and pain are called sensory nerves .... T F
9. Nerve points are not intended to be stimulated .... T F
10. There are 15 pairs of spinal nerves .... T F

ANSWERS

1—T	2—T	3—F	4—T	5—T
6—T	7—F	8—T	9—F	10—F

PART II — MATCHING TEST

Neuron   Optic nerve
Sympathetic system   Motor nerve
Sensory nerve   Facial nerve
Cerebro-spinal system   12 pairs
Trigeminal nerve   31 pairs

1. Consists of the brain, spinal cord, spinal nerves and cranial nerves ....(.........................)
2. Controls the involuntary muscles which affect respiration, circulation and digestion ....(.........................)
3. Carries impulses from a nerve center to a muscle ....(.........................)
4. A nerve cell ....(.........................)
5. The chief sensory nerve of the face ....(.........................)
6. A nerve which controls the sense of sight ....(.........................)
7. A nerve carrying sensations to a nerve center ....(.........................)
8. A nerve which controls facial expression ....(.........................)
9. Number of cranial nerves ....(.........................)
10. Number of spinal nerves ....(.........................)

ANSWERS

1—Cerebro-spinal system	6—Optic nerve
2—Sympathetic system	7—Sensory nerve
3—Motor nerve	8—Facial nerve
4—Neuron	9—12 pairs
5—Trigeminal nerve	10—31 pairs

PART III — MATCHING TEST

Scalp area at base of skull	Lower side of nose
Forehead and temple	Side of neck
Behind ear	Temple and ear
Forehead and scalp	Upper part of cheek
Lower lip and chin	Side of nose and mouth

1. Supra-orbital ....(.............................. .. ..)
2. Cervical ....(..)
3. Mental ....(. ....)
4. Infra-orbital ....(........... ....)
5. Auriculo-temporal ... . (...)
6. Lesser occipital . ...(............... ....)
7. Zygomatic ....(. ... .)
8. Temporal ....(...)
9. Posterior auricular ....(... .. ..)
10 Nasal .... (... .)

ANSWERS

1—Forehead and scalp	6—Scalp area at base of skull
2—Side of neck	7—Upper part of cheek
3—Lower lip and chin	8—Forehead and temple
4—Side of nose and mouth	9—Behind ear
5—Temple and ear	10—Lower side of nose

PART IV — CLASSIFICATION TEST

Directions: Classify the following cerebral nerves. Insert the correct nerves under the proper headings.

Facial	Optic	Oculomotor
Trifacial	Acoustic	Abducent
Olfactory	Vagus	Accessory

1. Sensory Nerves:	2. Motor Nerves:	3. Sensory-Motor:
....	....	------------------------------------
....	....	....
....	... .	------------------------------------

ANSWERS

1—Olfactory, optic, acoustic
2—Oculomotor, accessory, abducent
3—Trifacial, facial, vagus

CIRCULATION

PART I — TRUE OR FALSE TEST

1. The blood vascular system controls the circulation of blood .... T F
2. The supra-orbital artery supplies the back of the head ... T F
3. From 8 to 10 pints of blood circulates in the body of an adult person .... T F
4. Lymph reaches parts of the body not reached by the blood .... T F
5. General circulation carries the blood from the heart to the lungs .... T F
6. The blood carries oxygen to the cells and carbon dioxide from them .... T F
7. Arteries always carry the impure blood .... T F
8. The vascular system consists of the heart and blood vessels (arteries, veins and capillaries) .... T F
9. Red blood cells fight germs in the blood .... T F
10. Arteries, veins and capillaries are blood vessels .... T F

ANSWERS

1—T	2—F	3—T	4—T	5—F
6—T	7—F	8—T	9—F	10—T

PART II — MATCHING TEST

Auricles   Ventricles
General circulation Vein
Vascular   Plasma
White blood cells   Red blood cells
Jugular vein   Lymph
Carotid arteries   Capillary
Pulmonary circulation

1. The smallest blood vessel ....(.......................)
2. Upper chambers of the heart ....(........................)
3. Blood cells which carry oxygen .. ..(........................)
4. Blood circulation throughout the body . ...(........................)
- 5. Main arteries supplying the head, face and neck (........................)
6. The fluid part of the blood ....(........................)
7. Blood cells which destroy pathogenic bacteria ....(........................)
8. The lower chambers of the heart .. ..(........................)
9. A fluid derived from blood plasma ....(........................)
10. Blood circulation from the heart to the lungs . ..(........................)

ANSWERS

1—Capillary	6—Plasma
2—Auricles	7—White blood cells
3—Red blood cells	8—Ventricles
4—General circulation	9—Lymph
5—Carotid arteries	10—Pulmonary circulation

PART III — MATCHING TEST

Back of head	Forehead
Chin and lower lip	Side of nose
Orbicularis oculi	Upper lip
Scalp above and back of ear	Crown and side of head
Eye socket and forehead	Lower lip

1. Frontal ....(...)
2. Posterior auricular ....(...)
3. Submental ....(...)
4. Supra-orbital ....(...)
5. Angular ....(...)
6. Superior labial ....(...)
7. Occipital ....(...)
8. Parietal ....(...)
9. Inferior labial ....(...)
10. Orbital ....(...)

ANSWERS

1—Forehead	6—Upper lip
2—Scalp above and back of ear	7—Back of head
3—Chin and lower lip	8—Crown and side of head
4—Eye socket and forehead	9—Lower lip
5—Side of nose	10—Orbicularis oculi

PART IV — MATCHING TEST

Auricles	Hemoglobin	Veins
Ventricles	Lymphatics	Pericardium

1. A membrane enclosing the heart ....(..................)
2. Vessels which convey lymph ....(..................)
3. Upper cavities of the heart ....(..................)
4. Blood vessels containing valves ....(..................)
5. Coloring matter of red corpuscles ....(..................)
6. Lower cavities of the heart ....(..................)

ANSWERS

1—Pericardium	3—Auricles	5—Hemoglobin
2—Lymphatics	4—Veins	6—Ventricles

PART V — MATCHING TEST

Frontal	Superior labial
Parietal	Transverse facial
Posterior auricular	

1. Crown and side of head ....(..................)
2. Upper lip and septum of nose ....(..................)
3. Masseter muscle ....(..................)
4. Forehead ....(..................)
5. Scalp, back of ear ....(..................)

ANSWERS

1—Parietal	4—Frontal
2—Superior labial	5—Posterior auricular
3—Transverse facial	

SKIN, HAIR AND GLANDS

PART I — TRUE OR FALSE TEST

1. The subcutaneous tissue of the skin lies directly beneath the corium .... T F
2. Corium, derma and true skin are the same .... T F
3. The skin is an external non-flexible covering of the body T F
4. Dermatology is the study of the hair .... T F
5. The appendages of the skin are the nails, hair, sebaceous and sudoriferous glands .... T F
6. Skin absorbs water readily .... T F
7. Health, age and occupation have no influence on the texture of the skin .... T F
8. The skin is the organ of protection, absorption, elimination, heat regulation, and sensation .... T F
9. The skin is the seat of the organ of touch .... T F
10. The sebaceous glands secrete sebum .... T F
11. The blood vessels which nourish the hair are located in the hair papilla .... T F
12. When the blood supply is cut off, the growth of hair is stopped .... T F
13. Under normal conditions hair grows about one-half inch a month .... T F
14. Sebum cools the skin .... T F
15. Hair will grow again even though the papilla has been destroyed .... T F
16. There are more hairs than follicles .... T F
17. After a hair has fallen out, new hair will appear in about three days .... T F
18. Hair has no blood vessels .... T F
19. The average life of a hair is from seven to eight years T F
20. The health of the hair depends on the health of the body T F

ANSWERS

1—T	2—T	3—F	4—F	5—T
6—F	7—F	8—T	9—T	10—T
11—T	12—T	13—T	14—F	15—F
16—F	17—F	18—T	19—F	20—T

PART II — MATCHING TEST

Sudoriferous glands   Subcutaneous tissue
Melanin   Sebaceous glands
Derma   Papilla
Epidermis   Follicle
Stratum corneum   Perspiration
Sebum

1. The outer layer of the skin ....(....................)
2. The fatty tissue of the skin ....(....................)
3. The true layer of the skin ....(....................)
4. Glands which secrete sebum ....(....................)
5. An excretion which cools the skin by evaporation (....................)
6. Cone-shaped elevation which nourishes the hair (....................)
7. Glands which produce perspiration . ...(....................)
8. The coloring pigment in the skin ....(....................)
9. A product secreted by the oil glands .. ..(.. ....)
10. The horny layer of the epidermis ....(....................)

ANSWERS

1—Epidermis   6—Papilla
2—Subcutaneous tissue   7—Sudoriferous glands
3—Derma   8—Melanin
4—Sebaceous glands   9—Sebum
5—Perspiration   10—Stratum corneum

PART III — INSERTION TEST

Touch   Melanin   Granulosum
Eyelids   Skin   Corneum
Germinativum   Arrector pili   Limited
Lucidum   Blood   Unlimited
Nervous   Duct

1. The actively growing layer of the skin is called the stratum
....
2. The excretion of sweat is under the control of the ....
system.
3. Attached to the hair follicle is the .... muscle.
4. The skin is thinnest on the ....
5. The coloring matter of the skin and hair is known as ....
6. The sweat and oil glands of the skin are .... type of
glands.
7. The stratum .... is continually being shed and replaced.
8. The skin has .... powers of absorption through its pores.
9. The largest organ of the body is the ....
10. The skin has nerve endings which respond to heat, cold and
....
11. The largest amount of .... is found in the skin.

ANSWERS

1—Germinativum	5—Melanin	9—Skin
2—Nervous	6—Duct	10—Touch
3—Arrector pili	7—Corneum	11—Blood
4—Eyelids	8—Limited	

PART IV — MATCHING TEST

Papillary layer	Hirsute
Stratum corneum	Stratum germinativum
Dermis	Keratin
Stratum lucidum	Follicle
Subcutaneous tissue	Cortex
Papilla	

1. Clear layer of the epidermis ....(.........................)

2. Skin layer containing elastic fibers ....(.... ....)

3. Fatty tissue of the skin ....(.........................)

4. Layer of epidermis containing keratin ....(............. ....)

5. Layer of dermis containing tactile corpuscles ....(.........................)

6. A horny substance found in hair ....(.........................)

7. A tube-like depression extending into the dermis(.........................)

8. Hair layer containing pigment ....(............. ....)

9. Hairy ....(.........................)

10. Cone-like elevation at the base of hair follicle.. (..... ....)

11. Basal layer of epidermis ....(.........................)

ANSWERS

1—Stratum lucidum	7—Follicle
2—Dermis	8—Cortex
3—Subcutaneous tissue	9—Hirsute
4—Stratum corneum	10—Papilla
5—Papillary layer	11—Stratum germinativum
6—Keratin	

SKIN, SCALP AND HAIR DISEASES

` PART I — TRUE OR FALSE TEST

1. Trichophytosis is the term applied to ringworm of the scalp .... T F
2. Gray hair is best treated with safe hair dyes .... T F
3. Anthrax may be treated by a barber .... T F
4. Regular alopecia treatments alternated with hot oil treatments will correct canities .... T F
5. Scabies refers to head lice .... T F
6. Tinea tonsurans is ringworm of the scalp .... T F
7. Keloid is a wartlike growth commonly located in the eyelids .... T F
8. A communicable disease is one that can be transmitted from person to person .... T F
9. Alopecia areata is baldness at time of birth . ... T F
10. Pityriasis is the term applied to an excessively oily condition of the scalp .... T F
11. Canities is caused by fever, shock, nervousness, or old age .... T F
12. Eczema is a contagious, parasitic disease of the skin, with crust formations, emitting a mousy odor .... T F
13. Symptoms of alopecia areata and alopecia senilis are the same .... T F
14. Pediculosis capitis is a scaly condition of the scalp .... T F
15. A tight scalp is favorable to the growth of hair .... T F
16. Skin friction may cause the formation of a callous .... T F
17. The skin cannot function properly if the pores are clogged with dust, creams or sebum .... T F
18. If the skin has a tendency to be very dry, soap should be used regularly .... T F
19. Acne is a chronic inflammation of the sebaceous glands of the skin .... T F
20. No hair brushing is required when treating a dry scalp T F
21. Long neglected dandruff frequently leads to baldness .... T F
22. Pityriasis steatoides is also known as greasy or waxy dandruff .... T F
23. The symptoms of pityriasis capitis simplex are itching scalp and dry dandruff .... T F
24. Dandruff is considered a disease if the shedding of scales is excessive .... T F
25. Oily foods tend to aggravate a dry condition of the skin T F
26. Acne rosacea affects the sweat glands .... T F
27. Anidrosis means the same as excessive perspiration .... T F
28. In many cases the early stages of baldness can be corrected by proper treatment .... T F
29. The cause of eczema is unknown .... T F
30. Ringworm is a non-contagious disease .... T F

ANSWERS

1—T	2—T	3—F	4—F	5—F
6—T	7—F	8—T	9—F	10—F
11—T	12—F	13—F	14—F	15—F
16—T	17—T	18—F	19—T	20—F
21—T	22—T	23—T	24—T	25—F
26—F	27—F	28—T	29—T	30—F

PART II — MATCHING TEST

Comedones	Hyperidrosis	Canities
Pityriasis	Papule	Acne
Seborrhea	Eczema	Pustule

1. A chronic inflammatory disease of the skin occurring in or around a sebaceous gland .... (............ ... .)

2. A condition characterized by an excessive discharge of sebum .... (...... ... .)

3. Blackheads .... (... ....)

4. Excessive perspiration .... (. ... ...)

5. A lesion which contains pus .. ..(..... ....)

ANSWERS

1—Acne	3—Comedones	5—Pustule
2—Seborrhea	4—Hyperidrosis	

PART III — INSERTION TEST

baldness	bromidrosis	greasy
gray	skin	non-contagious
contagious	pus	follicle
chronic	contagious	acute
dry	dermatitis	

1. Alopecia means ....

2. Canities means . ... hair.

3. Foul smelling perspiration is known as ....

4. Dermatology deals with diseases of the ....

5. Dandruff may occur in a .... or .... form.

6. A pustule is an elevation of the skin having an inflamed base containing ....

7. A tumor is a .... skin lesion.

8. A disease of long duration is known as a .... disease.

9. Inflammation of the skin is called ....

10. A boil is an infection of a hair ....

ANSWERS

1—baldness	4—skin	7—non-contagious
2—gray	5—dry, greasy	8—chronic
3—bromidrosis	6—pus	9—dermatitis
		10—follicle

PART IV — MATCHING TEST

Scar	Fissure	Tumor
Ulcer	Vesicle	

1. Deep crack in the skin .... (........................)
2. A blister .... (........................)
3. External swelling .... (........................)
4. Open lesion having pus ....(. ....)
5. Healed wound or healed ulcer .... (............ ....)

ANSWERS

1—Fissure	3—Tumor	5—Scar
2—Vesicle	4—Ulcer	

PART V — MATCHING TEST

Asteatosis	Acne pustulosa	Acne vulgaris
Seborrhea	Acne indurata	

1. The common pimple .... (........................)
2. Excessive discharge of sebum .... (........................)
3. Deep-seated hardened lesions .... (........................)
4. Dry skin due to senile changes .... (........................)
5. Pimples containing pus ....(........................)

ANSWERS

1—Acne vulgaris	3—Acne indurata	5—Acne pustulosa
2—Seborrhea	4—Asteatosis	

ELECTRICITY AND LIGHT THERAPY

PART I — TRUE OR FALSE TEST

1. An alternating current flows first in one direction and then in the opposite direction .... T F
2. High-frequency treatments may be given after an alcoholic tonic has been applied .... T F
3. Infra-red rays are purely heat rays ... . T F
4. Ultra-violet rays are chemical rays . .. . T F
5. Electricity may be transmitted to the customers through the use of the vibrator . ... T F
6. High-frequency is an oscillating current which is stimulating .... T F
7. A closed circuit is one in which a current is continually flowing .... T F
8. It is unnecessary to sterilize electrodes used with high-frequency .... T F
9. An insulator conveys an electrical current .... T F
10. Only first degree sunburn has cosmetic value .... T F
11. An ohm is a unit of current resistance .... T F
12. The infra-red rays have a chemical effect .. .. T F
13. To obtain the most benefit from ultra-violet rays, the skin must be free of creams or other cosmetics .... T F
14. Any substance which carries electricity freely is called a conductor .. .. T F
15. The customer's eyes should be protected with goggles when using ultra-violet rays .... T F

ANSWERS

1—T	2—F	3—T	4—T	5—F
6—T	7—T	8—F	9—F	10—T
11—T	12—F	13—T	14—T	15—T

PART II — MATCHING TEST

Conductor	Ultra-violet rays
Volt	Ampere
Infra-red rays	Non-conductor
High-frequency current	Ohm

1. A unit of electrical resistance ....(......... ....)

2. The strength of an electric current ....(..........................)

3. Rays emitted from a quartz lamp .... (..........................)

4. A unit of electrical pressure ....(..........................)

5. Rays which have a deep penetrating effect on

 the skin ....(........................ ..)

6. A substance which transmits electricity ....(..... ....)

ANSWERS

1—Ohm	4—Volt
2—Ampere	5—Infra-red rays
3—Ultra-violet rays	6—Conductor

SHAVING AND HAIRCUTTING

PART I — TRUE OR FALSE

1. The width of the razor should be about ⅝ of an inch   T   F
2. Steel razors are more durable than silver-plated ones....   T   F
3. The French type of shears has no finger brace ....   T   F
4. Shears having a gauge of 7 inches and a plain edge are preferred to other kinds ....   T   F
5. The number 1 cutting edge of a hair clipper is the smallest size available ....   T   F
6. A razor is never used for thinning or tapering the hair   T   F
7. Shaving cake soap or stick should never be used in common ....   T   F
8. A razor has a perfect edge when its teeth are coarse   T   F
9. A rotary movement is best in lathering the beard ....   T   F
10. Before shaving, use hot towels for a sensitive or chapped face ....   T   F
11. Ingrown hair is caused by close shaving ....   T   F
12. In giving a haircut it is not necessary to consider the customer's facial features ....   T   F
13. Alcohol may be used to sterilize clipper blades ....   T   F
14. Use a fresh neck strip and towel for each customer ....   T   F

ANSWERS

1—T	2—T	3—F	4—T	5—F
6—F	7—T	8—F	9—T	10—F
11—T	12—F	13—T	14—T	

PART II — MATCHING TEST

Thinning	Free hand	Ingrown hair
Singeing	Tapering	Clipping
Hone	Back hand	

1. Decreasing the amount of hair where it is too thick .. ..(.........................)

2. Burning the hair ends ....(................ ... ...)

3. Hair growing underneath the skin ....(... ....)

4. A shaving stroke used most frequently ....(............. ....)

5. An implement used to sharpen the dull edge of a razor ....(............. ... .)

ANSWERS

1—Thinning	4—Free hand
2—Singeing	5—Hone
3—Ingrown hair	

PART III — INSERTION TEST

fourteen	dull	test
steam	two	stropping
left	synthetic	0000
right	free	00
grain	back	

1. There are .... standard shaving areas.

2. A .... towel is usually applied before and after shaving.

3. Shaving strokes are made with the .... of the hair.

4. The .... side of the face is usually shaved first.

5. A number .... cutting blade on a hair clipper gives the shortest cut.

6. A .... hone is a fast cutting hone.

7. The .... edge of the razor requires honing and stropping.

8. The .... hand stroke is used most often in face shaving.

9. Always .... a razor after honing or stropping.

10. The purpose of .... a razor before shaving is to make its edge smooth.

ANSWERS

1—fourteen	4—right	7—dull
2—steam	5—0000	8—free
3—grain	6—synthetic	9—test
		10—stropping

FACIAL AND SCALP TREATMENTS

PART I — TRUE OR FALSE TEST

1. Facial or scalp treatments are not to be given if a communicable disease is recognized in a customer .... T F

2. The barber gives massage treatments only to the head, face and neck .... T F

3. Dry hair requires more frequent shampooing than oily hair .... T F

4. Firm kneading or fast tapping movements help to reduce fatty tissue .... T F

5. A lanolin cream is best for a dry skin .... T F

6. An astringent lotion is recommended for an excessively dry skin .... T F

7. A clay pack is good for all types of skin except a dry skin .... T F

8. A hot oil mask is recommended for a dry skin .... T F

9. After extracting comedones, do not apply an antiseptic solution to the skin .... T F

10. Regular scalp massage will make a tight scalp flexible T F

11. Regular and systematic treatments for the skin or scalp are more effective than an occasional treatment .... T F

12. After an egg shampoo, use hot water to rinse the hair T F

13. The frequent use of strong soaps and alcoholic tonics will cause the hair to become dry .... T F

14. An acne facial may be given without the advice of a physician .... T F

15. Pure castile soap is good for a general shampoo .... T F

ANSWERS

1—T	2—T	3—F	4—T	5—T
6—F	7—T	8—T	9—F	10—T
11—T	12—F	13—T	14—F	15—T

PART II — MATCHING TEST

Dry hair	Sulphur ointment	Hard water
Soft water	Oily hair	Neutral
Alkaline	Boiling	Ultra-violet
Egg shampoo	Acid	Manipulations

1. Soap will not lather with ....(.........................)

2. Soap will form a lather with .... (.........................)

3. The easiest way to soften water is by . .. .(......... ....)

4. The best therapeutic rays for the treatment of dandruff ....(......... ....)

5. A medicinal ointment used in the treatment of alopecia ....(......... ....)

6. Hand movements ....(................ ... ..)

ANSWERS

| 1—Hard water | 3—Boiling | 5—Sulphur ointment |
| 2—Soft water | 4—Ultra-violet | 6—Manipulations |

PART III — INSERTION TEST

effleurage	stimulating	pressure
petrissage	hands	rotary
relaxing	face	shaking
nerves	skin	

1. Massage is applied either with the .... or with electric appliances.
2. Massage by the barber is usually limited to the regions of the head, ... and neck.
3. A kneading massage movement is known as ....
4. A stroking massage movement is applied in a slow, rhythmic manner without ....
5. .... massage movements are frequently used in scalp massage.
6. The .. .. are rested and soothed by massage.
7. Applying massage with an even rhythm produces a .... effect on the customer.
8. Vibration is described as a .... massage movement.
9. Friction stimulates the circulation and glandular activities of the ....
10. A stroking massage movement is also known as ....

ANSWERS

1—hands	4—pressure	7—relaxing
2—face	5—rotary	8—shaking
3—petrissage	6—nerves	9—skin
		10—effleurage

PART VI

GLOSSARY

*Used in connection with Barbering
relationship only.*

GLOSSARY

Compiled of words used in connection with barbering, defined in the sense of anatomical, medical, electrical, and barbering relationship only. Key to pronunciation will be found at bottom of each page.

A

abdomen (ăb-dō'měn): the belly.

abducent nerve (ăb-dū'sênt nûrv): the sixth cerebral nerve; a small motor nerve supplying the external rectus muscle of the eye

abductor (ăb-dŭk'těr): a muscle that draws a part away from the median line (opp., adductor).

abnormal (ăb-nôr'măl): irregular, contrary to the natural law or customary order.

abrasion (ă-brā'zhûn). scraping of skin.

abscess (ăb'sěs): an enclosed cavity containing pus.

absorption (ăb-sôrp'shûn)· assimilation of one body by another; act of absorbing.

accessory nerve (ăk-sěs'ō-rē nûrv): spinal accessory nerve; eleventh cerebral nerve; affects the sterno-cleido-mastoid and trapezius muscles of the neck and back.

acetic (ă-sět'ĭk): pertaining to vinegar; sour.

acid (ăs'ĭd). any chemical compound having a sour taste.

acid rinse (ăs'ĭd rĭns): a solution of water and lemon juice or vinegar.

acidosis (ăs-ĭ-dō'sĭs). a condition in which there is an excess of acid products in the blood or excreted in the urine.

acidum boricum (ăs'ĭ-dûm bôr'ĭ-kûm): boric acid.

acne (ăk'nē)· a skin disorder due to inflammatory changes of the sebaceous glands.

acne albida (ăl'bĭ-dă): milium; whitehead.

acne artificialis (ar-tĭ-fĭsh-ăl'ĭs): pimples due to external irritants or drugs take internally.

acne atrophica (ă-trŏf'ĭ-kă) acne in which the lesions leave a slight amount of scarring.

acne cachecticorum (kă-kěk-tĭ-kôr-ûm): pimples occurring in the subjects having anemia or some weakening body disease.

acne hypertrophica (hĭ-pěr-trŏf'ĭ-kă): pimples in which the lesions on healing leave conspicuous pits and scars.

acne indurata (ĭn-dū-ra'tă) deeply seated pimples with hard tubercles occurring chiefly on the back

acne keratosa (kěr-ă-tō'să). an eruption of papules consisting of horny plugs projecting from the hair follicles, accompanied by inflammation.

acne punctata (pŭnk-ta'tă). appear as red papules in which are usually found blackheads.

acne pustulosa (pŭs-tū-lō'să)· acne in which the pustular lesions predominate.

acne rosacea (rō-zā'shē-ă). a form of acne usually occurring around the nose and cheeks, due to congestion, in which the capillaries become dilated and sometimes broken.

acne simplex (sĭm'plěks). acne vulgaris; simple uncomplicated pimples.

acne vulgaris (vŭl-găr'ĭs): acne simplex; simple uncomplicated pimples.

acoustic (ă-kōos'tĭk): auditory; eighth cerebral nerve; controlling the sense of hearing

actinic (ăk-tĭn'ĭk): relating to the chemically active rays of the spectrum

activity (ăk-tĭv'ĭ-tē): natural or normal function or operation, physical motion or exercise of force.

acute (ă-kūt'). attended with severe symptoms, having a short and relatively short course.

ad (ăd). a prefix denoting to, toward, addition.

adductor (ă-dŭk'těr)· a muscle that draws a part toward the median line

adenoma sebaceum (ă-děn-ō'mă sē-bā'sē-ûm): small tumor of transparent appearance, originating in the sebaceous glands.

adipose tissue (tĭsh'û): fatty tissue, connective tissue containing fat cells; subcutaneous tissue.

adolescence (ăd-ô-lĕs'ĕns): state or process of growing from childhood to manhood or womanhood

adrenal (ăd-rē'năl)· an endocrine gland situated on the top of the kidneys.

adult (ă-dŭlt')· grown up to full age, size or strength.

aeration (ā-ēr-ā'shûn). the change of venous into arterial blood in the lungs.

aerobic (ā-ēr-ô'bĭk). unable to live without oxygen

aesthetic, esthetic (ĕs-thĕt'ĭk) relating to sensation, either mental or physical, appreciation of beauty and art.

afferent nerves (ă-fĕr'ĕnt nûrvz) convey stimulus from the external organs to the brain

affinity (â-fĭn-ĭ-tē)· attraction

agent (a'jĕnt). an active power which can produce a physical, chemical or medicinal effect

al (ăl). a word termination denoting belonging to, of, or pertaining to.

alae nasi (ā'lē nā'zī). the wing cartilage of the nose

albinism (ăl-bĭ-nĭz'm): congenital leucoderma or absence of coloring in the skin, hair and iris.

albino (ăl-bī'nō). a subject of albinism; a person with very little or no pigment in the skin, hair or iris.

alcohol (ăl'kô-hŏl). a readily evaporating colorless liquid with a pungent odor and burning taste; powerful stimulant and antiseptic

alimentary (ăl-ĭ-mĕn'tă-rē) nourishing; relating to food or nutrition.

alkali (ăl'kă-lī): an electropositive substance; capable of making soaps from fats; used to neutralize acids.

alkaline (ăl'ka-lĭn): having the properties of an alkali.

allergic (â-lûr'jĭk). sensitive to; susceptible.

allergy (ă'lûr-jē): a disorder due to extreme sensitivity to certain foods or chemicals.

alopecia (ăl-ô-pē'shē-ă): deficiency of hair; baldness

alopecia adnata (ăd-nă'tă): baldness at birth.

alopecia areata (ā-rē-ă'tă): baldness in spots or patches.

alopecia cicatrisata (sĭ-kă-trĭ-sa'tă): baldness in irregular spots or patches, due to shrinkage of the skin.

alopecia dynamica (dī-năm'ĭ-kă): loss of hair due to destruction of the hair follicle by ulceration or some other disease process

alopecia follicularis (fŏl-ĭk-ū-lăr'ĭs)· loss of hair due to inflamed hair follicles.

alopecia localis (lō-kā'lĭs) loss of hair occurring in patches on the course of a nerve at the site of an injury

alopecia maligna (mă-lĭg'nă). a term applied to any form of alopecia that is severe and persistent.

alopecia prematura (prē-mă-tū'ră)· baldness beginning before middle age.

alopecia seborrheica (sĕb-ôr-ē'ĭ-kă)· baldness caused by diseased sebaceous glands

alopecia senilis (sē-nĭl'ĭs): baldness occurring in old age

alopecia syphilitica (sĭf-ĭl-ĭt'ĭ'kă) loss of hair resulting from syphilis; usually a symptom of the second stage of the disease

alopecia universalis (ū-nĭ-vēr-să'lĭs): a condition manifested by general falling out of the hair of the body.

alum, alumen (ăl'ŭm, ă-lū'mĕn) sulphate of potassium and aluminum, an astringent; used as a styptic

amitosis (ăm-ĭ-tō'sĭs) cell multiplication by direct division of the nucleus in the cell.

ammonia (ă-mō'nē-ă): a colorless gas with a pungent odor; very soluble in water.

amperage (ăm-pâr'âj, ăm'pēr-âj) the strength of an electric current

ampere (ăm-pâr): the unit of measurement of strength of an electric current.

anabolism (ăn-âb'ô-lĭz'm). constructive metabolism; the process of assimilation of nutritive material and its change into living substance

analysis (ă-năl'ĭ-sĭs). a process by which the nature of a substance is recognized and its chemical composition determined.

anaphoresis (ăn-ă-fôr-ē'sĭs): the process of forcing liquids into the tissues from the negative toward the positive pole while using the galvanic current.

anatomy (ă-năt'ô-mē): the science of the gross structure of the body

ill; ōld, ôbey, ôrb, ŏdd, cônnect, sôft, fōōd, fŏŏt, ūse, ûnite, ûrn, ŭp, circûs; those

anemia, anaemia (ă-nē'mē-ă)· a condition in which the blood is deficient in red corpuscles, or in hemoglobin, or both.

anesthetic, anaesthetic (ăn-ĕs-thĕt'ĭk)· a substance administered to make the body incapable of feeling pain

angiology (ăn-jē-ŏl'ŏ-jē). the science of the blood vessels and lymphatics.

Angstrom (ăng'strŏm): a unit of measurement for the wave length of light

angular artery (ăng'ū-lăr ar'tĕr-ē)· supplies muscles and skin at side of nose.

anidrosis, anhidrosis (ăn-ĭ-drō'sĭs): a deficiency in perspiration.

aniline (ăn'ĭ-lĭn, -lēn): a product of coal tar used in the manufacture of artificial dyes.

anode (ăn'ōd) the positive terminal of an electric source.

anterior (ăn-tē'rē-ēr). situated before or in front of.

anthrax (ăn'thrăks). malignant pustule; gangrenous carbuncle-like lesion.

antibody (ăn'tĭ-bŏd-ĭ). a substance in the blood which builds resistance to disease.

antidote (ăn'tĭ-dōt): an agent preventing or counteracting the action of a poison.

anti-perspirant (ăn-tĭ-pĕr-spī'rănt)· a strong astringent liquid or cream used to stop the flow of perspiration in the region of the armpits, hands or feet.

antiseptic (ăn-tĭ-sĕp'tĭk). a chemical agent that kills or prevents the growth of bacteria

antitoxin (ăn-tĭ-tôk'sĭn): a substance in serum which binds and neutralizes toxin (poison).

aorta (ā-ôr'tă): the main arterial trunk leaving the heart, and carrying blood to the various arteries throughout the body.

apex (ā'pĕks)· the upper end of a lung or the heart.

aponeurosis (ăp-ō-nū-rō'sĭs): a broad, flat tendon; attachment of muscles.

appendage (ă-pĕn'dĕj): that which is attached to an organ, and is a part of it.

appendix (â-pĕn'dĭks): a small intestinal organ.

applicator (ăp'lĭ-kā-tēr): an instrument for the application of cosmetics or electricity to the body.

aqueous (ā'kwē-ŭs): watery; pertaining to water.

aromatic (ăr-ō-măt'ĭk): pertaining to or containing aroma; fragrant.

arrector pili (â-rĕk'tôr pī'lī): plural of arrectores pilorum.

arrectores pilorum (â-rĕk-tō'rēz pĭ-lôr'ûm): a minute involuntary muscle fiber in the skin inserted into the base of the hair follicle.

art (ärt): skill in performing any operation, intellectual or physical.

arterial (ar-tē'rē'âl): pertaining to an artery.

artery (ar'tĕr-ē): a vessel that conveys blood from the heart.

articulation (ar-tĭk-û-lā'shûn): joint; a connection between two or more bones.

asepsis (ă-sĕp'sĭs). a condition in which harmful bacteria are absent

assimilation (â-sĭm-ĭ-lā'shûn): the change of food into living tissue.

asteatosis (ăs-tē-â-tō'sĭs): a deficiency or absence of the sebaceous secretions.

astringent (ăs-trĭn'jênt). a substance or medicine that causes contraction of the tissues, and checks secretions.

athlete's foot (ăth'lēts fŏŏt): a fungus foot infection; ringworm of the foot

atom (ăt'ûm): the smallest part of an element capable of entering into the formation of a chemical compound

atrium (ăt'rē-ûm); pl, atria (-ă): the auricle of the heart.

atrophy (ăt'rō-fē)· a wasting away of the tissues of a part or of the entire body from lack of nutrition.

attollens aurem (ăt'ō-lĕns ō'rêm) auricularis superior; muscle that elevates the ear slightly.

attrahens aurem (ăt'ra-hĕns ō'rêm) auricularis anterior; muscle which pulls the ear forward slightly.

auditory (ō'dĭ-tô-rē): eighth cerebral nerve; controlling sense of hearing.

auricle (ō'rĭ-k'l): the external ear; one of the upper cavities of the heart.

auriculo-temporal (ō-rĭk-û-lō tĕm'pôr-âl): sensory nerve affecting the temple and external ear.

auricular (ō-rĭk'û-lăr): pertaining to the ear or cardiac auricle.

---

fāte, senâte, câre, ăm, finâl, arm, àsk, sofă; ēve, êvent, ĕnd, recênt, evêr; īce,

auto (ô'tô)· a prefix meaning self; of itself

autonomic nervous system (ô-tŏn'ô-mĭk nûrv'ŭs sĭs'tĕm)· the sympathetic nervous system; controls the involuntary muscles. '

axilla (ăk-sĭl'ă): the armpit.

axon (ăk'sŏn): a long nerve fiber extending from the cell body.

B

bacillus (bă-sĭl'ŭs); pl., bacilli (-ī). rod-like shaped bacterium.

bacteria (băk-tē'rē-ă): microbes, or germs

bactericide (băk-tē'rĭ-sīd). an agent that destroys bacteria.

bacteriology (băk-tē-rē-ŏl'ŏ-jē): the science which deals with bacteria.

bacterium (băk-tē'rē-ŭm), pl., bacteria (-ă) one-celled vegetable microorganism.

baldness (bôld'nĕss). a deficiency of hair; hair loss.

barber (bar'bĕr): one whose occupation is to shave or trim the beard, and to cut and dress the hair.

barber science (sī'ĕns): the study of the skin, scalp, beard and hair, and their treatments.

barber's itch (bar'bĕrz ĭch). tinea sycosis; ringworm of the beard; chronic inflammation of the hair follicles

basal layer (lā'ĕr): the layer of cells at base of epidermis closest to the dermis, stratum germinativum.

base (bās): the lower part or bottom; chief substance of a compound; an electropositive element that unites with an acid to form a salt.

battery (băt'ĕr-ē): an apparatus containing two or more cells, for generating electricity.

bayberry plant (bā'bĕr-ē plânt): the leaves of Myrcia acris yield oil of bay which is used to make bay rum.

bay rum (bā rŭm)· after shaving lotion; used as a tonic and astringent.

benign (bĕ-nīn): mild in character.

benzine (bĕn'zĕn)· an inflammable liquid derived from petroleum and used as a cleansing fluid.

Bernay tablets (bŭr'nā tăb'lĕts): a trade name; special tablets dissolved in water to be used as an antiseptic.

bi (bī): a prefix denoting two, twice, double.

bicarbonate of soda (bī-kar'bŏn-ât of sō'dă): baking soda; relieves burns, itching and insect bites Adding baking soda to the water in which instruments are to be boiled will keep them bright.

bichloride (bī-klō'rīd): a compound having two parts or equivalents of chlorine to one of the other element.

bile (bīl). a yellowish or greenish viscid fluid secreted by the liver; an aid to digestion.

binding posts (bīn'dĭng pōsts)· small metal posts in which are fitted the metal tips of the conducting cords.

biology (bī-ôl'ŏ-jē): the science of life and living things

birthmark (bûrth'mark): any mark which is present at birth, usually lasting; a form of nevus

blackhead (blăk'hĕd). a comedone; a plug of sebaceous matter.

bleach (blēch): to whiten or lighten.

bleached hair (blēcht hâr): hair from which the color has been wholly or partially removed by means of a bleaching solution.

bleaching solution (blēch'ĭng sŏ-lū-shŭn)· hydrogen peroxide with addition of ammonia.

bleb (blĕb): a blister of the skin filled with watery fluid.

blemish (blĕm'ĭsh): a mark, spot or defect, marring the appearance.

blister (blĭster): a vesicle; a collection of serous fluid causing an elevation of the skin.

blond; blonde (blŏnd): a person of fair complexion, with light hair and eyes

blood (blŭd): the nutritive fluid circulating through the arteries and veins.

blood poison (poi'z'n): an infection which gets into the blood stream.

ill; ōld, ôbey, ôrb, ŏdd, cônnect, sŏft, fōōd, fŏŏt; ūse, ûnite, ûrn, ŭp, circûs; those

blood vascular system (văs′kŭ-lăr sĭs′-těm): comprised of structures (the heart, arteries, veins and capillaries) which distribute blood throughout the body.

blood vessel (věs′êl): an artery, vein or capillary.

blue light (bloo līt): a therapeutic lamp used to soothe the nerves and ease pain.

bluing rinse (bloo′ĭng rĭns): a solution used to neutralize the unbecoming yellowish tinge on gray or white hair.

B.N.A. — meaning Basle Anatomical Nomenclature, a list of anatomical terms adopted by the German Anatomical Society in 1895.

bob (bŏb) a short haircut for women and children.

boil (boil)· a furuncle; a deep skin abscess which drains out onto the surface of the skin

boiling point (boil′ĭng point): 212° F. or 100° C. the temperature at which water begins to boil.

bone (bōn). os; the hard tissue forming the framework of the body

borax (bō′răks): sodium tetraborate; a white powder used as an antiseptic and cleansing agent.

boric acid (bō′rĭk ăs′ĭd)· used as an antiseptic dusting powder; in liquid form as an eye wash.

brain (brān). that part of the central nervous system contained in the cranial cavity.

brilliantine (brĭl-yân-tēn′) an oily composition that imparts luster to the hair

bristle (brĭs″l): short, stiff hairs found on brushes.

brittle (brĭt″l): easily broken, fragile.

bromidrosis (brō-mĭ-drō′sĭs) perspiration which smells foul.

bronchus (brŏn′kŭs), pl., **bronchi** (-kī)· the main branch of the wind pipe.

brow (brou): the forehead

brunette (broo-nĕt): a person having brown or olive skin, brown or black hair and eyes.

buccal nerve (bŭk′âl nûrv)· a motor nerve affecting the buccinator and the orbicularis oris muscle.

buccinator (bŭk′sĭ-nā-těr)· a thin, flat muscle of the cheek, shaped like a trumpet.

bulla (bool′ă, bŭl′ă): a large bleb or blister.

C

calamine lotion (kăl′ă-mīn lō′shûn)· zinc carbonate in alcohol used for the treatment of dermatitis in its various forms.

calcium (kăl′sē-ŭm): a brilliant silvery-white metal; enters into the composition of bone.

callous, callus (kăl′ŭs): skin which has become hardened, thick-skinned.

calory, calorie (kăl′ō-rē): a unit of heat.

cancellous (kăn′sê-lŭs): having a porous or spongy structure.

cancer (kăn′sĕr) a harmful growth, especially one attended with great pain and ulceration.

caninus (kăn-nīn′ŭs)· the levator anguli oris muscle which lifts the angle of mouth and help to keep it closed.

canitics (kă-nĭt′ĭks). the science which treats of canities.

canities (kă-nĭsh′ĭ-ēz): grayness or whiteness of the hair.

canities, accidental (ăk-sĭ-dĕn′tâl): grayness of hair caused by fright.

canities, congenital (kŏn-jĕn′ĭ-tâl). a type of gray hair transmitted by heredity as in albinism.

canities, premature (prē-mă-tūr′): grayness of hair at an early age.

canitics, senile (sē′nīl, -nĭl) grayness of hair in old age.

capillary (kăp′ĭ-lâ-rē): any one of the minute blood vessels which connect the arteries and veins; hair-like.

caput (kā′pût); poss, **capitis** (kăp′ĭ-tĭs): pertaining to the head.

carbohydrate (kăr-bō-hī′drāt) an organic substance containing carbon, hydrogen, and oxygen; such as starches and cellulose.

carbolic acid (kăr-bŏl′ĭk ăs′ĭd)· phenol; used in dilute solution as an antiseptic.

carbon (kàr'bôn): coal; an elementary substance in nature which is found in all organic compounds, charcoal, and lampblack

carbon-arc lamp (kàr'bôn ark lămp): an instrument which produces ultra-violet rays.

carbon dioxide (dī-ŏk'sīd) carbonic acid gas; product of the combustion of carbon with a free supply of air.

carbon monoxide (mŏn-ŏk'sīd). a colorless, odorless and poisonous gas

carbuncle (kàr'bŭn-k'l): a large enclosed inflammation of the deep skin tissue, similar to a furuncle, but much more extensive.

cardiac (kàr'dē-ăk) pertaining to the heart

carotid (kă-rŏt'īd): the principal artery of the neck.

cartilage (kar'tĭ-làj): gristle; a non-vascular connective tissue softer than bone.

castile soap (kăs'tēl sōp): a fine, hard, white soap containing olive oil and other oils; originally came from Castile, Spain.

catabolism (kă-tăb'ô-lĭz'm): chemical changes which involve the breaking down process within the cells.

cataphoresis (kă-tăf-ô-rē'sĭs). the process of forcing medicinal substances into the deeper tissues, using the positive pole of the galvanic current.

cathode (kăth'ōd)· the negative pole or electrode of a constant electric current.

cation (kăt' īon): an ion carrying a charge of positive electricity.

caustic (kôs'tĭk). an agent that burns and chars tissue.

cavity (kăv'ī-tē): a hollow space

cell (sĕl): a minute mass of protoplasm forming the structural unit of every organized body

cellular (sĕl'û-lăr): consisting of or pertaining to cells.

cellulose (sĕl'û-lōs): a carbohydrate, such as vegetable fiber.

centigrade (sĕn'tĭ-grād)· consisting of 100 degrees; of or pertaining to centigrade thermometer

centrosome (sĕn'trô-sōm). a cellular body which controls the division of the cell.

cerebellum (sĕr-ê-bĕl'ûm)· the posterior and lower part of the brain.

cerebral (sĕr'ê-brâl): pertaining to the cerebrum.

cerebrospinal system (sĕr-ê-brô'spī'nâl sĭs'tĕm). consists of the brain, spinal cord, spinal nerves and the cranial nerves.

cerebrum (sĕr'ê-brûm): the superior and larger part of the brain.

chancre (shăn'kĕr): the primary lesion of syphilis.

chemical (kĕm'ī-kâl)· relating to chemistry.

chemical dye remover (dī rê-mōōv'ĕr): a dye remover containing a chemical solvent.

chemistry (kĕm'ĭs-trē): the science dealing with the composition of substances, their reactions and the changes resulting from the formation and decomposition of compounds.

chloasma (klô-ăz'mă). large brown irregular patches on the skin, such as liver spots.

chlorazene (klō'ră-zēne)· a trade term; a chemical used for preparing an antiseptic or disinfectant.

chloro-zol (klō'rô-zōl)· a trade name; a special tablet used for preparing an antiseptic or disinfectant

cholesterin; cholesterol (kô-lĕs'tĕr-ĭn; -ōl): a waxy alcohol found in animal tissues; present in lanolin.

chromosome (krō'mô-sōm): tiny dark-stained bodies found in the nucleus of the cell; transmits hereditary characteristics in cell division.

chromatin (krō'mă-tĭn): a substance found in the nucleus of a cell.

chromidrosis (krō-mĭ-drō'sĭs): the excretion of colored sweat.

chronic (krŏn'ĭk): long-continued, the reverse of acute.

chrysarobin (krĭs-ă-rō'bĭn)· a powerful parasiticide; used in the treatment of various forms of tinea.

chyle (kīl): a creamy fluid taken up by the lacteals from the intestine during digestion.

chyme (kīm). food reduced to a liquid form in the process of digestion

cicatrix (sĭ-kā'trĭks, sĭk'ă-trĭks), pl., cicatrices (sĭk-ă-trī'sēz): the skin or film which forms over a wound, later contracting to form a scar.

cilia (sĭl'ī-ă). the eyelashes; microscopic hair-like extensions which assist bacteria in locomotion.

circuit (cûr'kĭt)· the path of an electric current

circuit, broken (brō'kĕn): caused by anything which changes the current from its regular circuit.

circuit, closed (klōz'd): a circuit in which a current is continually flowing.

circuit, complete (kŏm-plēt)· the path of an electric current in actual operation.

circuit, ground (ground). electricity in which one pole is used to deliver current and the other pole is connected to a ground (waterpipe or radiator)

circuit, open (ō'pĕn): a circuit through which the flow of current is interrupted.

circuit, short (shôrt): caused by anything which changes the current from its regular circuit.

circulation (sûr-kŭ-lā'shŭn): the passage of blood throughout the body.

circulation, general (jĕn'ēr-ăl). blood circulation from the heart throughout the body and back again

circulation, pulmonary (pŭl'mō-nâ-rē): blood circulation from the heart to the lungs and back to the heart.

citric acid (sĭt'rĭk ăs'ĭd): acid found in the lemon, orange, grapefruit; used for making a lemon rinse.

clavicle (klăv'ĭ-k'l): collar bone, joining the sternum and scapula.

clay (klā): an earthy substance containing kaolin, etc. and used for facial packs.

cleido (klī'dō). prefix meaning pertaining to the clavicle (collar bone).

clot (klŏt). a mass or lump of coagulated blood

club cutting (klŭb kŭt'ĭng): cutting the hair straight off without thinning or slithering

coagulate (kō-ăg'ŭ-lāt): to clot, to change a fluid into a soft jelly-like solid.

coccus (kŏk'ŭs); pl., **cocci** (kŏk'sī): spherical cell bacterium.

coiffeur (kwa-fûr') a male hairdresser

coiffeuse (kwa-fûz'). a female hairdresser.

coiffure (kwà-fūr'): an arrangement or styling of the hair.

color rinse (kŭl'ēr rĭns): a rinse which gives a temporary tint to the hair.

comb (kōm): an instrument used to dress, comb and arrange the hair.

combustion (kŏm-bŭs'chŭn). the rapid burning of any substance.

comedo; comedone (kŏm'ē-dō; -dŏn): blackhead; a worm-like mass in an obstructed sebaceous duct.

communicable (kŏ-mū'nĭ-kà-b'l): able to be communicated; transferable.

compact tissue (kŏm-păkt' tĭsh'ū): a dense, hard type of bony tissue

complexion (kŏm-plĕk'shŭn). hue or general appearance of the skin, especially the face.

composition (kŏm-pō-zĭsh'ŭn) the quality of being put together.

compound henna (kŏm'pound hĕn'ä)· Egyptian henna to which has been added one or more metallic preparations.

compressor (kŏm-prĕs'ēr): a muscle that presses, an instrument for applying pressure on a blood vessel to prevent loss of blood

concentrated (kŏn'sĕn-trăt-ĕd): condensed; increasing the strength by diminishing the bulk of a substance

conducting cords (kŏn-dŭkt'ĭng kôrdz). insulated copper wires which convey the current from the wall plate to the customer and operator.

conductor (kŏn-dŭk'tēr): any substance which will attract or allow a current to flow through it easily.

congeal (kŏn-jēl): to change from a fluid to a solid state.

congenital (kŏn-jĕn'ĭ-tăl)· existing at birth; born with

congestion (kŏn-jĕs'chŭn)· overfullness of the capillary and other blood vessels in any locality or organ.

connecting cords (kŏn-ĕkt'ĭng kôrdz). the insulated strands of copper wires which join together the apparatus and the commercial electric current

connective (kŏ-nĕk'tĭv). connecting, joining

constitutional (kŏn-stĭ-tū-shŭn-ăl): belonging to or affecting the physical or vital powers of an individual.

contact (kŏn'tăkt): bringing together so as to touch.

contagion (kăn-tā'jŭn) transmission of specific diseases by contact.

fāte, senâte, câre, ăm, fīnâl, ärm, àsk, sofä; ēve, ĕvent, ĕnd, recênt, evēr; īce,

contagiosa impetigo (kŏn-tā-jē-ō'sä ĭm-pĕt-ĭ-gō): a form of impetigo marked by flat vesicles that first become pustular, then crusted.

contagious (kŏn-tā'jŭs): acquired by contact.

contamination (kŏn-tăm-ĭ-nā'shŭn): pollution; soiling with infectious matter.

contour (kŏn'tōor): the outline of a figure or body.

contour of the hair: shape of the hair, straight, curly or wavy.

contra (kŏn'trä): a prefix denoting against; opposite; contrary.

contraction (kŏn-trăk'shŭn). having power to become shorter; the act of shrinking, drawing together.

converter (kŭn-vŭr'tēr): an apparatus used to change the direct current to alternating current.

copious (kō'pē-ŭs): large in amount.

copper (kŏp'ēr): a metallic element, being a good conductor of heat and electricity.

core (kōr)· the heart or most vital part of anything.

corium (kō'rē-ŭm): the derma or true skin.

cornification (kŏr-nĭ-fĭ-kā'shŭn): the process of becoming a horny substance or tissue.

coronary (kŭr'ô-nâ-rē): relating to a crown; encircling as a vessel or nerve.

corpuscles, red (kŏr'pŭs-'l rĕd): blood cells whose function is to carry oxygen to the cells.

corpuscles, white (whĭt): blood cells whose function is to destroy disease germs.

corrode (kô-rōd'): to destroy a metallic substance by chemical action.

corrosive sublimate (kô-rō'sĭv sŭb'lĭ-māt): an antiseptic, similar to mercury bichloride.

corrugations (kŏr-ōō-gā'shŭns). alternate ridges and furrows; wrinkles.

corrugator; corrugator supercilii (kŏr'-ōō-gā-tēr sū-pēr-sĭl'ē-ī): draws the eyebrows inward and downward, thus causing vertical wrinkles above the nose.

cortex (kŏr'tĕks): the second layer of the hair.

cortical (kŏr'tĭ-kâl): pertaining to the cortex

cosmetic dermatology (kŏz-mĕt'ĭk dûr-mă-tŏl'ô-jē): a branch of dermatology devoted to improving the health and beauty of the skin, hair and nails.

cosmetic therapy (thēr'ă-pē): a term used by some State Boards to designate the practice of cosmetology; cosmetic treatment for skin, hair or nail disorders.

cosmetics (kŏz-mĕt'ĭks). any external application intended to beautify the complexion, skin, hair or nails.

costal breathing (kŏs'tâl brĕth'ĭng). shallow breathing involving the use of the ribs.

cowlick (kou'lĭk): a tuft of hair forming a whorl.

cranial (krā'nē-âl): of or pertaining to the cranium.

cranium (krā'nē-ŭm)· the bones of the head excluding bones of the face; bony case for the brain

cream (krēm)· a semi-solid cosmetic.

cresol (krē'sŏl): a colorless, oily liquid or solid derived from coal tar and wood tar and used as a disinfectant

crown of the head (kroun): the top part of the head.

curd (kûrd): soap residue found on the hair after an unsatisfactory shampoo.

curd soap (sōp): a white soap of curdy texture, usually containing free alkali.

cure (kūr): to take care of; to heal.

current, alternating; A.C. (kŭr'ĕnt, ăl-tēr-nāt-ĭng): an interrupted current.

current, D'arsonval (d'-ár'sôn-vâl)· a high-frequency current of low voltage and high amperage.

current, direct; D.C. (dĭ-rĕkt'): an uninterrupted and even-flowing current.

current, electric (ê-lĕk'trĭk): electricity in motion, or moving within a conductor.

current, faradic (fâ-răd'ĭk): an induced interrupted current whose action is mechanical.

current, galvanic (găl-văn'ĭk). a direct constant current having a positive and negative pole and producing a chemical action

ĭll, ōld, ôbey, ôrb, ŏdd, cônnect, sôft, fōod, fŏŏt; ūse, ūnite, ûrn, ŭp, circŭs, those

current, high-frequency; Tesla (hĭ-frē-kwên-sē, tĕs'lä). an electric current of medium voltage and medium amperage.

current, sinusoidal (sĭn-û-soi'dâl): an induced interrupted current somewhat similar to faradic current.

curriculum (kû-rĭk'û-lŭm): the course of study in a school.

cutaneous (kû-tā'nē-ûs): pertaining to the skin.

cuticle (kū'tĭ-k'l). epidermis; the very thin outer layer of the skin or hair.

cutis (kū'tĭs): the derma or true skin.

cycle (sī'k'l): circle; a complete wave of an alternating current.

cyst (sĭst). a closed abnormally developed sac containing fluid

cytoplasm (sī'tô-plăz'm): the protoplasm of the cell body, exclusive of the nucleus.

D

dandruff (dăn'drôf): pityriasis; scurf or scales formed in excess upon the scalp.

de (dē): a prefix denoting from; down or away

decomposition (dē-kŏm-pô-zĭsh'ûn): act or process of separating the parts of a substance.

deficiency (dē-fĭsh'ĕn-sē). a lacking; something wanting.

deltoid (dĕl'toid). a muscle of the shoulder.

dense (dĕns): close; thick; heavy.

deodorant (dē-ō'dēr-ânt): a substance that removes or conceals offensive odors.

depilatory (dē-pĭl'ä-tô-rē)· a substance used to dissolve or remove the hair.

deportment (dē-pōrt'mĕnt): manner of conduct or behavior.

depressor (dē-prĕs'ēr): that which presses or draws down; a muscle that depresses

depressor alae nasi (ā'lē nā'sī): depressor septi; a muscle which contracts the opening of the nostril.

depressor anguli oris (ăng'û-lī ōr'ĭs): triangularis, a muscle that depresses the corner of the mouth

depressor labii inferioris (lā'bē-ī ĭn-fē-rē-ōr'ĭs): quadratus labii inferioris; a muscle that depresses lower lip down and a little to one side.

derivative (dē-rĭv'ä-tĭv): anything obtained from another substance.

derma (dûr'mä): the true skin; the corium; the sensitive layer of the skin below the epidermis.

dermal (dûr'mâl). pertaining to the skin.

dermatician (dûr-mă-tĭsh'ân): one skilled in the treatment of the skin

dermatitis (dûr-mä-tī'tĭs): inflammation of the skin.

dermatitis combustiones (kŏm-bŭs-tĭ-ō'nēs)· a type of dermatitis produced by extreme heat

dermatitis medicamentosa (mē-dĭk-a-mĕn-tō'sà): a type of dermatitis caused by the internal use of medicines, such as bromides.

dermatitis seborrheica (sĕb-ô-rē'ĭ-kà). a type of dermatitis found co-existent with seborrhea.

dermatitis venenata (vē-nē-nä'tà). inflammation of the skin caused by the action of an irritant substance such as hair dye.

dermatologist (dûr-mă-tŏl'ô-jĭst). a specialist who understands the science of treating the skin and its diseases.

dermatology (dûr-mă-tŏl'ô-jē): the science which treats of the skin and its diseases.

dermatosis (dûr-mà-tō'sĭs): any disease of the skin

dermis, derma (dûr'mĭs, dûr'mă): the layer below the epidermis; the corium or true skin.

detergent (dē-tûr'jĕnt)· an agent that cleanses the skin.

device (dē-vīs'). an apparatus for a particular use and purpose.

dexterity (dĕks-tĕr'ĭ-tē) skill and ease in using the hands.

di (dī): a prefix denoting two-fold; double; twice; separation or reversal

dia (dī'ă). a prefix denoting through; apart, asunder; between.

diagnosis (dī-ăg-nō'sĭs)· the recognition of a disease from its symptoms

fāte, senåte, câre, ăm, final, arm, ask, sofă, ēve, ĕvent, ĕnd, recênt, evêr; īce,

diaphragm (dī'ȧ-frăm). a muscular wall which separates the chest from the abdomen.

diathermy (dī'ȧ-thûr-mē): an instrument capable of generating a high-frequency current and elevating of temperature in the deep tissues

diet (dī'ĕt). a course of food selected with reference to a particular state of health.

digestion (dī-jĕs'chŭn): the process of converting food into a form which can be readily absorbed by the body.

digits (dĭj'ĭts). fingers or toes

dilatator; dilator (dī-lā-tȧ'-tẽr; dĭ-; dī-lā'tẽr; dĭ-)· that which expands or enlarges a cavity or an opening

dilator naris anterior (nā'rĭs ăn-te'rē-ẽr). a muscle which expands the opening of the nostril.

dilute (dĭ-lūt'; dī-)· to make thinner by mixing, especially with water.

diphtheria (dĭf-thē'rē-ȧ). an infectious disease involving the air passages, and the throat.

diplococcus (dī-plô-kŏk'ŭs): a coccus occurring in pairs; bacterium causing pneumonia.

dis (dĭs): a prefix denoting apart; away; asunder; between.

discharge (dĭs-charj)· the escape or flowing away of the contents of a cavity

disease (dĭ-zēz)· a pathologic condition of any part or organ of the body, or of the mind

disease carrier (kăr'ĭ-ẽr): a healthy person capable of transmitting disease germs to another person.

disinfectant (dĭs-ĭn-fĕk'tȧnt) an agent used for destroying germs.

dispensary (dĭs-pĕn'sa-rĭ): a place where medicines or other supplies are prepared and dispensed

dissolve (dĭ-zŏlv). to make a solution of; to break up

distal (dĭs'tȧl). farthest from the center or median line.

dormant (dôr'mȧnt). inactive, asleep.

dorsal (dôr'sȧl): pertaining to the back.

duct (dŭkt): a passage or canal for fluids

dye (dī)· to stain or color.

dye remover (rê-mōōv'ẽr): a chemical liquid used to remove old dye from the hair.

dynamo (dī'nȧ-mō): a machine for changing mechanical energy into electrical power.

E

ecto (ĕk'tô)· a prefix denoting without; outside; external.

eczema (ĕk'zē-mȧ). an inflammatory itching disease of the skin.

efferent (ĕf'ẽr-ĕnt): carrying outward, as efferent nerves carrying impulses away from the central nervous system.

efficiency (ĕ-fĭsh'ĕn-sē): usefulness; quality or degree of being able to produce results.

effleurage (ĕ-flû-razh'): a stroking movement in massage.

Egyptian henna (ê-jĭp'shân hĕn'ȧ): a pure vegetable hair dye

elasticity (ê-lăs'tĭs'ĭ-tē): the quality of being elastic.

electrical (ê-lĕk'trĭ-kȧl): consisting of, containing, producing, or operated by electricity.

electricity (ê-lĕk-trĭs'ĭ-tē): a form of energy, which when in motion, exhibits magnetic, chemical or thermal effects.

electricity, frictional (frĭk'shôn-âl): a kind of electricity produced by rubbing certain objects together.

electricity, induced or inductive (ĭn-dūst or ĭn-dŭk'tĭv)· a kind of electricity produced by nearness to an electrified body.

electricity, magnetic (măg-nĕt'ĭk): a kind of electricity developed by bringing a conductor near the poles of a magnet.

electricity, static (stăt'ĭk): frictional electricity.

electricity, voltaic (vŏl-tā'ĭk): galvanic or chemical electricity.

electrification (ê-lĕk'trĭ-fĭ-kā'shŭn): the application of electricity to the body by holding an electrode in the hand and charging the body with electricity

electrode (ê-lĕk'trōd): an applicator for directing the use of electricity on a customer.

ĭll; ōld, ôbey, ôrb, ŏdd, cônnect, sôft, fōōd, fŏŏt; ūse, ûnite, ûrn, ŭp, circŭs; those

electrology (ē-lĕk-trŏl'ō-jē): science in relation to electricity.

electrolysis (ē-lĕk-trŏl'ĭ-sĭs): decomposition of a chemical compound or body tissues by means of electricity.

electrolytic cup (ē-lĕk-trŏ-lĭt'ĭk kŭp). an appliance used to cleanse the skin, before giving a massage.

electron (ē-lĕk'trŏn): an extremely minute body or charge of negative electricity.

electropositive (ē-lĕk"trŏ-pŏz'ĭ-tĭv): relating to or charged with positive electricity.

element (ĕl'ē-mĕnt): a simple substance, one which is incapable of being split up into other substances

elimination (ē-lĭm-ĭ-nā'shŭn): act of expelling or excreting.

embellish (ĕm-bĕl'ĭsh): to make beautiful or decorate

embryo (ĕm'brē-o): in the first stages of development; a bud.

emollient (ē-mŏl'yĕnt). an agent that softens or soothes the surface of the skin.

emotion (ē-mō'shŭn): mental excitement.

emulsion (ē-mŭl'shŭn)· a milky fluid obtained by suspending oil in water.

endo (ĕn'dō): a prefix denoting inner; within.

endocrine (ĕn'dō-krīn)· any internal secretion or hormone.

endosteum (ĕn-dŏs'tē-ŭm): the membrane covering the inner surface of bone in the medullary cavity.

energy (ĕn'ēr'jē): power or capacity for performing work.

environment (ĕn-vī'rŭn-mĕnt): the surrounding conditions.

enzyme (ĕn'zīm) a complex organic substance which affects the rate of chemical reactions

epi (ĕp-ĭ): a prefix denoting upon: beside.

epicranium (ĕp-ĭ-krān'nĭ-ŭm): the structure covering the cranium.

epicranius (ĕp-ĭ-krā'nē-ŭs)· the occipito-frontalis; the scalp muscle

epidemic (ĕp-ĭ-dĕm'ĭk)· common to many people; a prevailing disease.

epidermis (ĕp-ĭ-dŭr'mĭs): the outer epithelial portion of the skin.

epithelium (ĕp-ĭ-thē'lē'ŭm): a cellular tissue or membrane, covering a free surface or lining a cavity.

eponychium (ĕp-ō-nĭk'ē-ŭm): the extension of excess cuticle at base of nail.

erector (ē-rĕk'tēr): an elevating muscle.

eruption (ē-rŭp'shŭn): a skin lesion due to a disease, marked by redness or papular condition, or both

erysipelas (ĕr-ĭ-sĭp'ē-lĕs): an acute infectious disease accompanied by a spreading inflammation of the skin and mucous membrane.

erythema (ĕr-ĭ-thē'mă)· a superficial blush or redness of the skin.

erythrocyte (ē-rĭth'rō-sīt) a red blood cell, red corpuscle

eschar (ĕs'kar). a dry slough, crust, or scab following a burn.

esophagus; oesophagus (ē-sŏf'ă-gŭs): the canal leading from the pharynx to the stomach

esthetic; aesthetic (ĕs-thĕt'ĭk)· relating to sensation, either mental or physical.

ethics (ĕth'ĭks): principles of good character and proper conduct.

ethmoid (ĕth'moid): a bone forming part of the walls of the nasal cavity.

etiology (ē-tē-ŏl'ō-jē)· the science of the causes of disease

evaporation (ē-văp-ō-rā'shŭn)· change from liquid to vapor form.

ex (ĕks)· a prefix denoting out of; from; away from.

excitation (ĕk-sĭ-tā'shŭn): the act of stimulating or irritating.

excoriation (ĕks-kō-rē-ā'shŭn): act of stripping or wearing off the skin; an abrasion.

excretion (ĕks-krē'shŭn) that which is thrown off or eliminated from the body.

exercise (ĕk'sĕr-sīz) putting muscles into action.

exfoliation (ĕks-fō-lē-ā'shŭn): the process of throwing off scales from the skin, as in dandruff

exhalation (ĕks-ha-lā'shŭn): the act of breathing outward.

exhaustion (ĕg-zŏs'chŭn): loss of vital and nervous power from fatigue or disease.

expansion (ĕks-păn'shŭn). distention; dilation or swelling.

expert (ĕks'pûrt): an experienced person; one who has special knowledge or skill in a particular subject.

fāte, senâte, câre, ăm, finâl, àrm, àsk, sofà; ēve, ĕvent, ĕnd, recênt, evēr; īce,

extensibility (ĕks-tĕn-sĭ-bĭl'ĭ-tĭ): capable of being extended or stretched.

extensor (ĕks-tĕn'sôr). a muscle which serves to extend or straighten out a limb or part

exterior (ĕks-tē'rē-ĕr): outside.

external (ĕks-tûr'năl) pertaining to the outside

externus (ĕks-tûr'nŭs): external; pertaining to the outside

extremity (ĕks-trĕm'ĭ-tē): the distant end or part of any organ; a hand or foot.

exudation (ĕks-û-dā'shŭn)· act of discharging from a body through pores or cuts as sweat, moisture or other liquid; oozing out.

eye (ī): the organ of vision.

eyeball (ī-bôl)· the globe of the eye.

eyebrow (ī'brou)· the hair, skin and tissue above the eye

eyelashes (ī'lĕsh-ês). the hair of the eyelids.

eyelid (ī'lĭd): the protective covering of the eyeball.

F

facial (fā'shăl)· pertaining to the face; the seventh cerebral nerve.

Fahrenheit (fa'rĕn-hīt): pertaining to the Fahrenheit thermometer or scale, water freezes at 32° F. and boils at 212° F.

faradism (făr'ă-dĭz'm)· a form of electrical treatment used for stimulating activity of the tissues

fascia (făsh'ē-ă): a sheet of connective tissue covering the muscles and separating their layers.

fat (făt): a greasy, soft-solid material found in animal tissue.

fatigue (fă-tēg'). body or mental exhaustion.

favus (fā'vŭs): a contagious parasitic disease of the skin, with crusts.

feather edge (fĕth'ĕr ĕj): a haircutting term; a very thin fringe of hair resembling the edge of a feather.

fetid (fĕt'ĭd; fā'tĭd) having a foul smell; stinking.

fever (fē'vĕr): rise of body temperature.

fever blister (blĭs'tĕr): an acute skin disease characterized by the presence of vesicles over an inflammatory base; herpes simplex.

fiber; fibre (fī'bĕr): a slender thread or filament; thread-like in structure.

fibrin (fī'brĭn): the active agent in coagulation of the blood.

fibrous (fī'brŭs): containing, consisting of, or like fibers.

finesse (fĭ-nĕs)· delicate skill

finger (fĭn'gĕr): one of the digits of the hand.

fissure (fĭsh'ûr): a narrow opening made by separation of parts; a furrow; a slit.

flabby (flăb'ē): lacking firmness; flaccid

flagella (flă-jĕl'a): slender hair-like parts which permit movement in certain bacteria

flexible (flĕk'sĭ-b'l): that which may be bent; not stiff.

flexor (flĕk'sôr). a muscle that bends or flexes a part or a joint.

florid (flŏr'ĭd): flushed with red

fluid (floo'ĭd). a non-solid liquid

foam (fōm): white bubbles forming on the surface of a liquid as a result of mixing or decomposition

folliculitis (fŏ-lĭk-û-lī'tĭs). an inflammation of any follicle

foramen (fō-rā'mĕn): a passage or opening through a bone or membrane.

formaldehyde (fôr-măl'dĕ-hīd). a pungent gas possessing powerful disinfectant properties.

formalin (fôr'mă-lĭn)· a 37% to 40% solution of formaldehyde

formula (fôr'mû-la): a prescribed method or rule; a recipe or prescription.

fossa (fŏs'ă): pl., fossae (-ē): a depression, furrow or sinus, below the level of the surface of a part.

fragilitas crinium (fră-jĭl'ĭ-tăs krī'nēûm)· brittleness of the hair.

frayed (frād): worn away by friction or use.

freckle (frĕk''l): a yellow or brown spot on the skin; lentigo.

free edge (frē ĕj). part of the nail-body extending over the finger tip.

frequency (frē'kwên-sē)· the number of complete cycles of current produced by an alternating current generator per second. Standard frequencies are 25 and 60 cycles per second

friction (frĭk'shŭn)· the resistance met in rubbing one body on another.

frontal (frŭn'tâl). in front; relating to the forehead; the bone of the forehead.

frontalis (frŏn-tā'lĭs): anterior portion of the epicranius, muscle of the scalp.

fulling (fŏŏl'ĭng)· a massage movement in which the limb is rolled back and forth between the hands.

fumigate (fū'mĭ-gāt): disinfect by the action of smoke or fumes

function (fŭnk'shŭn). a normal or special action of a part.

fundus (fŭn'dŭs): the bottom or lowest part of a sac or hollow organ.

fungus (fŭn'gŭs): a vegetable parasite; a spongy growth of diseased tissue on the body

furrow (fŭr'ō): a groove, wrinkle

furuncle (fū-rŭn'k'l): a boil.

fuse (fūz)· a special device which prevents excessive current from passing through a circuit

G

galea (gā'lê-ă): the aponeurotic portion of the occipito-frontalis muscle.

galvanism (găl'vă-nĭz'm) a constant current of electricity the action of which is chemical.

ganglion (găn'glē-ân), pl., ganglia (-ă): bundles of nerve cells in the brain, in organs of special sense, or forming units of the sympathetic nervous system.

gangrene (găn-grēn'). the dying of tissue due to interference with local nutrition

gastric juice (găs'trĭk jōōs)· the digestive fluid secreted by the glands of the stomach.

generator (jĕn'ĕr-ā-tĕr). a machine for changing mechanical energy into electrical energy, a dynamo, an apparatus for producing heat.

germ (jûrm). a bacillus, a microbe

germicide (jûr'mĭ-sīd). any chemical, especially a solution that will destroy germs

germinative layer (jûr-mĭ-nā'tĭv lā'ĕr). stratum germinativum; the deepest layer of the epidermis resting on the corium.

germitabs (jûr'mĭ-tăbs): a trade name; special tablets, which, when dissolved in water, form an antiseptic solution.

gland (glănd). a secretory organ of the body.

glossopharyngeal (glŏs-ô-fâ-rĭn'jē-âl). pertaining to the tongue and pharynx, the ninth cerebral nerve.

glycerin; glycerine (glĭs'ĕr-ĭn): sweet oily fluid, used as an application for roughened and chapped skin, also used as a solvent.

gonococcus (gŏn-ô-kŏk'ŭs), pl., gonococci (-sē). the germ causing gonorrhea.

gonorrhea (gŏn-ô-rē'ă). a contagious disease of the sex organs

granular layer (grăn'û-lăr lā'ĕr): the stratum granulosum of the skin.

granules (grăn'ūlz): small grains; small pills.

granulosum (grăn'û-lōs'ûm): granular layer of the epidermis

great auricular (grāt o-rĭk'û-lăr): a nerve affecting the face, ear and skin behind the ear.

greater occipital (grăt'ĕr ôk-sĭp'ĕ-tâl)· nerve affecting the scalp and back of the head as far up as the top of the head

gristle (grĭs''l): cartilage

groom (grōōm)· to make neat or tidy

ground wire (ground wīr). a wire which connects an electric current to a ground (waterpipe or radiator).

gumma (gŭm'ă). the gummy tumor in the tertiary stage of syphilis

·

---

fāte, senâte, câre, ăm, finâl, àrm, àsk, sofă; ēve, ĕvent, ĕnd, recênt, evêr; īce,

H

habit (hăb'ĭt). an acquired tendency to repetition.

hacking (hăk'ĭng): a chopping stroke made with the edge of the hand in massage

hair (hâr)· pilus, a slender thread-like outgrowth of the skin and scalp.

hair bobbing (bŏb'ĭng): the term commonly applied to the cutting of women's and children's hair.

hair bulb (bŭlb). the lower extremity of the hair.

hair clipping (klĭp'ĭng)· removing the hair by the use of hair clippers; removing split hair ends of the hair with the scissors

haircutting (hâr'kŭt'ĭng)· cutting and molding the hair into a becoming style.

hair dressing (hâr drĕs'ĭng): art of arranging the hair into various becoming shapes or styles.

hair dyeing (dī'ĭng): to give the hair new and permanent color by impregnating it with a coloring agent.

hair follicle (fŏl'ĭ-k'l): the depression in the skin containing the root of the hair

hairline (hâr'līn): the edge of the scalp at the brow or neck where the hair growth begins

hair papilla (hâr pă-pĭl'ă)· a small cone-shaped elevation at the bottom of the hair follicle.

hair pressing (prĕs'ĭng). a method of straightening curly or kinky hair by means of a heated iron or comb

hair pressing oil (oil): an oily or waxy mixture used in hair pressing.

hair restorer (rê-stŏr'ĕr): a preparation containing a metallic dye

hair root (rōōt): that part of the hair contained within the follicle.

hair shaft (shăft): the portion of the hair which projects beyond the skin.

hair shaping (shāp'ĭng): the art of haircutting.

hair straightener (strāt'n-ĕr): a physical or chemical agent used in straightening kinky or over-curly hair.

hair test (tĕst)· a sampling of how the hair will react to a particular treatment.

hair tint (tĭnt): to give a coloring to the hair, color or shade of hair.

hair trim (trĭm)· trimming, cutting the hair lightly over the already existing formed lines

halitosis (hăl''ĭ-tō'sĭs): offensive odor from the mouth; foul breath

hamamelis (hăm-ă-mē'lĭs). a shrub of eastern North America; witch-hazel is an extract of this plant, and is used as an astringent

hangnail (hăng'nāl): a tearing up of a strip of epidermis at the side of the nail; agnail.

hard water (härd wŏ'tĕr): water containing certain minerals, does not lather with soap.

Haversian canals (hă-vûr'shân kă-nălz'): small channels in bone tissue which contain minute blood vessels.

health (hĕlth)· state of being hale or sound in body and mind

heart (hart): a hollow muscular organ which, by contracting regularly keeps up the circulation of the blood

hematidrosis; hemidrosis (hĕm''ă-tĭ-drō'sĭs, hĕm-ĭ-drō'sĭs): the excretion of sweat stained with blood or blood coloring.

hematocyte (hĕ'mă-tō-sīt): a blood corpuscle.

hemi (hĕm'ĭ): a prefix signifying half.

hemoglobin; haemoglobin (hē''mō-glō'bĭn): the coloring matter of the red blood cell.

hemorrhage (hĕm'ô-râj)· bleeding; a flow of blood, especially when profuse

henna (hĕn'ă). the leaves of an Asiatic plant used as a dye to impart a reddish tint.

henna, compound (kŏm'pound)· Egyptian henna to which has been added one or more metallic preparations.

henna, white (whīt). a mixture of magnesium carbonate, peroxide and ammonia used in giving a bleach retouch.

heredity (hê-rĕd'ĭ-tĭ)· the transfer of qualities or disease from parents to offspring.

herpes (hûr'pēz): an inflammatory disease of the skin having small vesicles in clusters.

ĭll; ōld, ȯbey, ôrb, ŏdd, cȯnnect, sȯft, fōōd, fŏŏt; ūse, ûnite, ûrn, ŭp, circûs, **those**

herpes simplex (sĭm'plĕks): fever blister; cold sore

hidrosis (hĭ-drō'sĭs). abnormally profuse sweating

high-frequency, tesla (hī-frē'kwĕn-sē, tĕs'lă)· violet ray; an electric current of medium voltage and medium amperage.

hirsute (hûr'sūt; hĕr-sūt'), hirsuties.

hirsuties (hûr-sū'shĭ-ēz); hypertrichosis, growth of an unusual amount of hair in unusual locations, as on the face of women or the back of men; hairy; superfluous hair.

histology (hĭs-tŏl'ō-jē): the science of the minute structure of organic tissues, microscopic anatomy.

hives (hīvz). urticaria; a skin eruption

hormone (hôr'mōn): a chemical substance formed in one organ or part of the body and carried in the blood to another organ or part which it stimulates to functional activity.

humidity (hū-mĭd'ĭ-tĭ). moisture; dampness.

hydro (hī'drō): a prefix denoting water; hydrogen.

hydrocystoma (hĭd-rō-sĭs-tō'mă): a variety of sudamina appearing on the face.

hydrogen (hī'drō-jĕn) a gaseous element, lighter than any other known substance.

hydrogen peroxide (pĕr-ok'sīd): a powerful oxidizing and bleaching agent; in liquid form is used as an antiseptic.

hygiene (hī-jĕn): the science of preserving health.

hygroscopic (hī-grō'skŏp'ĭk). readily absorbing and holding moisture.

hyoid (hī'-oid). the "u" shaped bone at the base of the tongue.

hyperemia (hī''pĕr-ē'mē-ă): the presence of an excessive quantity of blood in a part of the body.

hyperhidrosis, hyperidrosis (hī''pĕr-ĭ-drō'sĭs): excessive sweating.

hypersecretion (hī''pĕr-sē-krē'shŭn): excessive secretion.

hypertrophy (hī''pĕr-trō'fē): abnormal increase in the size or a part of an organ; overgrowth.

hypo (hī'pō): a prefix denoting under; beneath, lower state of oxidation

hypodermic (hī''pō-dûr'mĭk): beneath the skin; a liquid injection into the subcutaneous tissues.

hypoglossal (hī''pō-glŏs'ăl)· under the tongue; the twelfth cerebral nerve

I

idiosyncrasy (ĭd-ē-ō-sĭn'kră-sē): an individual characteristic due to the action of certain drugs or substances in certain food.

imbrications of hair: tiny overlapping scales found on the hair cuticle.

immerse (ĭ-mûrs'): to plunge into; dip into a liquid.

immiscible (ĭ-mĭs'ĭ-b'l). a liquid that will not mix with another liquid.

immunity (ĭ-mūn'ĭ-tē): resistant to disease.

impetigo (ĭm-pē-tī'gō): an eruption of pustules, which soon rupture or become crusted, occurring chiefly on the face around the mouth and the nostrils.

impetigo contagiosa (kŏn-tā''jē-ō'să): scrum-pox; a contagious disease, characterized by an eruption of flat vesicles and pustules.

implement (ĭm'plē-mĕnt): an instrument or tool used by man to accomplish a given work.

in (ĭn): a prefix denoting not; negative, within; inside.

incandescent (ĭn-kăn-dĕs'ĕnt): giving forth light and heat.

incubation (ĭn-kū-bā'shŭn): the period of a disease between the implanting of the contagion and the development of the symptoms

index (ĭn'dĕks): the forefinger, the pointing finger.

induction (ĭn-dŭk'shŭn): the transfer of electricity from a current to a magnetized object.

inert (ĭn-ûrt): inactive.

infection (ĭn-fĕk'shŭn): the invasion of the body tissues by disease germs.

infection, general (jĕn'ĕr-ĕl): the result of the disease germs gaining entrance into the blood stream and thereby circulating throughout the entire body.

infection, local (lō'kăl): confined to only certain portions of the body, such as an abscess.

---

fāte, senâte, câre, ăm, finâl, arm, ȧsk, sofä; ēve, ēvent, ĕnd, recênt, evêr, īce,

infectious (ĭn-fĕk′shŭs): capable of spreading infection.

inferior (ĭn-fē′rē-ēr)· situated lower down, or nearer the bottom or base.

inferioris (ĭn-fē″rē-ŏr′ĭs): below; lower.

inflammation (ĭn-flă-mā′shŭn)· the reaction of the body to irritation with accompanying redness, pain, heat, and swelling.

influenza (ĭn-flōō-ĕn′ză). a contagious epidemic catarrhal fever, with great weakness and varying symptoms.

infra (ĭn′fră): a prefix denoting below; lower.

infra-mandibular (ĭn″fră-măn-dĭb′ū-lăr): below the lower jaw.

infra-mental (mĕn′tăl). below the chin.

infra-orbital (ôr′bĭ-tăl): below the orbit; nerve affecting the skin of lower eyelid, side of nose, upper lip, mouth and their glands.

infra-red (ĭn″fră-rĕd): pertaining to that part of the spectrum lying outside of the visible spectrum and below the red rays

infra-trochlear (trŏk′lē-ăr): nerve affecting the membrane and skin of the nose.

ingrown hair (ĭn′grŏn hâr): a wild hair that has grown underneath the skin, thereby causing an infection.

ingrown nail (ĭn′grŏn nāl). the growth of the nail into the flesh instead of toward the tip of the finger or toe, thereby causing an infection

inhalation (ĭn-hă-lā′shŭn): the inbreathing of air or other vapors.

innervation (ĭn-ēr-vā′shŭn). distribution of the nerves in a part.

inoculation (ĭn-ŏk-ū-lā′shŭn): the process by which protective agents are introduced into the body.

inorganic (ĭn-ôr-găn′ĭk): composed of matter not relating to living organisms.

insanitary; unsanitary (ĭ-săn′ĭ-tă-rē); ŭn-); not sanitary or healthful; injurious to health; unclean.

insoluble (ĭn-sŏl′ū-b′l). incapable of being dissolved or very difficult to dissolve.

instantaneous (ĭn-stân-tā′nĕ-ŭs): acting immediately.

insulator (ĭn′sū-lā-tēr): a non-conducting material or substance. Materials used to cover electric wires.

insurance (ĭn-shōōr′ăns): protection against loss, damage or injury.

integument (ĭn-tĕg′ū-mĕnt): a covering, especially the skin

inter (ĭn′tēr): a prefix denoting amid; between; among.

intercellular (ĭn-tēr-sĕl′ū-lăr): between or among cells

interior (ĭn-tē′rē-ēr): inside

internal (ĭn-tûr′năl): pertaining to the inside; inner part.

internus (ĭn-tûr′nŭs)· internal; pertaining to the inside.

interosseous (ĭn-tēr-ŏs′ê-ŭs). lying between or connecting bones

intestine (ĭn-tĕs′tĭn): the digestive tube from the stomach to the anus

invasion (ĭn-vā′zhŭn)· the beginning of a disease

involuntary muscle (ĭn-vŏl′ŭn-tă-rē mŭs′l): function without the action of the will.

iodine (ī′ô-dĭn; -dīn)· a non-metallic element used as an antiseptic for cuts, bruises, etc

ion (ī′ŏn): an atom or group of atoms carrying an electric charge

ionization (ī-ŏn-ĭ-zā′shŭn)· the separating of a substance into ions.

irradiation (ĭ-rā″dĭ-ā′shŭn)· the process of exposing an object to the natural or artificial sunlight.

irritability (ĭr-ĭ-ta-bĭl′ĭ-tĭ) readily excited or stimulated

irritant (ĭr′ĭ-tănt). causing irritation; an irritating agent; a stimulus.

ive (ĭv): a word ending meaning relating or belonging to, such as active

ize (īz): a word ending forming verbs, such as sterilize.

J

jowl (jōl): the hanging part of a double chin.

joint (joint): a connection between two or more bones.

jugular (jōō′gū-lăr): pertaining to the neck or throat; the large vein in the neck.

ĭll; ōld, ôbey, ôrb, ŏdd, cônnect, sôft, fōōd, fŏŏt; ūse, ûnite, ûrn, ŭp, circŭs; those

K

keloid (kē′loid): a fibrous growth arising from irritation and usually from a scar.

keratin (kĕr′ă-tĭn) the principal constituent of horny tissues, hair, nails and feathers

kidney (kĭd′nē)· a glandular organ which excretes urine.

kilowatt (kĭl′ŏ-wŏt): one thousand watts of electricity.

kinky (kĭnk′ĭ): very curly hair

knead (nēd): to work and press with the hands as in massage.

knowledge (nŏl′ĕj): instruction; learning; practical skill.

L

laboratory (lăb′ŏ-ră-tŏ-rē): a room containing apparatus for conducting experiments

lachrymal; lacrimal (lăk′rĭ-măl) pertaining to tears or weeping; bone at front part of inner wall of the orbit

lacteals (lăk′tē-ălz)· any one of the lymphatics of the small intestines that take up the chyle

lanolin (lăn′ŏ-lĭn)· purified wool fat.

lanugo (lă-nū′gō): the fine hair which covers most of the body.

larkspur (lark′spûr): the seeds of the Delphinium plant; its tincture is used to treat head lice.

larynx (lăr′ĭnks): the upper part of the trachea or wind pipe; the organ of voice production.

lateral (lăt′ĕr-ăl). on the side.

lather (lăth′ĕr). froth made by mixing soap and water.

latissimus dorsi (la-tĭs′ĭ-mŭs dôr′sī). a broad, flat superficial muscle of the back

laxative (lăk′sa-tĭv). a medicinal agent which relieves constipation

layer cutting (lā′ĕr kŭt′ĭng): tapering and thinning the hair by dividing it into many thin layers

lemon rinse (lĕm′ŭn rĭns). a product containing lemon juice or citric acid; used to lighten the color of the hair.

lentigo (lĕn-tī′gō)· pl., **lentigines** (lĕn-tĭ-jī′nēz): a freckle; spot or coloration in the skin.

lesion (lē′zhŭn) a structural tissue change caused by injury or disease.

lesser (smaller) occipital (lĕs′ĕr ŏk-sĭp′ĭ-tăl)· the nerve supplying scalp area at the base of the skull.

leuco (lū′kŏ): a prefix denoting white; colorless

leucocyte (lū′kŏ-sīt): a white corpuscle; white blood cell.

leucoderma (lū-kŏ-dûr′mă): abnormal white patches on the skin; absence of color in the skin.

leuconychia (lū-kŏ-nĭk′ē-ă) a whitish discoloration of nails; white spots

levator (lĕ-vā′tôr): a muscle that elevates a part

levator anguli oris (ăng′û-lī ŏr′ĭs). caninus; muscle that raises the angle of mouth and helps to keep it closed.

levator labii superioris (lā′bē-ī sū-pē-rē-ŏr′ĭs): quadratus labii superioris; muscle that elevates and draws back upper lip and dilates the nostril.

levator palpebrae superioris (păl′pĕ-brē): muscle that raises upper eyelid

ligament (lĭg′ă-mĕnt): a tough band of fibrous tissue, serving to support bones at the joints

light therapy (līt thĕr′ă-pē)· the application of light rays for treatment of diseases.

liquefy (lĭk′wē-fī): to reduce to the liquid state; said of both solids and gases.

liquid (lĭk′wĭd). flowing like water; a fluid that is not solid or gaseous.

liquor cresolis compound (lĭk′ĕr krē′sŏl′ĭs kŏm′pound). a powerful germicide

listerine (lĭs-tĕr-ēn′). a trade name; a mild antiseptic in liquid form

litmus paper (lĭt′mŭs pā′pĕr): strip of paper containing a blue coloring matter that is reddened by acids and turned blue again by alkalies.

liver (lĭv′ĕr) an internal organ which secretes bile for digestion.

liver spots (lĭv′ĕr spŏts) the lesions of chloasma

locomotion (lŏ-kŏ-mŏ′shŭn): animal movement

lotion (lŏ′shŭn) a liquid solution used for bathing the skin.

---

louse (lous); pl., lice (līs): pediculus; an animal parasite infesting the hairs of the head.

lubricant (lū'brĭ-kȧnt): anything that makes things smooth and slippery, such as oil.

lung (lŭng) one of the two organs of respiration.

lunula (lū'nû-lȧ): the half moon-shaped area at the base of the nail.

lymph (lĭmf): a clear yellowish or light straw colored fluid.

lymphatic system (lĭm-făt'ĭk sĭs'těm)· consists of lymph flowing through the lymph spaces, lymph vessels, lacteals, and lymph nodes or glands.

lysol (lī'sōl): a trade name, a disinfectant and antiseptic; a mixture of soaps and phenols.

M

macroscopic (măk-rô-skŏp'ĭk). visible to the unaided eye

macula (măk'û-lȧ); pl., maculae (-lē). a spot or discoloration level with skin, a freckle; macule.

magnet (măg'nět)· an instrument having the power to attract iron bodies.

magnify (măg'nĭ-fī): to increase the size or importance of

malar (mā'lȧr). of or pertaining to the cheek, the cheek bone

malignant (mȧ-lĭg'nȧnt). resistant to treatment; growing worse; occurring in severe form.

malnutrition (măl-nû-trĭsh'ûn) poor nutrition resulting from the eating of improper foods or faulty assimilation.

malpighian (măl-pĭg'ê-ȧn): stratum mucosum, the deeper portion of the epidermis.

management (măn'ȧj-mênt). directing; carrying on; control.

mandible (măn'dĭ-b'l). the lower jaw bone

mandibular nerve (măn-dĭb'û-lȧr nûrv): branch of the fifth cerebral nerve which supplies the temple, auricle of ear, lower lip, lower part of face and muscles of mastication.

manipulation (mȧ-nĭp-û-lā'shûn)· act or process of treating, working or operating with the hands or by mechanical means, especially with skill.

manus (mā'nûs), pl, mani (-nī): the hand.

marrow (măr'ō)· a soft fatty substance filling the cavities of bone.

mask (mask): a special cosmetic formula used to beautify the face

massage (mȧ-sazh')· systematic manipulations of body tissues with the hands and/or mechanical or electrical appliances.

masseter (mȧ-sē'těr): a chewer; the muscle which closes the jaws.

masseur (mȧ-sûr')· a man who practices massage

masseuse (mȧ-sûz'): a woman who practices massage.

mastication (măs-tĭ-kā'shûn): the act of chewing.

mastoid process (măs'toyd prŏs'ěs): a conical nipple-like projection of the temporal bone.

matter (măt'ěr): pus; a substance that occupies space and has weight.

maxilla (măk-sĭ'lȧ): jaw bone

maxilla, inferior (ĭn-fē'rē-ēr) lower jaw bone or mandible

maxilla, superior (sû-pē'rē-ēr): upper jaw bone.

mechanical (mè-kan'ĭ-kȧl): relating to a machine; performed by means of some apparatus not manual.

medial; median (mē'dē-ȧl; -ȧn): pertaining to the middle.

medicine (měd'ĭ-sĭn): a drug; the art of preventing or curing disease.

medius (mē'dē-ûs). the middle finger.

medulla (mè-dŭl'ȧ): the marrow in the various bone cavities; pith of the hair.

medulla oblongata (ŏb-lŏn-gä'tȧ). the lowest, or posterior part of the brain, continuous with the spinal cord.

medullary space (měd'û-lȧ-rē spȧs): the cavity through the shaft of the long bones

mega (měg'ȧ)· a prefix denoting great; extended, powerful; a million

melanin (měl'ȧ-nĭn). the dark or black coloring which imparts various shades of coloring to skin and hair.

membrane (měm'brān) a thin layer of tissue, serving as a covering.

mental nerve (měn'tȧl nûrv): a nerve which supplies the skin of the lower lip and chin.

mentalis (měn-tā'lĭs): the muscle that elevates and pushes up the lower lip.

mercurochrome (měr-kū'rô-krōm). a trade name; a germicide.

mercury bichloride (mûr'kû-rē bī-klō'-rĭd): a powerful germicide, poisonous and also corrosive to metal

mercury cyanide (sī'ā-nĭd): a powerful germicide, very poisonous.

meso (měs'ô). a prefix denoting in the middle; intermediate.

meta (mět'ā). a prefix signifying over; beyond; among.

metabolism (mě-tăb'ô-lĭz'm). the constructive and destructive life processes of the cell

metacarpus (mět-ă-kär'pŭs). the bones of the palm of the hand.

metatarsus (mět-a-tar'sŭs): the bones which make up the instep of the foot.

metallic (mě-tăl'ĭk): relating to, or resembling metal.

meter (mē'tēr): an instrument used for measuring; a measure of length, the basis of the metric system

metric (mět'rĭk)· pertaining to the meter as a standard of measurement.

micro (mī'krô): a prefix denoting very small; slight; millionth part of.

microbe (mī'krōb). a micro-organism; a minute one-celled vegetable bacterium.

micrococcus (mī-krô-kŏk'ŭs): a minute bacterial cell having a spherical shape.

micro-organism (mī"krô-ôr'gân-ĭz'm)· microscopic plant or animal cell; a bacterium.

microscope (mī'krô-skōp): an instrument for making enlarged views of minute objects.

mid (mĭd)· a prefix denoting the middle part.

milliampere (mĭl-ē-ăm-pâr): one thousandth of an ampere.

milliamperemeter (-mē'tēr). an electrical instrument which registers the amount of current required for a given treatment.

miliaria (mĭl-ē-ā'rē-ă). an eruption of minute blisters at the mouths of the sweat glands.

miliaria rubra (rōōb'rā). prickly heat; burning and itching usually caused by exposure to excessive heat.

miliary fever (mĭl'ē-ă-rē fē'vēr): sweating sickness; an infectious disease characterized by fever, profuse sweating and sudamina.

milium (mĭl'ē-ûm); pl, **milia** (-ă): a small whitish pimple due to a retention of sebum, beneath the epidermis; a whitehead.

mineral (mĭn'ēr-âl): any inorganic material found in the earth's crust

minor (mĭn'ēr)· smaller; lesser; under age.

mitosis (mĭ-tō'sĭs)· indirect nuclear division, the usual process of reproduction of the human cells.

mobility (mô-bĭl'ĭ-tĭ): being easily moved.

mode (mōd)· fashion; way; style.

mold; mould (mōld): to form into a particular shape.

mole (mōl): a small brownish spot on the skin.

molecule (mŏl'ê-kūl): the smallest possible unit of existence of any substance

monilethrix (mô-nĭl'ê-thrĭks)· a condition in which the hairs show bead-like enlargements along the shaft and become brittle; beaded hair.

morbid (môr'bĭd): diseased.

motile (mō'tĭl): having the power of movement, as certain bacteria

motor nerves (mō'tēr nûrvz): carry impulses from nerve centers to muscles for certain motions.

motor oculi (ŏk'û-lī): oculomotor; third cerebral nerve, the nerve controlling most of the eye muscles

mucous membrane (mū-kŭs měm'-brăn): a membrane secreting mucus

mucus (mū'kŭs): the clear thick secretion which lubricates the mucous membranes found at natural openings of the body.

mug (mŭg): a cup used for shaving soap

muscle (mŭs''l): the contractile tissue of the body by which movement is accomplished.

muscle oil (oil): an oil, vegetable or mineral, in which either lecithin or cholesterin is dissolved; used in conjunction with massage to relieve fatigue and sore muscles.

fāte, senâte, câre, ăm, finâl, ärm, ásk, sofă; ēve, ěvent, ěnd, recênt, evēr; īce,

muscle strapping (străp'ĭng): a heavy massage treatment used to reduce fatty deposits

muscle tone (tōn): the normal degree of tension in a healthy muscle.

myology (mī-ŏl'ŏ-jē): the science of the function, structure, and diseases of muscles.

N

naevus; nevus (nē'vŭs); pl., naevi; nevi (vī) a birthmark; a congenital skin blemish.

nail (nāl): unguis; the horny protective plate located at the end of the finger or toe

nail-bed (bĕd): that portion of the skin on which the body of the nail rests

nail-body (bŏd'ē) the horny nail blade resting upon the nail-bed.

nail-fold (fōld)· nail-wall.

nail-grooves (grōovz) the furrows between the nail-walls and the nail-bed

nail matrix (mā'trĭks): the portion of the nail-bed extending beneath the nail-root

nail-root (rōot): located at the base of the nail, imbedded underneath the skin.

nail-wall (wŏl): cuticle covering the sides and base of the nail body.

nape (năp): the back part of the neck.

naris (nā'rĭs); pl., nares (-rēz): a nostril

nasalis (nă-sā'lĭs)· a muscle of the nose.

nasociliary (nā-zŏ-sĭl'yă-rē): a nerve affecting the mucous membrane of the nose.

neck duster (nĕk dŭs'tĕr). a brush used to brush the hair from the neck after cutting, in most states its use is prohibited.

neck line (nĕk līn) in hair cutting, where the hair growth of the head ends and the neck begins; hair line.

negative (nĕg'ă-tĭv): the opposite of positive; expressing denial.

negative pole, N. or — (pōl): the pole from which negative current flows.

nerve (nûrv) a whitish cord, made up of bundles of nerve fibers, through which impulses are carried

nerve papillae (pă-pĭl'ē): a bundle of nerve tissue in the derma

nervous (nûr'vŭs) easily excited.

network (nĕt'wûrk): any system of lines crossing each other at certain intervals

neuritis (nū-rī'tĭs): inflammation of nerves.

neurology (nū-rŏl'ŏ-jē): the science of the structure, function and pathology of the nervous system

neuron (nū'rŏn) the unit of the nervous system, consisting of the nerve cell and its various processes.

neurosis (nū-rō'sĭs). a functional nervous disorder.

neutral (nū'trâl)· exhibiting no positive properties; indifferent; in chemistry, neither acid nor alkaline

neutralization (nū-trâl-ĭ-zā'shŭn). the rendering ineffective of any action or process; a chemical reaction between an acid and a base.

neutralizer (nū'trâl-īz-ēr)· an agent capable of neutralizing another substance.

nevus (nē'vŭs): a birthmark.

nit (nĭt). the egg of a louse, usually attached to a hair

nitrogen (nī'trŏ-jĕn): a colorless gaseous element, tasteless and odorless found in air and living tissue.

node (nōd). a knot or knob; a swelling; a knuckle or finger joint.

nodosa (nō-dōs'ă) having nodes or knot-like swellings

nodule (nŏd'ūl): a small node.

non (nŏn)· a prefix denoting not.

non-conductor (nŏn-kŏn-dŭk'tĕr)· any substance that resists the passage of electricity, light or heat towards or through it.

non-pathogenic (nŏn-păth-ŏ-jĕn'ĭk)· non-disease producing; growth promoting.

non-striated (strī'āt-ĕd): involuntary muscle function without the action of the will; consists of spindle shaped cells without striations; smooth muscle.

ĭll; ōld, ŏbey, ôrb, ŏdd, cônnect, sŏft, fōod, fŏot; ūse, ûnite, ûrn, ŭp, circûs; those

non-vascular (văs'kû-lăr): not supplied with blood vessels

nourishment (nŭr'ĭsh-mênt) anything which nourishes; nutriment; food.

noxious (nŏk'shŭs): harmful, poisonous.

nucleus (nū'klē-ûs); pl, **nuclei** (-ī). the active center of cells

nutrition (nû-trĭsh'ûn) the process of nourishment.

O

obese (ô-bēs): extremely fat.

oblique (ôb-lēk'; -līk); **obliquis** (-ûs); slanting, or inclined

obnoxious odor (ôb-nŏk'shûs ō-dĕr)· offensive; hateful.

occipital (ŏk-sĭp'ĭ-tāl) pertaining to the back part of the head; the bone which forms the back and lower part of the cranium.

occipito-frontalis (ŏk-sĭp'ĭ-tō-frŏn-tā'-lĭs): epicranius, the scalp muscle.

occiput (ŏk'sĭ-pŭt): the back of the head.

occupational disease (ŏk-û-pā'shûn-âl dĭ-zēz) due to certain kinds of employment, such as coming into contact with chemicals, dyes, etc

oculomotor (ŏk"û-lô-mō'tĕr): third cerebral nerve; controlling the motion of the eye.

oculus (ŏk'û-lûs). pl., **oculi** (lī): the eye.

odor (ō'dĕr). smell.

offensive (ô-fĕn'sĭv)· giving offense; disagreeable; obnoxious; distasteful.

ohm (ōm). a unit of measurement used to denote the amount of resistance in an electrical system or device.

Ohm's law (ōm's lô): the simple statement that the current in an electric circuit is equal to the pressure divided by the resistance.

oil (oil)· a greasy liquid.

ointment (oint'mênt): a fatty, medicated mixture used externally.

olfactory (ŏl-făk'tô-rē). relating to the sense of smell; first cerebral nerve, the special nerve of smell.

onychia (ô-nĭk'ē-ă). inflammation of the matrix of the nail with pus formation and shedding of the nail

onychophagy (ŏn-ĭ-kŏf'ă-jē) the habit of eating or biting the nails.

onychorrhexis (ŏn-ĭ-kô-rĕk'sĭs): abnormal brittleness of the nails with splitting of the free edge

onyx (ō-nĭks). a nail of the fingers or toes

opaque (ō-pāk): not transparent to light.

operator (ŏp'ĕr-ā-tĕr)· one who is able to perform correctly any service rendered professionally in the care of the face, hair, etc

ophthalmic (ŏf-thăl'mĭk): pertaining to the eye

optic (ŏp'tĭc). second cerebral nerve; the nerve of sight, pertaining to the eye, or to vision.

optimistic (ŏp-tĭ-mĭs'tĭk): hoping for the best.

orbicular (ŏr-bĭk'û-lăr)· circular; a muscle whose fibers are circularly arranged.

orbicularis oculi (ŏk'û-lī): orbicularis palpebrarum; the ring muscle of the eye.

orbicularis oris (ŏr-bĭk'û-lă'rĭs ō'rĭs): orbicular muscle; muscle of the mouth

orbit (ŏr'bĭt)· the bony cavity of the eyeball; the eye-socket.

organ (ŏr-gân): any part of the body exercising a specific function.

organic (ŏr-găn'ĭk): relating to an organ, pertaining to substances derived from living organisms.

organism (ŏr'gân-ĭz'm). any living being, either animal or vegetable.

orifice (ŏr'ĭ-fĭs)· a mouth; an opening

origin (ŏr'ĭ-jĭn): the beginning; the starting point of a nerve; the place of attachment of a muscle to a bone.

oris (ō'rĭs). pertaining to the mouth; an opening

orris root (ŏr'ĭs rōot)· a special powder used to give a dry shampoo

os (ŏs): a bone

osis (ō'sĭs): a word ending denoting an abnormal or a diseased condition.

fāte, senâte, câre, ăm, finâl, arm, ȧsk, sofă, ēve, ĕvent, ĕnd, recênt, evêr; īce,

osmidrosis (ŏs-mĭ-drō'sĭs, ŏz-)· bromidrosis, foul smelling perspiration.

osmosis (ŏs-mō'sĭs ŏz-): the passage of fluids and solution through a membrane or other porous substance

osseous; osseus (ŏs'ē-ŭs): bony.

osteology (ŏs-tē-ŏl'ō-jē): science of the anatomy, structure, and function of bones.

Oudin current (ōō'dĭn kŭr'rĕnt): high frequency current of high voltage and low amperage.

oxidation (ŏk-sĭ-dā'shŭn). the act of combining oxygen with another substance.

oxygen (ŏk'sĭ-jĕn)· a gaseous element, essential to animal and plant life.

oxygenation (ŏk"sĭ-jĕ-nā'shŭn): combination with oxygen as the blood passes through the lungs.

P

pack (păk)· a special cosmetic formula used to beautify the face.

palate (păl'ăt)· the roof of the mouth and the floor of the nose

palatine bones (bōnz): situated at the back part of the nasal fossae.

palmar (păl'măr)· referring to the palm of the hand.

palpebra (păl'pē-bră); pl , palpebrae (-brē)· eyelid.

palpebrarum (păl-pē-bră'rŭm): of or pertaining to the eyelids.

pancreas (păn'krē-ăs)· a gland connected with the digestive tract

papilla, hair (pă-pĭl'ă, hâr)· a small cone-shaped elevation at the bottom of the hair follicle in the dermis.

papillary layer (păp'ĭ-lă-rē lā'ēr). the outer layer of the dermis.

papular (păp'ū-lăr). characterized by papules.

papule (păp'ūl)· a pimple; a small, enclosed elevation on the skin containing no fluid.

para (pă'ră)· a prefix denoting alongside of; beyond; beside; against, near.

para-phenylene-diamine (păr-ă-fēn'-ĭ-lĕn-dĭ-ăm'ĭn; dī'ă-mēn) an aniline derivative used in hair dyeing

parasite (păr'ă-sĭt): a vegetable or animal organism which lives on or in another organism, and draws its nourishment therefrom.

parasiticide (păr-ă-sĭt'ĭ-sīd): a substance that destroys parasites.

parietal (pă-rī'ē-tăl). pertaining to the wall of a cavity; a bone at the side of the head.

paronychia (păr-ō-nĭk'ē-ă)· felon; an inflammation of the tissues surrounding the nail.

parotid (pă-rŏt'ĭd): near the ear; a gland near the ear.

patch test (păch tĕst). a skin test used to determine individual reaction to a chemical substance.

pathogenic (păth-ō-jĕn'ĭk) causing disease, disease producing.

pathology (păth-ŏl'ō-jē). the science which treats of modification of the structural and functional changes caused by disease.

patron (pā'trŭn)· the person to whom service is rendered.

pediculosis capitis (pē-dĭk"ū-lō'sĭs kăp'ĭ-tĭs)· lousiness of the hair of the head.

percussion (pĕr-kŭsh'ŭn) a form of massage consisting of repeated blows or taps of varying force.

pH symbol for hydrogen-ion concentration, the relative degree of acidity or alkalinity.

peri (pĕr'ĭ-): a prefix denoting about; near; around.

periosteum (pĕr-ĭ-ŏs'tē-ŭm): the fibrous membrane covering the surface of the bones.

peripheral system (pē-rĭf'ēr-ăl sĭs-tĕm)· consists of the nerve endings in the skin and sense organs

peroxide rinse (rĭns). it is used to lighten the color of the hair

personality (pûr-sŭn-ăl'ĭ-tĭ): the sum total of physical and mental qualities in a person.

perspiration (pûr'spĭ-rā'shŭn): sweat; the fluid excreted from the sweat glands of the skin.

petrissage (pĕt-rĭ-sàj). the kneading movement in massage.

petrolatum (pĕt-rō-lā'tŭm). petroleum jelly; vaseline; a purified, yellow mixture of semi-solid hydrocarbons obtained from petroleum.

petroleum (pē-trō'lē-um): an oily liquid coming from the earth.

ĭll, ōld, ôbey, ôrb, ŏdd, cônnect, sŏft, fōōd, fŏŏt; ūse, ûnite, ûrn, ŭp, circŭs; those

phagocyte (făg'ō-sīt): a cell possessing the property of ingesting bacteria, particles, and other harmful cells.

phalanx (fā'lănks), pl, phalanges (fă-lăn'jēz). the long bone of the finger or toe.

pharynx (făr'inks). the upper portion of the digestive tube, behind the nose and mouth.

phenol (fē'nōl). carbolic acid, caustic poison; in dilute solution is used as an antiseptic and disinfectant

phoresis (fō-rē'sĭs)· the process of introducing solutions into the tissues through the skin by the use of galvanic current.

phosphorus (fŏs'fôr-ŭs). a chemical element found in the bones, muscles and the nerves.

phyma (fī'mă): pl., phymata (fī'mă-tă): an enclosed swelling on the skin larger than a tubercle.

physic (fĭz'ĭk): a medicine, especially a laxative; drugs in general

physical (fĭz'ĭ-kăl): relating to the body, as distinguished from the mind.

physics (fĭz'ĭks). the branch of science that deals with matter and motion and comprises the study of light, heat, electricity, sound and mechanics.

physiology (fĭz-ē-ŏl'ō-jē): the science of functions of living things.

pigment (pĭg'mênt): any organic coloring matter, as that of the red blood cells, of the hair, skin and iris

pigmentation (pĭg″mên-tā'shŭn). the deposition of coloring in the skin or tissues

pilus (pī'lŭs), pl, pili (-lī): hair.

pimple (pĭm'p'l)· any small pointed elevation of the skin; a papule or small pustule

pit (pĭt) a surface depression or hollow.

pith (pĭth) the marrow of bones; the center of the hair.

pituitary (pĭ-tū'ĭ-tĕr-ē): a ductless gland located at the base of the brain.

pityriasis (pĭt-ĭ-rī'ă-sĭs). dandruff; an inflammation of the skin characterized by the formation and flaking of fine branny scales.

pityriasis capitis simplex (kăp'ĭ-tĭs sĭm'plĕks): a scalp inflammation marked by dry dandruff or branny scales.

pityriasis pilaris (pĭ-lă-rĭs): characterized by an eruption of papules surrounding the hair follicles, each papule pierced by a hair, and tipped with a horny plug or scale.

pityriasis steatoides (stê-ă-toy'dēz): a scalp inflammation marked by fatty type of dandruff characterized by yellowish to brownish waxy scales or crusts on the scalp.

plasma (plăz'mă): the fluid part of the blood and lymph.

platelets (plăt'lĕts). blood cells which aid in the formation of clots

platysma (plă-tĭz'mă): a broad thin muscle of the neck.

pledget (plĕj'ĕt): a compress or small flat mass of lint, absorbent cotton, or the like.

plexus (plĕk'sŭs): a network of nerves or veins.

pluck (plŭk): to pull with sudden force.

pneumogastric nerve (nū-mō-găs'trĭk nûrv). vagus nerve; tenth cerebral nerve

poise (poiz): the manner in which the head or body is carried

poison (poi'z'n): a substance, which when taken internally, is injurious to health, or dangerous to life.

poison ivy (ī'vĭ). a harmful plant which is poisonous to the touch.

polarity (pō-lăr'ĭ-tē): the property of having two opposite poles, as that possessed by a magnet or galvanic current.

pollex (pŏl'ĕks). the thumb.

pomade (pō-mād', -mad')· a medicated ointment for the hair.

pomphus (pŏm'fŭs): a whitish or pinkish elevation of the skin; a wheal.

pore (pôr): a small opening of the sweat glands of the skin.

porous (pō'rŭs). full of pores.

portable (pôr'ta-b'l): easily carried.

positive (pŏz'ĭ-tĭv)· not negative, the presence of abnormal condition, having a relative high potential in electricity.

positive pole, P. or + (pōl)· the pole from which positive electricity flows post (pōst): a prefix denoting back; after.

posterior (pŏs-tē'rē-ēr): situated behind; coming after or behind.

posterior auricular (ô-rĭk'û-lăr)· a nerve which supplies muscles behind the ear and at base of the skull

posture (pŏs'tûr) the position of the body as a whole.

potassium hydroxide (hĭ-drŏk'sīd): a powerful alkali, used in the manufacture of soft soaps.

potential (pô-tĕn'shâl). indicating possibility; electric pressure enabling it to do work under suitable conditions.

powder (pou'dĕr)· a dry mass of extremely fine particles

precaution (prē-kô'shŭn): to warn or advise beforehand.

predisposition (prē-dĭs-pô-zĭsh'ûn)· a condition of special susceptibility to disease; allergy.

preventive (prē-vĕn'tĭv). a prophylactic, warding off disease

primary (prī'mă-rē): first; primitive

procerus (prô-sē'rûs). pyramidalis nasi muscle

process (prŏ'sĕss). a course of development; a projecting part.

profession (prô-fĕsh'ûn): vocation, those engaged in work which requires special knowledge to serve the public in a particular art.

progressive dyes (prô-grĕs'ĭv dīz): hair restorers requiring time to oxidize; color develops gradually.

prophylactic (prô-fĭ-lăk'tĭk): preventing disease, relating to prophylaxis

prophylaxis (prô-fĭ-lăk'sĭs) prevention of disease.

proportion (prô-pŏr'shûn): comparative relation of one thing to another.

protection (prô-tĕk'shûn): the act of shielding from injury.

protein (prô'tē-ĭn) a complex organic substance present in all living tissues, both animal and vegetable, necessary in the diet.

protoplasm (prô'tô-plăz'm): the material basis of life, a substance found in all living cells.

protozoa (prô-tô-zō'ă) a class of animal organisms

proximal (prŏk'sĭm-ăl)· nearest.

psoriasis (sô-rī'ă-sĭs): a skin disease with enclosed red patches, covered with adherent white scales

psychic (sī'kĭk). relating to the mind.

psychology (sī-kŏl'ô-jē)· the science of the mind and its operations.

pterygium (tē-rĭj'ē-ŭm). a forward growth of the eponychium with adherence to the surface of the nail.

pterygoideus (tĕr-ĭ-goid'ē-ûs): internus and externus muscle between mandible and cheek bone, draws mandible forward.

puberty (pū'bĕr-tē)· the period of life in which the organs of reproduction are developed.

pulse (pŭls): the rhythmical dilation of an artery

purification (pū-rĭ-fĭ-kā'shŭn) the act of cleaning or removing foreign matter.

pus (pŭs)· a fluid product of inflammation, consisting of a liquid containing leucocytes, dead cells and tissue elements.

pustule (pŭs'tūl) an inflamed pimple containing pus.

pyogenic (pī-ô-jĕn'ĭk): pus forming

pyramidalis nasi (pĭ-răm-ĭ-dā'lĭs nā-sī): procerus; muscle of the nose.

Q

quadratus labii superioris kwŏd-rā'tûs lā'bē-ī sû-pē"rē-ŏr'ĭs). a muscle of the upper lip.

quality (kwŏl'ĭ-tĭ): distinctive kind trait, or character.

quarantine (kwŏr'ân-tēn): the keeping of a person away from others to prevent spread of a contagious disease.

·   —

ĭll; ōld, ôbey, ôrb, ŏdd, cônnect, sŏft, fōōd, fŏŏt; ûse, ûnite, ûrn, ŭp, circûs; those

R

radiation (rā-dĭ-ā'shŭn): the process of giving off light or heat rays.

rash (răsh) a skin eruption having little or no elevation.

receptacle (rē-sĕp'tá-k'l): a utensil used for storage.

reconditioning treatment (rē-kôn-dĭ-shŭn-ĭng trēt'mĕnt): a treatment to bring the hair back to a healthy condition, cream or oil treatment

rectifier (rĕk'tĭ-fī-ĕr): an apparatus to change an alternating current of electricity into a direct current.

rectus (rĕk'tûs): in a straight line; the name of small muscle of the eye

reflex (rē'flĕks). an involuntary nerve reaction.

relaxation (rē-lăk-sā'shŭn)· the act of being loose and less tense.

reproductive (rē-prō-dŭk'tĭv): pertaining to reproduction or the process by which plants and animals give rise to offspring.

research (rē-sûrch'): a careful search for facts or principles.

residue (rĕz'ĭ-dū): that which remains after a part is taken; remainder.

resilient (rē-zĭl'ĭ-ĕnt). elastic.

resistance (rē-zĭs'tâns): opposition; in electricity the opposition of a substance to the passage through it of an electric current

respiration (rĕs-pĭ-rā'shŭn)· the act of breathing; the process of inhaling air into the lungs and expelling it.

respiratory system (rē-spīr'ă-tō-rē sĭs'tem): consists of the nose, pharynx, larynx, trachea, bronchi and lungs which assist in breathing

retouch (rē'-tŭch): application of hair dye or bleach to new growth of hair.

retrahens aurem (rē'trā-hĕnz ôr'ĕm): auricularis posterior, a muscle back of the ear.

rhagades (răg'ă-dēz) cracks, fissures or chaps on the skin

rheostat (rē-ō-stăt) a resistance coil; an instrument used to regulate the strength of an electric current.

rhythm (rĭth'm). regular recurring movements.

rickettsia (rĭk-ĕt'sĭ-a) a type of pathogenic microorganism, capable of producing typhus fever

ringed hair (rĭngd hăr). a variety of canities in which the hair appears white or colored in rings.

ringworm (rĭng'wûrm) a vegetable parasitic disease of the skin and its appendages which appears in circular lesions and is contagious.

rinse (rĭns): to cleanse with a second or repeated application of water after washing, a prepared rinse water

risorius (rĭ-zôr'ē-ûs): muscle at the corner of the mouth.

rolling (rō'ĭng): massage movement in which tissues are pressed and twisted.

root (rōōt)· in anatomy the base; the foundation or beginning of any part

rotary (rō'ta-rĭ): circular motion of the fingers as in massage.

S

Sabouraud Rousseau (să'bōō-rō rōō'-sō): a discoverer of a 24-hour skin test used in hair dyeing to determine whether or not a patron can tolerate an aniline derivative hair dye.

sage tea rinse (sāj tē rĭns): given to darken the hair.

saline (sā'lĭn): salty; containing salt.

saliva (să-lī'vă)· the secretion of the salivary glands.

salivary gland (săl'ĭ-vă-rē glănd)· the gland in the mouth secreting saliva

salt (sôlt): the union of a base with an acid.

sanitary (săn'ĭ-tă-rē): pertaining to cleanliness, promoting health

sanitation (săn-ĭ-tā'shŭn): the use of methods to bring about favorable conditions of health

saponification (să-pŏn'ĭ-fĭ-kā'shŭn). act, process or result of changing into soap.

saprophyte (săp'rŏ-fīt): a microorganism which grows normally on dead matter, as distinguished from a parasite.

saturate (săt'ū-rāt). to cause to become soaked.

scab (skăb): a crust formed on the surface of a sore

fāte, senâte, câre, ăm, finâl, ärm, ásk, sofă; ēve, ĕvent, ĕnd, recênt, evēr; īce,

scabies (skā'bǐ-ez) a skin disease caused by an animal parasite, attended with intense itching; the itch.

scale (skāl) any thin plate of horny epidermis; regular markings used as a standard in measuring and weighing.

scalp (skǎlp) the skin covering of the cranium.

scalpial (skǎl'pē-âl): the technical term for general all around treatment of the scalp

scapula (skǎp'û-lǎ). the shoulder blade; a large flat triangular bone of the shoulder

scar (skar): a mark remaining after a wound has healed

scarf skin (skǎrf skǐn) epidermis.

science (sī'ēns)· knowledge duly arranged and systematized.

scientific (sī-ên-tǐf'ǐk) pertaining to, or used in science

scrum-pox (skrŭm'pŏks): impetigo contagiosa.

scurf (skûrf) thin dry scales or scabs on the body especially on the scalp, dandruff.

sebaceous (sē-bā'shûs): oily; fatty.

sebaceous cyst (sǐst): an enlarged oily or fatty sac.

sebaceous glands (glǎndz): oil glands of the skin

seborrhea (sēb-ô-rē'ǎ): over-action of the sebaceous glands.

seborrhea oleosa (ō-lē-ō'sǎ): excessive oiliness of the skin, particularly the forehead and nose.

seborrhea sicca (sǐk'ǎ)· dandruff; pityriasis.

sebum (sē'bŭm): the fatty or oily secretions of the sebaceous glands.

secondary (sĕk'ûn-dâ-rē). second in order.

secretion (sē-krē'shûn): a product manufactured by a gland for a useful purpose

sectioning (sĕk'shûn-ǐng): dividing the hair into separate parts.

segment (sĕg'mênt): to divide and redivide into small equal parts

selector switch (sē-lĕk'tēr swǐch). an apparatus used to select the kind of current desired for a treatment.

senility (sē-nǐl'ǐ-tē): quality or state of being old.

sensation (sĕn-sā'shûn). a feeling or impression arising as a result of the stimulation of an afferent nerve.

sensitive (sĕn'sǐ-tǐv)· easily affected by outside influences

sensory nerve (sĕn'sô-rē nûrv). afferent nerve; a nerve carrying sensations.

sepsis (sĕp'sǐs): the presence of various pus forming and other harmful organisms, or their toxins, in the blood or tissues.

septic (sĕp'tǐk): relating to or caused by sepsis

septum (sĕp'tûm): a dividing wall; a partition

serous (sē'rûs): relating to, or containing serum

serratus anterior (sē-rā'tûs ǎn-tē'rē-ēr)· a muscle of the chest assisting in breathing and in raising the arm.

sewage (sū'âj) the waste matter, solid and liquid, passing through a sewer.

shaft (shǎft)· slender stem-like structure; the long slender part of the hair above the scalp.

shampoo (shǎm-pōō). to subject the scalp and hair to washing and rubbing with some cleansing agent such as soap and water.

sheen (shēn). gloss; brightness

shingling (shǐng'lǐng)· cutting a woman's hair close to the nape of the neck and gradually longer toward the crown

short wave (shôrt wāv) a form of high-frequency current used in permanent hair removal

singeing (sǐnj'ǐng) process of lightly burning hair ends with a lighted wax taper

sinus (sī'nûs): a cavity or depression; a hollow in bone or other tissue.

skeletal muscles (skĕl'ē-tâl mŭsT'z). muscles connected to the skeleton.

skeleton (skĕl'ē-tûn): the bony framework of the body.

skin (skǐn)· the external covering of the body. -

skull (skŭl): the bony case or the framework of the head.

sleek (slēk). to render smooth, soft, and glossy.

ǐll; ōld, ôbey, ôrb, ŏdd, cônnect, sôft, fōōd, fŏŏt; ūse, ûnite, ûrn, ŭp, circûs; those

slithering (slĭth'ĕr-ĭng). tapering the hair to graduated lengths with scissors.

slough (slŭf): to separate as dead matter from living tissues; to discard.

small pox (smŏl pŏks): a contagious skin disease resulting in the production of pock marks.

snarls (snarlz)· tangles, as of hair.

soap (sōp): compound of fatty acid with an alkaline base.

soapless shampoo (sōp'lĕs shăm-pōō): a shampoo made with sulfonated oil, alcohol, mineral oil and water; this type of shampoo does not foam, and is usually slightly acid in reaction.

socket (sŏk'ĕt): a cavity in which a movable part is inserted.

sodium bicarbonate (sō-dē-ŭm bĭ-kar-bŏn-àt): baking soda, bicarbonate of soda, it relieves burns and insect bites.

sodium carbonate (kár'bŏn-àt): washing soda; used to prevent rusting of metallic instruments when added to boiling water.

sodium hydroxide (hī-drŏk'sīd). powerful alkali used in the manufacture of hard soaps.

soft water (sŏft wôtĕr) water which readily lathers with soap.

soluble (sŏl'û-b'l): capable of being dissolved.

solution (sō-lū'shûn)· the act or process by which a substance is absorbed into a liquid.

solvent (sŏl'vĕnt): an agent capable of dissolving substances.

sparsely (spars'lē)· pertaining to the hair, thinly scattered.

spatula (spăt'û-là): a flexible, knife-like implement for removing creams from jars.

specialist (spĕsh'ă-lĭst). one who devotes himself to some special branch of learning, art, or business

spectrum (spĕk'trŭm): the band of rainbow colors produced by decomposing light by means of a prism.

spermaceti (spûr-mă-sĕt'ē) an animal wax; used to give firmness to creams.

sphenoid (sfē'noid): wedge-shaped; a bone in the cranium.

spinal (spī'nâl). pertaining to the spine or vertebral column

spinal accessory (ăk-sĕs'ō-rē): eleventh cerebral nerve.

spinal column (kŏl'ŭm): the backbone or vertebral column.

spinal cord (kôrd): the portion of the central nervous system contained within the spinal, or vertebral canal

spinal nerves (nûrz)· the nerves arising from the spinal cord.

spine (spīn): a short process of bone; the backbone.

spirillum (spī-rĭl'ŭm); pl., spirilla (-ă): curved bacterium.

spirochaeta pallida (spī-rô-kē'ta păl'-ĭ-dă)· pathogenic bacteria responsible for syphilis.

spongy (spŭn'jē): like a sponge; porous

spore (spŏr): a tiny bacterial body having a protective covering to withstand unfavorable conditions

spray (sprā)· to discharge liquid in the form of fine vapor.

squama (skwā'mă): an epidermic scale made up of thin, flat cells.

staphylococcus (stăf-ĭ-lô-kŏk'ûs): coccus which is grouped in clusters like a bunch of grapes, found in pustules and boils

steamer, facial (stĕm'ĕr fā'shâl): an apparatus, used in place of hot towels, for steaming the scalp or face.

steatoma (stē-ă-tō'mă). a sebaceous cyst; a fatty tumor

sterile (stĕr'īl). barren; free from all living organisms.

sterilization (stĕr-ĭ-lĭ-zā'shŭn): the process of making sterile; the destruction of germs.

sterilizer (stĕr'-ĭ-lĭ-zĕr)· an agent or receptacle for sterilization.

sterilizer, wet (wĕt). a receptacle containing a disinfectant for the purpose of sterilizing implements.

sterilizer, cabinet or dry (kăb'ĭ-nĕt or drī): a closed receptacle containing chemical vapors to keep sterilized objects ready for use.

sterno-cleido-mastoideus (stûr"nō-klī-dŏ-măs-toid'ē-ûs): a muscle of the neck which depresses and rotates the head.

sternomastoid (stûr-nô-măs'toid)· pertaining to the sternum and the mastoid process

stimulant (stĭm'û-lânt): an agent that arouses functional activity.

stimulation (stĭm-û-lā'shŭn) act of arousing increased functional activity.

stimulus (stĭm'ū-lŭs)· an agent which causes stimulation.

stomach (stŭm'ŭk)· the dilated portion of the alimentary canal, in which the first process of digestion takes place

strand (strănd): a fiber, hair or the like

stratum (strā'tŭm); pl., strata (-ă) layer of tissue.

stratum corneum (kôr'nē-ŭm): horny layer of the epidermis.

stratum germinativum (jûr-mĭ-nā'tĭv-ŭm): the deepest layer of the epidermis resting on the corium

stratum granulosum (grăn-ū-lō'sŭm): granular layer of the epidermis.

stratum lucidum (lū'sĭ-dŭm)· clear layer of the epidermis

stratum muscosum (mū-kō'sŭm)· mucous or malpighian layer of the epidermis

streptococcus (strĕp-tō-kŏk'ŭs): pus-forming bacteria that grow in chains; found in erysipelas and blood poisoning

striated (strī'āt-ĕd): marked with parallel lines or bands, striped; voluntary muscle

stroking (strōk'ĭng): a gliding movement over a surface; to pass the finger or any instrument gently over a surface; effleurage.

structure (strŭk'tûr) organization; manner of building or form

sty, stye (stī); pl., sties, styes (stīz): inflammation of one of the sebaceous glands of the eyelid.

styptic (stĭp'tĭk). an agent causing contraction of living tissue used to stop bleeding; an astringent

sub (sŭb): a prefix denoting under; below.

subcutaneous (sŭb-kū-tā'nē-ŭs): under the skin.

submental artery (sŭb-mĕn'tăl är'tēr-ē). supplies blood to the chin and lower lip

substance (sŭb'stăns): matter; material.

sudamen (sū-dā'mĕn), pl, sudamina sū-dăm'ĭ-nă) a disorder of the sweat glands with obstruction of their ducts.

sudor (sū'dôr)· sweat, perspiration.

sudoriferous glands (sū-dōr-ĭf'ēr-ŭs glăndz): sweat glands of the skin.

sulfonated oil (sŭl'fŭn-āt-ĕd oil): an organic substance prepared by the chemical combination of oils with sulphuric acid; has a slightly acid reaction and mixes with water; used as a base in soapless shampoos.

sulphur (sŭl'fûr): a chemical element whose compounds are used in certain scalp ointments

sunburn (sŭn'bûrn): inflammation of the skin caused by excessive exposure to the sun.

sunlight (sŭn'līt)· the light rays coming from the sun.

suntan (sŭn'tăn): a brownish coloring of the skin as a result of sun exposure.

super (sū'pēr)· a prefix denoting over; above; beyond

supercilium (sū'pēr-sĭl'ē-ŭm); pl., supercilia (-ă). the eyebrow.

superficial cervical (sū-pēr-fĭsh'ăl sûr'-vĭ-kăl): a nerve which supplies the muscle and skin at back of head and neck

superior (sū-pē'rē-ēr). higher; upper; better or of more value.

suppuration (sŭp-ū-rā'shŭn)· the formation of pus.

supra (sū'pră): a prefix denoting on top of, above, over, beyond, besides; more than.

supra-orbital (sū-pră-âr'bĭ-tăl): above the orbit or eye.

susceptible (sū-sĕp'tĭ-b'l): capable of being influenced or easily acted on.

sycosis (sī-kō'sĭs): a chronic pustular inflammation of the hair follicles.

sycosis barbae (bar'bē): a chronic inflammation of the hair follicles of the beard; folliculitis barbae.

symbol (sĭm'bŏl): a mark representing an atom of an element or a molecule of a radical.

sympathetic nervous system (sĭm-pă-thĕt'ĭk nûr'vŭs sĭs'tĕm)· controls the involuntary muscles which affect respiration, circulation and digestion.

symptom (sĭm'tŭm): a change in the body or its functions which indicates disease.

symptom, objective (ŏb-jĕk'tĭv): that which can be seen, as in pimples, pustules, etc.

symptom, subjective (sŭb-jĕk'tĭv)· that which can be felt, as in itching.

ĭll; ōld, ōbey, ôrb, ŏdd, cônnect, sôft, fōōd, fŏŏt, ūse, ûnite, ûrn, ŭp, circûs; those

synthetic (sĭn-thĕt'ĭk): made artificially by the union of two or more substances

syphilis (sĭf'ĭ-lĭs): a chronic, infectious venereal disease.

system (sĭs'tĕm): a group of organs which especially contribute toward one of the more important vital functions.

systematic (sĭs-tĕm-ăt'ĭk)· proceeding according to system or regular method.

systemic (sĭs-tĕm'ĭk)· pertaining to a system or to the body as a whole.

T

tactile corpuscle (tăk'tĭl kôr'pŭs-'l) touch nerve endings found within the skin.

tan (tăn): sunburn; pigmentation of the skin from exposure to the sun

tannic acid (tăn'ĭk ăs'ĭd)· a plant extract used as an astringent

taper (tā'pĕr): regularly narrowed to a point.

tapotement (ta-pôt-man')· a massage movement using a short, quick slapping or tapping movement.

tapping (tăp'ĭng): a massage movement; striking lightly with the partly flexed fingers.

taut (tôt): tensely stretched, not slack.

technic; technique (tĕk'nĭk; tĕk'nēk). manner of performance; a skill; a process.

technical (tĕk'nĭ-kâl): relating to a technic.

temperature (tĕm'pĕr-ă-tôr): the degree of heat or cold

temple (tĕm'pl). the flattened space on the side of the forehead.

temporal bone (tĕmp'ŏ-rǎl bōn)· the bone at the side of the skull

temporalis (tĕm-pô-rā'lĭs). the temporal muscle.

tendon (tĕn'dŭn): fibrous cord or band connecting muscle with bone

tension (tĕn'shŭn)· stress caused by stretching or pulling.

tepid (tĕp'ĭd): neither hot nor cold; lukewarm; about blood heat.

terminal (tûr'mĭ-nâl)· of or pertaining to the end or extremity.

tertiary (tûr'shē-ă-rē) third in order.

testes (tĕs'tēs): the male reproductive glands.

test, hair dye (tĕst, hâr dī) a test made upon the scalp, behind the ear, or in the bend of the arm, for predisposition to the dye agent used; a test to determine the reaction of the

dye upon the sample strand, regarding both color and breakage.

texture of hair (hăr). the general quality and feel of the hair.

texture of skin (skĭn): the general feel and appearance of the skin.

theory (thē'ŏ-rē): a reasoned and probable explanation.

therapeutic lamp (thĕr-ă-pū'tĭk lămp): an electrical apparatus producing any of the various rays of the spectrum; used for skin and scalp treatments.

therapy (thĕr'ă-pē): the science and art of healing.

thermal (thûr'mâl)· pertaining to heat

thermometer (thĕr-mŏm'ē-tēr) any device for measuring temperature.

thinning, hair (thĭn'ĭng)· decreasing the thickness of the hair where it is too heavy

thorax (thō'răks). the part of the body between the neck and the abdomen; the chest.

thrombocyte (thrŏm'bŏ-sĭt) a blood platelet which aids in clotting

thyroid gland (thī'roid glănd)· a large ductless gland situated in the neck.

tinea (tĭn'ē-ă): a skin disease, especially ringworm.

tinea barbae (bar'bē)· tinea sycosis.

tinea capitis (kăp'ĭ-tĭs). tinea tonsurans; ringworm of the scalp

tinea favosa (fā-vō'să). favus, honey comb ringworm.

tinea sycosis (sĭ-kō'sĭs): parasitic sycosis; ringworm of the beard; barber's itch.

tinea tonsurans (tŏn-sū'rănz): tinea capitis, ringworm of the scalp

tinea unguium (ŭn'gwē-ŭm) ringworm of the nail.

tint (tĭnt) to color the hair by means of hair dye, color rinse, or hair tint.

fāte, senâte, câre, ăm, finâl, arm, ȧsk, sofă; ēve, ĕvent, ĕnd, recênt, evêr; īce,

tissue (tĭsh'û). a collection of similar cells which perform a particular function.

tissue, connective (kŏ-nĕk'tĭv): binding and supporting tissue.

tone (tōn). the normal activity or vigor of the body or its parts.

tonic (tŏn'ĭk) increasing the strength or tone of the body.

toupee (tōō-pē'). a small wig used to cover the top or crown of the head.

toxemia (tŏk-sē'mē-à): a form of blood poisoning.

toxic (tŏk'sĭk): due to, or of the nature of poison; poisonous.

toxin; toxine (tŏk'sĭn; -sēn) a poisonous substance of undetermined chemical nature, produced during the growth of harmful micro-organisms.

trachea (trā'kḗ-à; trà-kē'à): wind-pipe.

transformer (trăns-fôr'mẽr): used for the purpose of increasing or decreasing the voltage of the current used, it can only be used on an alternating current

transmission (trăns-mĭsh'ûn): passing on by anything, often said of disease.

transverse facial (trăns-vŭrs' fā'shàl)· an artery supplying the masseter muscle.

trapezius (trà-pē'zē-ûs)· muscle that draws the head backward and sideways

tremor (trē'mŏr; trĕm'ôr). an involuntary trembling or shaking

Treponema pallidum (trĕp-ŏ-nē'mà păl'ĭ-dûm): the pathogenic parasite of syphilis.

triangularis (trī-ăn-gû-lā'rĭs) depressor anguli oris; a muscle that pulls down corner of the mouth

trichology (trī-kŏl'ô-jē): the science of the care of the hair.

trichonosus (trĭk-ô-nō'sûs)· any disease of the hair.

trichophyton (trī-kŏf'ĭ-tŏn). a fungus parasite responsible for ringworm.

trichophytosis (trī-kŏf-ĭ-tō'sĭs). ringworm of the skin and scalp, due to growth of a fungus parasite

trichoptilosis (trī-kŏp-tĭ-lō'sĭs). a splitting of the hair ends, giving them a feathery appearance.

trichorrhexis (trĭk-ô-rĕk'sĭs)· brittleness of the hair.

trichosis (trī-kō'sĭs). any disease or abnormal growth of hair

trifacial (trī-fā'shàl): the fifth cerebral nerve, trigeminus nerve.

trigeminal (trī-jĕm'ĭ-nàl)· relating to the fifth cerebral or trigeminal nerve.

true skin (trōō skĭn): the corium.

tubercle (tū'bĕr-k'l): a rounded, solid elevation on the skin or membrane.

tumor (tū'mẽr). a swelling; an abnormal enlargement; a mass of new tissue which persists and grows independently of its surrounding structures, and which has no physiological use.

turbinal; turbinate (tûr'bĭ-nàl; -nāt): a bone in the nose.

tweezers (twēz'ẽrs)· a pair of small forceps to remove or extract hair.

U

ulcer (ŭl'sẽr) an open sore not caused by a wound.

ulna (ŭl'nà): the inner and larger bone of the forearm

ultra (ŭl'trà): a prefix denoting beyond; on the other side, excessively

ultra-violet (ŭl'trà-vī'ô-lĕt): invisible rays of the spectrum which are beyond the violet rays.

un (ŭn): a prefix denoting not; contrary.

unguis (ŭn'gwĭs); pl., ungues (gwēz): the nail of a finger or toe.

unguium, tinea (ŭn'gwē-ŭm tĭn'ē-à). ringworm of the nails

unit (ū'nĭt)· a single thing or value

United States Pharmacopeia (û-nĭt'ĕd stāts fár-ma-kô-pē'ya)· an official book of drug and medicinal standards.

unsanitary (ŭn-săn'ĭ-tâ-rē): not sanitary, injurious to health

uridrosis (ū-rĭ-drō'sĭs) the presence of urea in sweat

urine (ū'rĭn): the fluid secreted - by the kidneys.

urticaria (ûr-tĭ-kā'rē-à): a skin disease in which wheals and severe itching develops; hives; nettle rash

ĭll, ōld, ôbey, ôrb, ŏdd, cônnect, sŏft, fōōd, fŏŏt; ūse, ūnite, ûrn, ŭp, circûs; those

V

vaccination (văk-sĭ-nā′shŭn): injection of the virus of cowpox, or vaccina as a means of producing resistance against small pox.

vagus (vā′gŭs). pneumogastric nerve; tenth cerebral nerve.

valve (vălv). a structure which temporarily closes a passage or opening or permits flow in one direction only.

vapor (vā′pēr): the gaseous state of a liquid or solid.

vascular (văs′kū-lăr)· supplied with or pertaining to blood or lymph vessels.

vaseline (văs′ê-lĭn; ēn): a trade name; petrolatum; a semi-solid greasy or oily mixture of hydrocarbons obtained from petroleum.

vaso-constrictor (văs-ō-kŏn-strĭk′tēr): a nerve which, when stimulated, causes narrowing of blood vessels

vaso-dilator (văs-ō-dĭ-lā′tēr): a nerve which, when stimulated, causes expansion of the blood vessels.

vegetable dyes (věj′ê-tà-b′l dīz) comprised of Egyptian henna, indigo, and camomile used as hair dyes or hair rinses.

vein; vena (văn; vē′nà): a blood vessel carrying blood toward the heart.

vena cava (kā′và)· one of the large veins which carry the blood to the right auricle of the heart.

venereal (vê-nē′rê-âl): pertaining to a disease arising from unlawful sexual indulgence with an infected person.

ventilate (věn′tĭ-lāt)· to renew the air in a place

ventricle (věn′trĭ-k′l): a small cavity; particularly in the brain or heart.

vermin (vûr′mĭn): parasitic insects, as lice and bedbugs.

verruca (vě-rōō′kà)· a wart; small growths covered by thickened epidermis.

vertebra (vûr-tê-brǎ); pl, vertebrae (brē): a bony segment of the spinal column.

vertex (vûr′těks): the crown or top of the head.

vesicle (věs′ĭ-k′l): a small blister or sac; a small elevation on the skin.

vessel (věs″l): tube or canal in which blood, lymph, or other fluid is contained and circulated

vibration (vī-brā′shŭn)· shaking; a to and fro massage movement.

vibrator (vī′-brā-tēr): an electrically driven massage apparatus causing a swinging, shaking sensation on the body, producing stimulation.

vibrissae (vī-brĭs′a)· stiff hairs in the nostrils.

vibroid (vī′broid): a vibratory movement in massage.

vinegar (vĭn′ê-gēr)· formed by fermentation of wine, cider, etc.; it contains acetic acid, used as a rinse to remove soap curds from the hair

violet-ray (vī′ō-lět rā) high-frequency; Tesla; an electric current of medium voltage and medium amperage.

virgin hair (vûr′jĭn hăr): normal hair which has had no previous bleaching or dyeing treatments

virulent (vĭr′ōō-lênt)· extremely poisonous.

virus (vī′rûs)· poison; the specific poison of an infectious disease.

vitality (vī-tăl′ĭ-tē) the state or quality of being vital; power of enduring or of continuing

vitamin (vī′-tà-mĭn): one of a group of organic substances present in a very small quantity in natural foodstuffs, which are essential to normal metabolism, and the lack of which in the diet causes deficiency diseases.

vitiligo (vĭt-ĭ-lī′gŏ). milky-white spots of the skin, common in negroes.

vogue (vōg)· fashion, custom, style.

volatile (vŏl′à-tĭl). easily evaporating; diffusing freely, not permanent

volt (vōlt): the unit of electromotive force.

voltage (vōl′tàj) electrical potential difference expressed in volts.

volume (vŏl′ūm). space occupied, as measured in cubic units.

voluntary (vŏl′ŭn-tà-rē): under the control of the will.

vomer (vō′mēr): the thin plate of bone between the nostrils

W

wall plate (wôl plāt): an apparatus equipped with indicators and controlling devices to produce various currents.

wall socket (sŏk'ĕt): a wall receptacle into which may be fitted the plug of an electrical appliance.

wart (wôrt): verruca; an enclosed overgrowth covered by thickened epidermis.

water (wô'tēr): a compound of oxygen and hydrogen.

water softener (sŏf"n-ēr): certain chemicals, such as the carbonate or phosphate of sodium, used to soften hard water to permit the lathering of soap.

watt (wĕt): the electrical unit of energy.

wattage (wŏt'åj): amount of electric power expressed in watts.

wen (wĕn): a sebaceous cyst, usually on the scalp.

wheal (whĕl): a raised ridge on the skin, usually caused by a blow, a bite of an insect, urticaria, or sting of a nettle.

whitehead (whīt'hĕd): milium.

wig (wĭg): an artificial covering for the head, consisting of hair interwoven by a kind of network.

windpipe (wĭnd'pīp): trachea.

witch hazel (wĭch hā'z'l): after-shaving lotion; an extract of the bark of the hamamelis shrub.

wrinkle (rĭnk'l): a small ridge or a furrow.

wrist electrode (rĭst ê-lĕk'trōd): an electrode connected to the wrist.

Z

zygoma (zī-gō'mă): a bone of the skull which extends along the upper and outer part of the face, below the eye; the malar or cheek bone.

zygomatic (zī-gô-măt'ĭk): pertaining to the zygoma; pertaining to the malar or cheek bone.

zygomaticus (zī-gô-măt'ĭ-kŭs): a muscle that raises angle of mouth backward and upward.

BIBLIOGRAPHY

In the preparation of this book, the following works have been consulted as authorities on the various phases of barbering treated herein. The student who seeks amplification of points covered briefly in this book will do well to refer to these sources:

Men's Hair Tinting and Bleaching
                    Anthony Colletti (Milady Publishing Corp.)
The Hair and Scalp—A. Savill, M A., M.B.
Electrotherapy and Light Therapy—Richard Kovacs, M.D.
Physical Treatment—James B. Mennell, M.A., M.D., B.C.
Morris' Human Anatomy—
                    J. Parsons Schaeffer, A.M., M.D., Ph.D., Sc.D.
Human Anatomy and Physiology—
                    N. D. Millard, R.N., M.A., and Barry G. King, Ph.D.
Modern Textbook of Barbering—
                    S. C. Thorpe (Milady Publishing Corp.)
Barber State Board Regulations—Milady Publishing Corp.
The Barbers' Manual—A. B. Moler.
Skin Deep—M. G. Phillips.
Anatomy and Physiology—Kimber, Gray, Stackpole and Leavell.
Gray's Anatomy—Charles Mayo Goss, M.D.
Normal Histology—William H. F. Addison.
Diseases of the Skin—Oliver S. Ormsby.
Electricity and Light—Noble M. Eberhart, M.D.
Electricity Manual—Glendora Stingley.
Care of the Skin and Health—Herman Goodman, M.D.
Sanitation, Hygiene, Bacteriology and Sterilization—
                    Herman Goodman, M.D.
Gould's Medical Dictionary—George M. Gould, A.M., M.D.
Stedman's Medical Dictionary—
                    Thomas Lathrop Stedman, A.M., M.D.
Standard Textbook of Cosmetology—
                    Constance V. Kibbe (Milady Publishing Corp.)
Baldness—Richard Muller, M.D.
Modern Cosmetics—E. G. Thomssen.

CPSIA information can be obtained
at www.ICGtesting.com
Printed in the USA
BVHW042126291121
622843BV00011B/509

9 781376 058734